GUIDE TO THE
FAMILY MEDICINE
CLERKSHIP

GUIDE TO THE
FAMILY MEDICINE CLERKSHIP

Editor
Susan Louisa Montauk, M.D.
Professor of Clinical Family Medicine
Department of Family Medicine
University of Cincinnati College of Medicine
Cincinnati, Ohio

Assistant Editors
Rick E. Ricer, M.D.
Director, Predoctoral Medical Education
Vice Chair for Education
Professor of Family Medicine
University of Cincinnati College of Medicine
Cincinnati, Ohio

Andrew T. Filak, Jr., M.D.
Associate Dean for Medical Education
Association Professor of Family Medicine
University of Cincinnati College of Medicine
Cincinnati, Ohio

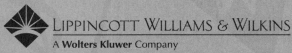
LIPPINCOTT WILLIAMS & WILKINS
A Wolters Kluwer Company
Philadelphia · Baltimore · New York · London
Buenos Aires · Hong Kong · Sydney · Tokyo

Editor: Elizabeth A. Nieginski
Editorial Director: Julie P. Scardiglia
Development Editors: Lisa Bolger and Bridget Blatteau
Managing Editor: Marette Magargle-Smith
Marketing Manager: Aimee Sirmon

01 02
1 2 3 4 5 6 7 8 9 10

Dedication

To Coulter Montauk Loeb, my younger son, for sharing his passion for computers and music, and for bringing me all of his Scientific Americans with pages of the medical stories he liked marked in the hopes that he might help me to write and edit.

To Benjamin Montauk Loeb, my elder son, for smiling with me once in a while even during adolescence, for sharing his poetry with me, and for identifying this book's title.

To Stan Loeb, my husband, for his many years of domestic engineering, growth, and caring that allowed us to raise our family and expand our love.

To all of my wonderful friends, family members, mentors, colleagues, students, and patients who have taught me so much about medicine, teaching, and unconditional love.

Contents

Contributors

Orson J. Austin, M.D.
Associate Professor of Clinical
  Family Medicine
Department of Family Medicine
University of Cincinnati College
  of Medicine
Cincinnati, Ohio

Todd S. Carran, M.D.
Adjunct Assistant Professor of
  Family Medicine
Department of Family Medicine
University of Cincinnati College
  of Medicine
Cincinnati, Ohio

Philip M. Diller, M.D., Ph.D.
Director, Family Medicine Residency
  Program
Associate Professor of Clinical
  Family Medicine
University of Cincinnati College
  of Medicine
Cincinnati, Ohio

Jill A. Foster, M.D.
Assistant Professor
Department of Nutrition Services
University of Alabama at
  Birmingham
Birmingham, Alabama

Timothy Freeman, M.D.
Assistant Professor of Clinical
  Family Medicine
Department of Family Medicine
University of Cincinnati College
  of Medicine
Cincinnati, Ohio

Jerry A. Friemoth, M.D.
Associate Professor of Clinical
  Family Medicine
Department of Family Medicine
University of Cincinnati College
  of Medicine
Cincinnati, Ohio

Bruce Gebhardt, M.D.
Assistant Professor of Clinical
  Family Medicine
Department of Family Medicine
University of Cincinnati College
  of Medicine
Cincinnati, Ohio

Lora Hasse, Ph.D.
Research Assistant Professor of
  Family Medicine
Department of Family Medicine
University of Cincinnati College
  of Medicine
Cincinnati, Ohio

Jeff Kirschman, M.D., M.S.

Occupational & Environmental
    Health
Guthrie Clinic
Sayre, Pennsylvania

Charles Margolis, M.D.

Vice Chairman, Clinical Affairs
Professor of Clinical Family
    Medicine
Department of Family Medicine
University of Cincinnati College
    of Medicine
Cincinnati, Ohio

Jennifer Margolis, M.D., F.A.A.P.

Volunteer Assistant Professor of
    Family Medicine
Department of Family Medicine
University of Cincinnati College
    of Medicine
Cincinnati, Ohio

Arvind Modawal, M.D., M.P.H., M.R.C.G.P.

Assistant Professor of Clinical
    Family Medicine
Department of Family Medicine
University of Cincinnati College
    of Medicine
Cincinnati, Ohio

Susan Louisa Montauk, M.D.

Professor of Clinical Family
    Medicine
Department of Family Medicine
University of Cincinnati College of
    Medicine
Cincinnati, Ohio

Edward Onusko, M.D.

Associate Residency Program
    Director
Family Practice Residency Program
Clinton Memorial Hospital
Wilmington, Ohio

Assistant Professor of Clinical
    Family Medicine
Department of Family Medicine
University of Cincinnati College
    of Medicine
Cincinnati, Ohio

Erik Powell, M.D., M.S.

Volunteer Assistant Professor of
    Family Medicine
Department of Family Medicine
University of Cincinnati College
    of Medicine
Cincinnati, Ohio

Rick E. Ricer, M.D.

Vice Chairman for Education
Professor of Family Medicine
Department of Family Medicine
University of Cincinnati College
    of Medicine
Cincinnati, Ohio

Maria M. Sandvig, M.D.

Volunteer Assistant Professor of
    Family Medicine
Department of Family Medicine
University of Cincinnati College
    of Medicine
Cincinnati, Ohio

James Short, Ph.D.
Field Service Assistant Professor of
Family Medicine
Department of Family Medicine
University of Cincinnati College
of Medicine
Cincinnati, Ohio

Robert Smith, M.D.
Professor Emeritus & Founding
Director
Department of Family Medicine
University of Cincinnati College
of Medicine
Cincinnati, Ohio

**Douglas R. Smucker, M.D.,
M.P.H.**
Director, Research Division
Associate Professor of Family
Medicine
Department of Family Medicine
University of Cincinnati College
of Medicine
Cincinnati, Ohio

Jeffrey Susman, M.D.
Professor and Chair
Department of Family Medicine
University of Cincinnati College
of Medicine
Cincinnati, Ohio

**Barbara Bowman Tobias,
M.D.**
Associate Professor of Clinical
Family Medicine
Department of Family Medicine
University of Cincinnati College
of Medicine
Cincinnati, Ohio

Gregg Warshaw, M.D.
Director, Office of Geriatric Medi-
cine
Professor of Family Medicine
Department of Family Medicine
University of Cincinnati College of
Medicine
Cincinnati, Ohio

Therese Zink, M.D., M.P.H.
Assistant Professor of Clinical Fam-
ily Medicine
Department of Family Medicine
University of Cincinnati College of
Medicine
Cincinnati, Ohio

Preface

During 1 day of a family medicine clerkship, a medical student may see a 47-year-old diabetic with end-stage renal disease; an abused mother of five; a 7-year-old with streptococcal pharyngitis; two women with depression, one of whom also has acute low back pain; a 68-year-old man with gastroenteritis; a young boy whose acne is raging; and a newborn in for a well check. The *Guide to the Family Medicine Clerkship* was developed for such an experience.

Perhaps the following "history and physical" can help explain what is in store for you when you purchase this book.

HISTORY AND PHYSICAL

Chief Complaint

A student-friendly pocket guide was needed to enhance our students' clerkship experience.

History of Present Illness

Although there are several excellent resources for family physicians as well as for residents and students of the specialty, none of these resources are written in a standardized format that is easy to access during patient care and at the level of third-year medical students. Students admitted to being frustrated with not having a primary user-friendly, up-to-date publication for their family medicine clerkship. Preceptors admitted to their frustration with a lack of standardized information.

Family History

The *Guide to the Family Medicine Clerkship* comes from a large family. Twenty-four faculty members wrote on the top 10 diagnoses seen in a family practice as well as on several other relevant topics. Contributors were chosen based on their knowledge of family medicine, their skills, their subexpertise within the field of family medicine, their literary and teaching pursuits, and their experience with medical students.

Social History

Just as teamwork made the family medicine clerkship at the University of Cincinnati College of Medicine the highest rated third-year clerkship for several years, it was teamwork that first gave rise to the notion of designing a guide that students could take home for study and use as a quick, on-site reference. Department chairpersons were supportive and colleagues encouraged that the successful product be shared, so the major publisher of medical texts for students (Lippincott Williams & Wilkins) was contacted and added to the extensive support system.

Review of Systems

Students and family medicine clerkship directors from other areas of the country were hired throughout the development of *Guide to the Family Medicine Clerkship* to critique format and content.

Pertinent positives

- User friendly
- Pocket sized (i.e., lab coat pocket)
- Up-to-date information
- Well written

Pertinent negatives

- Minimal extraneous information
- Does not assume students know too little or too much

Physical Examination

The chapter format of *Guide to the Family Medicine Clerkship* contains the following notable findings:

 Introduction—a succinct description of key aspects of each topic

Terminology—short definitions of many of the medical terms used in the chapter

 Background—a brief narrative on why the topic is important in family medicine

 Prevention—a discussion of primary and secondary prevention techniques

 Diagnosis—a detailed description of what to ask about and look for in a family practice encounter

Differential Diagnoses—a list of what diagnoses to rule out

 Therapy—a discussion of what nonpharmacologic therapies help, which medications are indicated, why these medications help, and possible side effects

 Consults—an explanation of when a consult should be considered and which specialty should be consulted

Miscellaneous pertinent positive physical findings unique to *Guide to the Family Medicine Clerkship* include separate sections in each chapter on:

 Special Populations—important information specific to the diagnosis and treatment of children, seniors, and pregnant women

 Complementary/Alternative Medicine—significant information on therapies outside of mainstream medicine for each topic in addition to an appendix devoted to introducing the reader to complementary and alternative medicine techniques

Additional helpful features include:

- **Note Boxes**—highlight knowledge particularly important when seeing patients in a family practice setting
- **Icons**—clearly designate all of the main topic headings to allow the reader to access desired facts in a timely manner

Impression

- *Guide to the Family Medicine Clerkship* allows easy access to information relevant to clerking in a family practice outpatient office.
- Students who purchase *Guide to the Family Medicine Clerkship* will have the knowledge necessary to successfully focus their encounters with family practice patients.
- *Guide to the Family Medicine Clerkship* is an invaluable, student-tested resource for the family medicine clerkship.

Plan

Medical students should purchase their own copy of *Guide to the Family Medicine Clerkship* before starting their first primary care clerkship.

On a more personal note, may your experience in family medicine be a good one. If you can share in even a small portion of the exciting challenges, poignant discoveries, and joyful moments many of us experience daily as family physicians, I know you will have a good clerkship!

Acknowledgments

A book like this could never have happened without the efforts of many. I would like to thank all of the people who helped to make my dream possible, including:

- **All of the contributing authors** for their perseverance and flexibility, which allowed the format to grow and adapt with reviewer and editor feedback. With each change came a new challenge for each contributor, but higher quality for the reader.
- **Rick Ricer, MD** for editing in record time and for all of the guidance, warmth, caring, friendship, and support he exhibited throughout the project.
- **Andrew Filak, MD** for performing a miracle—finding time where none existed to help edit.
- **Barbara Mikulik, Ingrid White, and Lois Grimenstein** for their secretarial and administrative assistance.
- **Bridget Blatteau,** my editor, who guided the *Guide* as only an experienced and caring editor can.
- **Joseph Bateman, MD; Todd Carran, MD; Anna Daddabbo, MD; Timothy Freeman, MD; Erik Powell, MD; Rick Ricer, MD; and Maria Sandvig, MD,** my practice partners, for taking up the slack when my book schedule dictated I glue myself to the computer.
- **My department chairpersons, Alan K. David, MD** (chairperson from 1992 through September 1998); **Gregg Warshaw, MD** (interim chairperson from September 1998 through October 1999); and **Jeffrey L. Susman, MD** (chairperson from November 1999 to the present) for the support necessary to complete the *Guide* during a time of such departmental transition.
- **Nan Fox, PhD** who helped by critiquing some of the mental health issues, but also by being a superb psychologist for many of my patients in need and a special friend to me.
- **Tom D'Erminio and Doug Pentz, PhD** for their helpful critiques and education on mental health issues. Opal Riddle, MPT for pointing me toward a more wholistic approach to musculoskeletal care.
- **The dozens of medical students** whose honesty and commitment to excellence encouraged them to carefully identify ways to perfect the *Guide* for future colleagues as well as the current and future students who will encourage the positive evolution of the *Guide*.

Basic Principles

CHAPTER 1

What is Family Medicine?

Jeffrey Susman • Susan Louisa Montauk
• Rick E. Ricer

> *. . . yours is a higher and more sacred duty . . . you belong to the great army of quiet workers, physicians and priests, sisters and nurses, all over the world, the members to which is given the ministry of consolation in sorrow, need and sickness . . . that you may apply in your practice the best that is known in our art, and with the increase in your knowledge, may be an increase in that priceless endowment . . . that will make you under all circumstances true to yourselves, true to your high calling, and true to your fellow man.*
>
> —Osler

It is 8:30 on an unseasonably warm morning in January and you are seeing patients for the first time at your new practice. You are excited and happy to be in your own office and to be practicing medicine again after a several month hiatus prompted by a move to a new city after your residency.

You gulp a last sip of juice, fish your stethoscope out of your briefcase, and dive into the day's patients. Your first is a seven-year boy. The nursing note says "physical examination." After initial pleasantries, the real reason for the encounter unfolds: "My child has been limping."

In an instant you are more alert. A dozen thoughts race through your mind: Has he been febrile? Was there an injury? What about child abuse? What is this mother worried is going on? Have there been other symptoms? How did those patients I saw with osteomyelitis, a slipped capital femoral epiphysis, or Legg-Calve-Perthes disease present?

You visually reassess both patient and mother. When you walked in the room they were engaged in some form of make believe game. They seem to be getting along fine. You glance at the vital signs, especially the temperature. All normal. You watch the boy clamor up and down from the examination table with abandon. You begin to take the history.

Mom confirms that the past history is unremarkable. Chicken pox and otitis media, the usual childhood illnesses. Up to date with immunizations.

No trauma. Never been far from home. No particularly germane family or past history.

The limping, as it turns out, was for several days, several weeks ago. It wasn't preceded by a cold, fever or accompanied by any other symptoms. There are no constitutional signs and the child is behaving normally now.

The physical examination is also normal. No hip or knee problems. He jumps up and down off the examination table and, in response to your challenge to how fast he can run, tears down the hallway.

Still, you wonder. An overanxious mother? Are you missing a serious problem? Is there some other psychosocial issue? Or is it another of those inexplicable occurrences in family medicine? You discuss the normal findings and unlikely but potential problems. You explain "growing pains" but also advise her to carefully watch things. Your thoughts fly through the differential diagnosis again, particularly the most serious possibilities. You suggest they follow up in a week, or sooner if symptoms recur.

You watch as the boy skips down the hall. Then guided by his mother's hand, he slows down as they near the checkout desk. Both of them turn and smile. He waves. You return the gesture and find yourself smiling even after turning away. You're finally in practice!

INTRODUCTION

This chapter represents the interpretations of three family physicians. Although our interpretations regarding family medicine (Table 1–1) may reflect many of your preceptor's experiences, your preceptor may also find them quite unfamiliar. To corrupt an old adage, "When you've met one family physician, you've met one family physician." We are an incredibly diverse group.

For some of you, family medicine will be a life-long career. Those of you in other specialties will work with patients referred from family practices, providing consultation and, at times, ongoing care. Whatever your path, you should be familiar with the challenges faced by family physicians, when a referral will occur, and what information is needed when patients return to their family physicians.

Third-year medical school rotations allow a clinical framework to be placed on a sturdy and hard-earned foundation. Your family medicine rotation allows you to approach clinical situations from a biopsychosocial, outpatient perspective. During your rotation, allow yourself to better understand the perspectives and needs of the colleagues you will be working closely with over the years.

CORE CONCEPTS OF FAMILY MEDICINE

Family medicine, as all specialties, is based on core concepts. Although the scope of family medicine overlaps greatly with other specialties and the

TABLE 1–1. **Pearls of Wisdom Based on the Experiences of Three Family Physicians**

1. Prevention is the best medicine.
2. Anticipatory guidance is the best prevention.
3. Our most important tool is our relationship with our patients.
4. Outcomes should be matched to patient preferences, including end-of-life issues, benefits and harms of therapy, and effects of the plan of care on function and overall quality of life.
5. Consider the costs and values of intervention, implementing decisions only after ethical forethought.
6. The patient-doctor relationship is a vital component for wellness.
7. The family (i.e., the family of origin as well as the family chosen later in life) has a strong influence on both physical and mental health.
8. Patients deserve comprehensive care.
9. Continuity of care is essential and costs less in morbidity, mortality, and dollars.
10. Strive to be patient advocates at all times.
11. Medical care is best when delivered according to a patient-centered model.
12. Caring for patients with undifferentiated problems takes time, yet we must often formulate differential diagnoses and treatment plans based on limited information gathered in a limited amount of time. This takes skill and the acceptance that reality is uncertain, even for the most knowledgeable.
13. There are many important rewards for patient encounters.
14. Community resources are crucial to public health.
15. Understanding patients in a community, family, and cultural context is necessary for preeminent care.
16. Long-term treatment goals are necessary for optimal care.
17. Time management skills allow for implementation of the other core ideals.
18. The history of family medicine is one of reform, commitment, and humanism.
19. Strive to treat every patient with caring, empathy, and respect.
20. Treat the whole patient, not a disease process or organ system.
21. Both the physician's and the patient's health belief models alter the presentation and management of an illness.
22. Involving the patient and caregiver can greatly increase adherence.
23. Evidence-based medicine is the key to the scientific process and should always be a primary goal.
24. Science does not have all of the answers.

way that family physicians practice medicine is not fundamentally different from other physicians, family medicine has a foundation that is unique.

We refer patients for major surgeries and procedures as well as for in-depth management beyond our personal level of comfort. At the same time, we delve more deeply into many issues using a biopsychosocial model. We combine our clinical acumen with our knowledge of health beliefs, the social sciences (e.g., anthropology, sociology, psychology), psychiatry, and counseling. We deal with undifferentiated problems in patients in the early stages of diseases; therefore, we learn to deal with uncertainty and to make decisions based on limited information. Out of necessity, we often find ourselves choosing practicality over theory.

> **NOTE**
>
> Know what type of person has the disease process, not just what type of disease process the person has.

A WELL-BALANCED PROFESSION

Diversity

Family physicians often get excited by the range of human health and maladies, fascinated by the dynamic relationship between physicians and patients over time and enthralled with knowledge of a community. Many of us, eclectic by nature, were entranced with each new rotation as medical students—the joys of childbirth on the obstetrics and gynecology rotation, the intellectual challenges on the internal medicine wards, the raw excitement of the emergency room. Ultimately, there was only one choice that allowed the opportunity to continue to sample the full smorgasbord of medicine—family medicine.

The literature on family medicine education reflects the diversity of the specialty. The residency curricula guidelines range from obstetrics, cardiology, and AIDS to complementary and alternative medicine, culturally sensitive health care, and spirituality. Given the breadth of family medicine, it is not surprising to see a wide variation in practice style, scope, and special interests.

Some family physicians are "full-service doctors," walking with ease from the maternity suite to the intensive care unit to the clinical office on a daily basis. Others have pursued interest areas in geriatrics, sports medicine, or adolescent medicine. Family physicians are often the primary caretakers of the poor and underserved. We cross many boundaries because, as our interests mature and change, we have incredible latitude to pursue many special areas. Such freedom keeps the specialty of family medicine fresh and dynamic.

Challenge

Every specialty has its challenges, but several make family medicine particularly intriguing. Unlike many of our subspecialty colleagues, we see patients with undifferentiated problems. Some offer presentations foreign to most medical texts; for example, the patient with vague neck pain who turns out to have temporal arteritis or the patient with headaches who is a victim of family violence. Family physicians are experts at melding the science and art of medicine.

In one day we may motivate a patient to quit smoking, comfort a family who has lost a loved one, and educate our community about teen pregnancy. Daily, we are asked to make ethical judgments about allocating resources, truth telling, and placing limits on care while we struggle to promote patient autonomy through education and unconditional positive regard. While striving for an evidence-based approach to medicine, we concurrently improve our intuition, our sixth sense of the underlying truth that helps guide our science when facing unusual and potentially serious situations.

> *Science is not only a method for deriving quantitative data from carefully controlled experiments, it is also a faith—that nature is orderly, consistent, and ultimately rational . . . (it) is tautology, predictability and mathematical equivalence . . . (it) knows neither good nor evil and cannot comprehend uncaused effect, genuine novelty, hope, or even real surprise. But all of these nonscientific things are part of the human experience, even the experience of scientists.*
> —G. Gayle Stephens, MD

Continuity and Communication

Getting to know patients over a long period of time and caring for them in many different situations teaches us how to help them care for themselves. Discovering family dynamics and learning about our patients' hobbies and priorities gives us the foundation upon which to develop successful care plans. Translating information among our consultants, our patients, and our patients' families hones our communication skills. While the current landscape is changing—managed care, improved transportation and communication, a plethora of diverse health care providers—the relationship between most patients and their personal physicians remains special. It is this unique privilege that energizes the majority of us in family medicine.

MAXIMIZING YOUR FAMILY MEDICINE EXPERIENCES

So, how do you make the best use of your family medicine rotation? What can you do to experience first hand the combination of art and science that led to the formation of the American Academy of General Practitioners (1949) and the American Board of Family Practice (1969)? Consider the following suggestions:

- While working with a patient whose cultural and ethnic background is different from your own, explore the patient's health beliefs (i.e., the personal meaning of their illness).

- Learn about a patient's family by drawing a genogram. Try this on a complex patient and on an individual presenting for routine prevention.
- Act as a mirror, not an oracle. For example, for a patient with chronic obstructive pulmonary disease who continues to smoke, explore the barriers between smoking and cessation and acknowledge the difficult task the patient faces.
- Ask patients who have recently seen consultants if they understand everything clearly or if they still have critical questions that have not been answered.
- Think about how your life would transpire if committed to service and altruism (i.e., seeking earned respect, not self-aggrandizement).
- While striving for excellence, endeavor to remain humbled by the subtle recognition that you are human and therefore fallible, with limits to your knowledge and abilities.
- Above all, open your heart and your mind during your family medicine experience. Be open to the joys and sorrows of your patients. Reflect regularly on the scientific method, but also on lessons about humanity, for they too are essential to your calling.

CHAPTER 2

Changing Health Behaviors in a Family Practice

Douglas R. Smucker • Lora Hasse

OBJECTIVES

■ Understand how values and beliefs influence health-related decisions and behaviors in both patients and clinicians

■ Understand the basic components of the stages of change model (i.e., transtheoretical model)

■ Be able to use the stages of change model to help patients adopt beneficial health behaviors

■ Understand the basic components of the health belief model

■ Be able to use the health belief model in a family practice setting

INTRODUCTION

Although health practitioners can give directions and make recommendations, it is ultimately the patient's responsibility to follow through with the necessary actions. However, the choices that patients make are influenced by many complex factors, including personal, familial, spiritual, and social issues. Consequently, you will encounter patients who do not adhere to your recommendations. For example, patients often find it difficult to implement recommendations regarding diet, exercise, smoking cessation, and other lifestyle patterns. Patients may not take medications as instructed or they may fail to complete a simple, preventive task (e.g., screening mammogram).

Attempting to treat uncooperative patients can be frustrating and can lead to a cynical view of your ability to positively influence health behaviors. In fact, the thought of working through the complex issues unique to each patient during a 15-minute office visit can strongly influence your practitioner's belief system, making it easy to say, "Why even try?" However, hundreds of published studies have proved that with the right tools and knowledge you can have a positive influence on your patients' abilities to institute healthier lifestyle choices and to adhere to treatment recommendations.

PATIENT EDUCATION

Educating patients about healthy lifestyle habits and helping them to understand and follow through with treatment recommendations are the cornerstones of primary health care; therefore, patient education should be a priority for all family physicians. However, there are many barriers to providing optimal patient education in a busy family practice, including the time demands of caring for patients' illnesses, lack of financial reimbursement for patient education, and the belief that many patients will not be successful in making lifestyle changes.

Based on extensive review of the scientific literature, the United States Preventive Services Task Force (USPSTF) has provided recommendations regarding how to structure office practice and patient encounters to improve prevention and patient education. The *Guide to Clinical Preventive Services*, a report by the USPSTF, is an excellent source for guiding patient education efforts in a family practice office. The principles outlined by the USPSTF (Table 2–1) are important for success in educating patients about prevention as well as helping patients adhere to advice about taking medications and caring for acute and chronic illnesses.

Virtually every patient encounter should include some element of patient education. The family physician who uses a variety of strategies (e.g., verbal messages, printed materials, computerized information), organizes a sample system for education in the office, and involves staff in patient education efforts is most likely to be a successful patient educator.

> **NOTE**
>
> An important goal of the family medicine clerkship is to learn to go beyond a focus on "routine sick care" and to positively influence the health behaviors of patients.

CONTINUITY OF CARE

> **NOTE**
>
> Building a partnership with patients over time and understanding the perceptions, values, and beliefs that influence their health behaviors are the underlying principles of family practice that provide the foundation for helping patients to change.

When a patient and a physician have an ongoing, one-on-one relationship, both are better able to understand each other's values and perceptions about health-related behaviors. This understanding allows physicians to assist patients as they work to improve their health. It is in this context (i.e.,

TABLE 2–1. **Initial Steps Toward Improving Office-Based Patient Education**

√ Communicate the importance of healthy choices verbally, with patient education materials, and by writing out suggested lifestyle changes on a prescription slip

√ Involve staff in creating simple systems that promote patient education

√ Inform the patient of the purpose and expected results of your advice

√ Suggest small changes rather than large changes

√ Be specific in your instructions for behaviors to be changed

√ Get an explicit commitment for change from the patient

√ Monitor progress through a follow-up contract with the patient

Adapted with permission from *Guide to Clinical Preventive Services: Report of the United States Preventive Services Task Force,* 2nd ed. Baltimore, Williams & Wilkins, 1995.

continuity of care) that theories of health behavior are most beneficial, strengthening the physician's understanding of how to help patients change.

Although the family medicine clerkship does not allow for the development of ongoing patient–physician relationships, using theories of health behavior during your clerkship and discussing them with faculty and colleagues can have an important influence on your future abilities as a care provider.

BEHAVIORAL MODELS

Many theories that relate to positively influencing patient behavior have been proposed and studied. Two widely studied health behavior models are discussed in this chapter: the stages of change model and the health belief model.

Stages of Change Model

The stages of change model (Figure 2–1) describes the process of changing long-term behaviors and sustaining new behaviors (e.g., smoking cessation, starting an exercise program). The stages of change model recognizes that behavioral change often involves a temporal sequence of different processes and that successful patient education and support must acknowledge these processes and be stage specific.

The stages of change model recognizes five distinct stages related to behavior: precontemplation, contemplation, preparation, action, and maintenance. Based on these stages, the model assumes that:

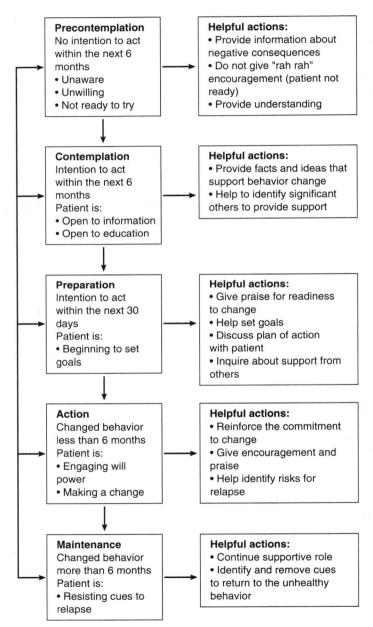

FIGURE 2–1. Stages of change model (i.e., transtheoretical model).

- Change is a process that unfolds over time through a sequence of the five stages
- Patients tend to remain in early stages without planned interventions
- Patients are most likely to progress through the stages if offered education and support specific to their current stage

The Health Belief Model

The health belief model, based on the work of Rosenstock and Becker, is one of the most popular conceptual frameworks used to explain change and maintenance of health-related behaviors. This model proposes that decisions about health-related behaviors involve a balance between a value (i.e., the desire to become well or avoid illness) and an expectation (i.e., whether or not an action will benefit a patient's health). The health belief model is most useful in describing patients' values and determining what motivates patients to make the decisions they do about medical care, diagnostic tests, and treatment options.

> **NOTE**
>
> The cultural and spiritual aspects of a patient's history contribute to the patient's opinions about preventive care and treatment of disease and often are the greatest influencing factors on health-related decisions.

The health belief model (Figure 2-2) suggests that individuals take action to ward off, screen for, or control unhealthy conditions if they believe:

- They are susceptible to the condition (perceived susceptibility)
- The condition has potentially serious consequences (perceived severity)
- An available course of action will help to reduce their susceptibility to or the severity of the condition (perceived benefits)
- The benefits of taking action outweigh the anticipated barriers (perceived barriers)

Perceived susceptibility

Perceived susceptibility refers to the patient's subjective perception of the risk of contracting an illness. The level of perceived susceptibility is reflected by the patient's willingness to accept the diagnosis, estimates of the risk of recurrence, and beliefs regarding susceptibility to illness in general. For example, a smoker who is convinced that he will "never" get cancer or emphysema because everyone in his family lives into their 90s may not try to quit smoking based on a low perceived susceptibility to the consequences of smoking.

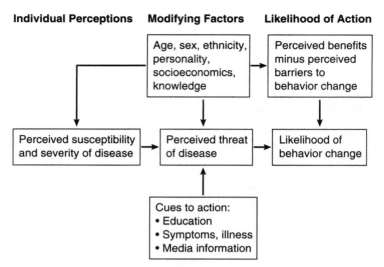

Individual Perceptions   **Modifying Factors**   **Likelihood of Action**

Age, sex, ethnicity, personality, socioeconomics, knowledge

Perceived benefits minus perceived barriers to behavior change

Perceived susceptibility and severity of disease

Perceived threat of disease

Likelihood of behavior change

Cues to action:
• Education
• Symptoms, illness
• Media information

FIGURE 2–2. Summary of the key variables in the health belief model. (Adapted with permission from Strecher VJ, Champion VL, Rosenstock IM: The Health Belief Model and Health Behavior. In *Handbook of Health Behavior Research: Personal and Social Determinants.* Edited by Gochman DS. New York, Plenum Press, 1997.)

Perceived severity

Perceived severity refers to the patient's feelings about the seriousness of contracting an illness or leaving it untreated. It includes perceptions of possible medical, clinical, and social consequences. For example, a patient with diabetes who frequently forgets to take her medicine and says, "I feel just as good when I don't take it, even when my sugar is 200," will likely have difficulty adhering to a medication regimen because of a low perceived severity of poorly controlled diabetes.

Perceived threat is the term often used to express the combined effects of the patient's level of perceived susceptibility and perceived severity.

Perceived benefits

Perceived benefits are the patient's beliefs about whether or not the recommended action or treatment will be effective in reducing the threat of disease. Factors that influence perceived benefits include non–health-related benefits (e.g., smoking cessation saves money). A patient could have a high level of perceived susceptibility and severity (i.e., perceived threat) but not take action unless the action is perceived as potentially effective. For example, a 19-year-old woman who "heard of someone who had Pap smears every year and still got cancer" is less likely to complete a visit for her first Pap smear because of low perceived benefit of screening for cervical cancer.

Perceived barriers

Perceived barriers are the potentially negative aspects of a particular action or impediments to undertaking the recommended behavior. Possible barriers include cost, danger, discomfort, inconvenience, and time. For example, an elderly patient who refuses a recommended flu vaccine because he "hates shots" has a perceived barrier to the vaccine.

SUMMARY

Knowledge and use of models, such as the stages of change model and the health belief model, can help you to be more successful in persuading patients to make healthy changes in behavior and to follow through with prevention and treatment recommendations. These models also can help alleviate the frustration that clinicians experience when patients do not follow through with changes that are mandatory for an improved quality of life.

CHAPTER 3

Prevention and Screening Guidelines for Adults

Rick E. Ricer • Orson Austin

OBJECTIVES

- Explain the concept of targeted preventive screening as the current standard of care
- Describe the role that an in-depth history (i.e., family history, risk factors, personal lifestyle issues) plays in appropriate preventive screening
- Compare and contrast the prevention recommendations from different organizations for specific disease processes
- Identify the strengths and weaknesses of various recommendations for screening and prevention

INTRODUCTION

For most of the last century, the annual physical was the accepted standard of care practiced by physicians, even for well patients. The written history of its institutionalization began in 1923 when the American Medical Association first referred to the healthy patient in a manual entitled, *Periodic Health Examination: A Manual for Physicians.* By 1940, a revision of the same manual suggested using the annual physical as a standard approach to healthy patients. Little changed over the next 30 years, and the annual physical became the de facto standard of care.

In the early 1970s, two family physicians (Frame and Carlson) were the first to challenge the accepted standards regarding the annual physical examination and to critically examine preventive screening (i.e., when to consider screening and the value of screening). Their findings supported history taking and counseling, but did not support annual physical examinations in asymptomatic patients with benign family histories and unremarkable past medical histories. Numerous other studies since Frame and Carlson have reached the same conclusion; history taking and targeted screening should replace the annual physical examination.

The criteria used by Frame and Carlson to evaluate screening tests for disease processes are the same criteria most relevant organizations use today. Currently, more than 100 national organizations have published recommendations on routine preventive screening. Many of the recommendations from these organizations conflict with each other. It is up to each physician (or medical student) to decide which guidelines she will follow for screening purposes. No one organization is considered the true standard of care.

Although many patients still expect the old standard, the current standard is the age-appropriate, focused preventive visit, an approach much more suitable to overall health. If healthy patients present for their annual physical, an initial explanation of this evolution is often warranted, emphasizing how focused prevention using extensive history taking is now done because it is much more beneficial than an all-encompassing, nonfocused physical.

> **NOTE**
>
> Reassure patients that studies have shown that a focus on their personal history, family history, lifestyle issues, and risk factors is the most important part of prevention; and prevention is the best medicine.

PREVENTION

Prevention needs to be tailored to the person's age, gender, and specific risks. It is a longitudinal and continuous process that changes as the patient ages. Not every preventive measure needs to be addressed during each visit. Rather, try to incorporate at least one preventive component in each acute care visit. One way to remember to incorporate prevention into your patient care routine is to use the SOAPP documentation method: subjective, objective, assessment, plan, prevention.

A Prevention History

Family history

The information obtained from a family history is critical for risk assessment, and risk assessment is critical for targeted screening. A genogram (Figure 3–1) can be used to identify and record information obtained as part of the family history (e.g., known chronic illnesses, cause of death), providing a later quick reference to help focus counseling and primary prevention issues. As we come to further understand the human genome, the genogram will become an increasingly more important tool in patient management.

Lifestyle issues

Questions about a patient's lifestyle are also extremely important. When a new patient presents to a physician it is helpful to explore some general

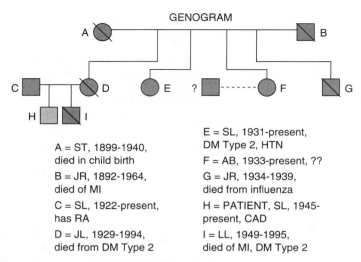

GENOGRAM

A = ST, 1899-1940,
died in child birth

B = JR, 1892-1964,
died of MI

C = SL, 1922-present,
has RA

D = JL, 1929-1994,
died from DM Type 2

E = SL, 1931-present,
DM Type 2, HTN

F = AB, 1933-present, ??

G = JR, 1934-1939,
died from influenza

H = PATIENT, SL, 1945-
present, CAD

I = LL, 1949-1995,
died of MI, DM Type 2

FIGURE 3–1. Example of a genogram.

social history issues. Following are samples of lifestyle topics that should be addressed during preventive visits.

Alcohol

- Does the patient currently drink alcohol?
- How much alcohol does the patient drink (be specific)?
- How would you classify the patient's use of alcohol (i.e., at risk or abuse)?

Contraception

- If the patient is sexually active, what does the patient use for contraception or for prevention of sexually transmitted diseases?

NOTE

Many women do not think of birth control as medication. Encourage all women who use birth control (i.e., pills or medroxyprogesterone injections) to mention these contraceptive methods when questioned about medications.

- If the patient is an adolescent, see Chapter 5.

Exercise

- Is the patient engaged in a regular exercise program?
- If so, what type of activity?
- What is the frequency, intensity, and duration of exercise?

Some physicians find it helpful to write an exercise prescription. One commonly used standard is a frequency of at least three times every week, a duration of at least 30 minutes, and an intensity geared at a target heart rate of 70% to 80% of the maximal heart rate. The equation for the target heart rate is: $(220 - \text{age})(70\%\text{--}80\%)$.

Health belief model (see Chapter 2)

- Does the patient believe that changing his lifestyle will actually prevent or delay future health problems?

History of abuse (see Chapter 22)

- Does the patient feel safe at home?
- Did the patient feel safe as a child?

Occupation

- What is the patient's current occupation?
- What types of jobs has the patient had in the past?
- Are there any job-related exposures or hazards?

Sexual activity

- How many sexual partners has the patient had, especially over the last 1 to 2 years?
  - □ The greater the number of partners, the greater the risk of sexually transmitted diseases.
- Is there a history of a sexually transmitted disease? If so, was it treated appropriately?

Sexual orientation

- Has the patient engaged in sexual activity with men, women, or both?
- Does the patient identify himself or herself as heterosexual, homosexual, or bisexual?

NOTE

Do not assume patients have had or intend to have heterosexual intercourse. Always ask if you are unsure about sexual orientation. Such information can greatly affect suggestions about future prevention and will strengthen the patient–doctor relationship.

Spirituality

- Does the patient have a spiritual belief system that may significantly impact on his health?

Tobacco

- Does the patient currently use or has she ever used tobacco products (i.e., cigarettes, cigars, snuff, chewing tobacco)?

Preventive Care

Preventive care includes immunizations [e.g., pneumococcal vaccine (Pneumovax), influenza virus vaccine], medications (e.g., hormone replacements, daily aspirin), screening programs for the early detection of disease processes (e.g., cancer), and education regarding lifestyle changes for healthy behaviors (see Chapter 2). Because immunization recommendations change frequently, you should refer to the website of the National Institutes of Health (see Appendix III) for the most recent update.

The United States Preventive Services Task Force (USPSTF), the Canadian Task Force, and the American Academy of Family Physicians are organizations that look at preventive care for both genders across the entire life span. Most organizations provide recommendations for their specific interest or specialty. Specific examples include the American Cancer Society (ACS) for cancer-related diseases, the American College of Obstetrics and Gynecology for women's health issues, and the American Academy of Pediatrics for children's issues. Tables 3–1 through 3–6 summarize the recommendations of the ACS and the USPSTF.

TABLE 3–1. **American Cancer Society Recommendations***

Cancer Type	Patient Age	Recommendations
Breast cancer	≥ 20 years	Monthly breast self-examination
	20–40 years	Clinical breast examination every 3 years
	≥ 40 years	Annual clinical breast examination and mammogram
Colorectal cancer	≥ 40 years	Annual digital rectal examination
	≥ 50 years	Annual fecal occult blood test; flexible sigmoidoscopy every 5 years, barium enema every 5–10 years, or colonoscopy every 10 years
Cervical cancer	18 years (or sexually active)	Pap smear and pelvic examination annually for 3 years, then less frequently
Endometrial cancer	Menopause	Endometrial biopsy sampling of high-risk women
Prostate cancer	≥ 50 years	Prostate-specific antigen test and digital rectal examination annually

*For asymptomatic patients, the American Cancer Society recommends a cancer checkup every 3 years from 20–40 years of age and then annually after 40 years of age. The examination should include the thyroid, oral cavity, skin, lymph nodes, testes, and ovaries.

TABLE 3–2. United States Preventive Services Task Force Recommendations for Adult Women

Age	Recommendations
18–24 years	Pap smear every 2 years, diphtheria-tetanus vaccine every 10 years, chlamydia screen every 2 years, hypertension screen every 2 years
25–44 years	Pap smear every 2 years, diphtheria-tetanus vaccine every 10 years, hypertension screen every 2 years
45–50 years	Pap smear every 2 years, cholesterol test every 5 years, diphtheria-tetanus vaccine every 10 years, hypertension screen every 2 years
51–65 years	Fecal occult blood test every year, diphtheria-tetanus vaccine every 10 years, sigmoidoscopy every 3–10 years, Pap smear every 2 years, mammogram every year, cholesterol test every 5 years
66–70 years	Pneumococcal vaccine once, influenza vaccine every year, diphtheria-tetanus vaccine every 10 years, mammogram every year, fecal occult blood test every year, sigmoidoscopy every 3–10 years
71–death	Influenza vaccine every year, sigmoidoscopy every 3–10 years, fecal occult blood test every year

SCREENING RECOMMENDATIONS

NOTE

Many suggested screening procedures and laboratory tests, even some recommended by highly respected organizations, are controversial.

TABLE 3–3. United States Preventive Services Task Force Recommendations for Adult Men

Age	Recommendations
21–34 years	Hypertension screen every 2 years, diphtheria-tetanus vaccine every 10 years
35–49 years	Hypertension screen every 2 years, diphtheria-tetanus vaccine every 10 years, cholesterol test every 5 years
50–64 years	Fecal occult blood test every year, sigmoidoscopy every 3–10 years, cholesterol test every 5 years, diphtheria-tetanus vaccine every 10 years
65–death	Fecal occult blood test every year, influenza vaccine every year, pneumococcal vaccine once, sigmoidoscopy every 3–10 years, diphtheria-tetanus vaccine every 10 years

TABLE 3–4. **Lifetime Items Recommended by the United States Preventive Services Task Force for Adults**

Items	Number Needed
Multivitamin with folate*	1 every day for 30 years
Smoke detector	3 in an average-size home
Batteries for smoke detector	1 every year for life for each smoke detector
Ipecac	1 ounce available at all times
Bike helmet	1 for every rider
Dental visit	1 visit every 6 months, annual x-ray
Toothpaste and floss	Enough for daily use
Toothbrush	1 every 3 months

*Men do not have to take a multivitamin with folate.

TABLE 3–5. **Medical Problems for Which the United States Preventive Services Task Force Found Insufficient Evidence for Routine Screening**

Abdominal aortic aneurysm	Coronary artery disease (by basic or stress electrocardiogram)
Carotid artery stenosis	
Dementia	Depression
Diabetes mellitus	Drug abuse
Family violence	Glaucoma
Oral cancer	Osteoporosis
Scoliosis	Skin cancer
Testicular cancer	Suicide
Asymptomatic bacteriuria	Youth violence

TABLE 3–6. **United States Preventive Services Task Force Recommendations for Office Counseling**

Prevent	Promote
Tobacco abuse	Physical activity
Motor vehicle accidents	Healthy diet
Household and recreational injuries	
Youth violence	
Sexually transmitted diseases	
Unintended pregnancy	
Dental and periodontal disease	
Low back pain	

Organizations determine what screening recommendations to offer based on one of two formats: literature review or expert opinion. Literature review recommendations are based on the relative strengths of study evidence. Findings are then assigned a "grade" that rates the need for a specific screening test. Organizations that use this format include the USPSTF and the Canadian Task Force.

Organizations that rely on expert opinion use a panel of experts to make recommendations for screening purposes. The recommendations are based on the judgment of the experts and their combined practice experience and knowledge. Many times these experts are specialists for the organization. The American Heart Association and the ACS use the expert opinion approach.

Cancer Screening Guidelines

> **NOTE**
>
> All recommendations for cancer screening are based on the screening of asymptomatic persons with no risk factors. If an individual has risk factors, more aggressive screening beginning at a younger age and occurring more frequently may be required.

Breast cancer

Incidence

Breast cancer is the leading cause of death among American women 40 to 55 years of age. According to the National Cancer Institute, the risk of developing breast cancer increases with age:

- 40 years of age = 1/217 chance
- 50 years of age = 1/50 chance
- 60 years of age = 1/24 chance

Risk factors

Risk factors for breast cancer include:

- Gender (female)
- Age
- Family history of breast cancer
- Previous breast cancer
- First pregnancy after 30 years of age
- Menarche before 12 years of age
- Menopause after 50 years of age
- Obesity
- High socioeconomic status
- History of ovarian or endometrial cancer
- Estrogen replacement therapy (controversial)

Screening guidelines

A summary of breast cancer screening guidelines can be found in Table 3–7.

> **NOTE**
>
> Currently, the most important screening method for breast cancer is mammography.

Colon cancer

Incidence

Colon cancer has the second highest mortality rate of any cancer in the United States. It effects men and women about equally.

Risk factors

Risk factors for colon cancer include:

- Family history of colon cancer, polyposis coli, or cancer family syndrome
- History of ulcerative colitis or adenomatous polyps
- History of colon, endometrial, ovarian, or breast cancer

Screening guidelines

A summary of colon cancer screening guidelines can be found in Table 3–8.

TABLE 3–7. **Breast Cancer Screening Guidelines**

Organization	Recommendations
USPSTF	Mammogram every 1–2 years from 50–70 years of age, with or without a clinical breast examination; there is insufficient evidence for or against performing clinical breast examination alone or for teaching breast self-examination also.
ACS	Breast self-examination monthly beginning at 20 years of age, clinical breast examination every 3 years from 20–40 years of age, and a mammogram and clinical breast examination every year after 40 years of age; no recommendation for when to stop screening
Canadian Task Force	Mammogram annually after 50 years of age, with clinical breast examination annually after 60 years of age
WHO	Does not support breast self-examination
ACP	Mammogram every 2 years from 50–70 years of age

ACP = American College of Physicians; ACS = American Cancer Society; USPSTF = United States Preventive Services Task Force; WHO = World Health Organization.

TABLE 3–8. **Colon Cancer Screening Guidelines**

Organization	Recommendations
USPSTF	Fecal occult blood test annually and sigmoidoscopy every 10 years beginning at 50 years of age; there is insufficient evidence for or against screening with digital rectal examination, colonoscopy, and barium enemas.
ACS	Fecal occult blood test annually beginning at 50 years of age (both sexes), digital rectal examination annually beginning at 40 years of age, and flexible sigmoidoscopy every 3–5 years (depending on risk) beginning at 50 years of age
Canadian Task Force	Does not recommend digital rectal examination or routine flexible sigmoidoscopy
ACP	Sigmoidoscopy, colonoscopy, or barium enema every 10 years from 50–70 years of age
American Association of Gastrointestinal Endoscopists	Colonoscopy can be used as a screening tool.
American Gastrological Association	Colonoscopy can be used as a screening tool.

ACP = American College of Physicians; ACS = American Cancer Society; USPSTF = United States Preventive Services Task Force.

Cervical cancer

Incidence

Carcinoma of the cervix is a common malignancy in women. With Pap smear screening, the incidence of cervical cancer in the United States has decreased from 30 cases per 100,000 in 1950 to less than 10 cases per 100,000 in 1995. However, there are still 15,700 new cases and 4900 cervical cancer–related deaths in the United States each year.

Risk factors

Risk factors for cervical cancer include:

- Lower socioeconomic status
- Intercourse at a young age (i.e., younger than 18 years)
- Multiple partners
- Human papilloma virus infection

NOTE

The risk of cervical cancer is virtually zero if the woman has never been sexually active.

TABLE 3–9. **Cervical Cancer Screening Guidelines***

Organization	Recommendations
USPSTF	Pap smear every 3 years for all women who are or who have been sexually active; stop Pap smears at 65 years of age if all previous Pap smears were normal
ACS†	Pap smear annually until three negative Pap smears are recorded, then less frequently‡; begin when woman becomes sexually active or 18 years of age, whichever comes first
Canadian Task Force	Pap smear annually until two negative Pap smears are recorded, then every 3 years until 69 years of age; begin when woman becomes sexually active or 18 years of age, whichever comes first

ACS = American Cancer Society; USPSTF = United States Preventive Services Task Force.
*No one recommendation for cervical cancer screening has been clearly shown to be superior.
†The recommendations of the National Cancer Institute, the American College of Obstetrics and Gynecology, and the American Medical Association are very similar to the recommendations of the ACS.
‡The ACS does not define "less frequently."

Screening guidelines

A summary of cervical cancer screening guidelines can be found in Table 3–9.

Prostate cancer

Incidence

Prostate cancer is the most common nonskin cancer in men. It is the second leading cause of death in men (after lung cancer) because prostate

TABLE 3–10. **Prostate Cancer Screening Guidelines***

Organization	Recommendations
USPSTF	Does not recommend digital rectal examination, transrectal ultrasound, or prostate-specific antigen test
ACS	
Colon cancer screening panel	Digital rectal examination annually after 40 years of age
Prostate cancer screening panel	Prostate examination and a prostate-specific antigen test annually after 50 years of age
Canadian Task Force	Digital rectal examination annually between 50 and 70 years of age; recommends against prostate-specific antigen test

ACS = American Cancer Society; USPSTF = United States Preventive Services Task Force.
*No one recommendation for prostate cancer screening has been clearly shown to be superior.

cancer that metastasizes beyond the prostate, although responsive to palliative therapy, is still essentially incurable. Fortunately, most prostate cancers are extremely slow growing. Although at least 25% of men older than 50 years of age and 33% of men older than 65 years of age have a focus of prostate cancer, only approximately 1 in every 300 actively metastasizes to cause death.

Risk factors

Risk factors for prostate cancer include:

- Age
- Race
- Family history of prostate cancer

Screening guidelines

A summary of prostate cancer screening guidelines can be found in Table 3–10.

Prevention and Screening Guidelines for Seniors

Arvind Modawal • Gregg Warshaw

INTRODUCTION

OBJECTIVES

- Describe prevention and healthy screening guidelines for the elderly
- Characterize and evaluate important components of functional status in the elderly
- Be aware of the major elements of home- and community-based support systems available to the elderly

Advancements in medical science and improvements in health care have made it possible for people to live longer, increasing the need for physicians to be aware of the special attributes and requirements of older persons. In the United States, life expectancy at birth is currently older than 75 years. Eradication of infection, immunizations, improvements in social and nutritional status, basic sanitation, and a public health emphasis on health promotion and disease prevention have all contributed to improved life expectancy.

The age at which a person can be called "old" or "senior" is arbitrary. Retirement cannot be used as the criteria for defining "old" because there is no standard age for retirement in the United States, and many older persons return to the work force after retirement. However, 65 years of age is an important landmark in the United States because Medicare and Social Security benefits have traditionally started at this age. Therefore, the prevention and screening guidelines in this chapter relate to persons older than 65 years of age.

Population-based measures have the largest impact on prevention of disease and promotion of health, yet medical models often emphasize a preventive strategy that focuses on the individual patient. Both of these approaches have advantages and disadvantages. This chapter is based on a model of prevention and screening that focuses on enhancement of functional status and maintenance of support systems in the context of the elderly, individual patient.

NORMAL AGING AND DISEASE

There is evidence that underutilization of senior-oriented preventive programs is partly due to misconceptions about normal aging. Normal aging is a predetermined biologic process, with associated changes in many organ systems. Many symptoms of disease (e.g., constipation, hearing and memory impairment) may be dismissed as part of normal aging; however, there may be easily identifiable, reversible factors responsible for these symptoms. Misinterpreting normal physiologic, age-related changes can lead to an inappropriate acceptance of unhealthy body changes and disease symptoms.

PREVENTION AND SCREENING GUIDELINES

Until recently, elderly populations were excluded from major clinical trials, such as those involving new strategies for prevention and treatment of cardiovascular disease and cancer. Therefore, there has been little data to help analyze conflicting recommendations regarding prevention and screening for seniors. Clinical trials now include more elderly people and provide important prevention information for this group of individuals. For example, it is now known that control of systolic hypertension and the use of warfarin anticoagulation in atrial fibrillation help to prevent cerebrovascular accidents in the elderly. Recent research has also contributed to osteoporosis prevention and treatment, including exercise interventions to prevent falls, balance and gait training to maintain mobility, reduction in the use of restraints, and environmental modifications.

Prevention and screening in the elderly should focus on the specific characteristics and needs of this unique population. Older persons generally follow healthier behavior patterns compared to the younger population in regards to accident prevention, dietary habits, smoking cessation, alcohol consumption, and blood pressure checks. Older persons also have, on average, a greater sense of autonomy, a greater reliance on complementary/alternative medicine therapies and over-the-counter products, and a greater belief in the ability of lifestyle modification to alter the risk of morbidity and prolong death. However, in the elderly population there is also a higher prevalence of malignant conditions, musculoskeletal problems, cardiovascular morbidity, and cognitive and sensory impairments. Therefore, it is important to establish separate guidelines for preventive screening and health maintenance for the elderly population.

Screening interventions in older persons are likely to give a higher yield (i.e., more true-positive results) than in their younger counterparts. Table 4–1 lists some of the preventive screening recommendations for seniors. Generally accepted and effective preventive interventions are listed in Table 4–2.

TABLE 4–1. **Preventive Screening Recommendations for Seniors 65 and Older**

Screening Procedure	Recommendation
Blood pressure	Check at least every 2 years
Breast examination and mammography	Annual mammography until 85 years of age
Pelvic examination and Pap smear	Discontinue if three adequate specimens in a row are normal
Cholesterol test	Base on patient's cardiovascular risk factors; may not be necessary
Rectal and prostate examinations, PSA	No specific recommendations
Visual acuity and glaucoma screen	Check acuity every 1–3 years; include glaucoma screen if there is a strong family history or African ancestry
Hearing acuity	Perform periodically*
Glucose monitoring	Perform fasting plasma glucose periodically if in a high-risk group
Thyroid function	Test TSH periodically if clinically justified
Dementia screening	Perform periodic mini-mental status examinations

PSA = prostate-specific antigen; TSH = thyroid-stimulating hormone.
*One-third of seniors older than 65 and one-half of seniors older than 85 have hearing loss.

TABLE 4–2. **Effective Preventive Interventions for Seniors**

Condition	Intervention
Cardiovascular disease	Physical exercise, hypertension management, aspirin prophylaxis
Cancer	Breast, colon, cervical, and skin cancer screening*
Infectious diseases	Pneumococcal and influenza vaccinations
Endocrine disease	Screen for diabetes and thyroid disorders via history taking
Dementia	Screen via history taking†
Polypharmacy	Screen periodically via history taking, reevaluate prescription and over-the-counter medications (include herbal and nutritional supplements)
Other (e.g., falls, vision, hearing, general safety)	Address during history taking

*Some elderly patients who have become irreversibly debilitated with a limited life expectancy have no interest in the therapies indicated for some cancers. For these patients, cancer screening becomes less significant and should not be offered without a thorough discussion.
†When possible, also question people who live with and care for the patient.

GOALS OF PREVENTION AND SCREENING IN THE ELDERLY

To be most effective, screening and prevention must have an impact on an elderly person's ability to live independently and avoid or postpone institutionalization. When life expectancy becomes limited, aggressive treatment approaches may not be indicated due to the increase in frailty and resultant inability to withstand treatment protocols. In such cases, injudicious use of screening is disruptive to lifestyle, expensive, time-consuming, and unnecessary because it will have only a marginal effect on quality and quantity of life. The health maintenance program should be adapted to the personal preference of the older individual. Advance directives (e.g., living wills) can help determine how aggressive one should be.

Enhancing Functional Status

There are certain interventions and outcome measures that may change with advancing age. For instance, as we become older, enhancing functional status (i.e., quality of life) may become more important relative to simply extending life (i.e., quantity of life).

Assessment of functional status

To determine functional status, it is necessary to assess:

- Activities of daily living (e.g., ability to get dressed, bathe, and prepare food)
- Motility and balance (e.g., timed get-up-and-go test)
  - □ To complete the timed get-up-and-go test, observe the patient getting up from a chair with a straight back, walking 10 feet, and returning to sit down in the chair.
  - □ Record the time taken to complete the test in seconds (normally 10 seconds). This correlates with independence in activities of daily living.
- Transportation options
  - □ As aging progresses, transportation often becomes more difficult because of the likelihood of increased physical impairment and decreased driving potential.
- Environmental hazards (e.g., mobile rugs)
- Iatrogenic hazards that may lead to falls (e.g., orthostasis from diuretics)
- Sensory deprivation from poor vision and deafness
- Urinary problems (e.g., incontinence, retention)
- Constipation
- Insomnia
- Sexual problems (e.g., erectile dysfunction, dyspareunia)
- Cognitive impairment and depression

NOTE

The inability to walk safely, cook, shop, or drive can rapidly cause de-conditioning and malnutrition as well as contribute to social isolation and depression.

Methods of enhancing functional status

General recommendations for enhancing functional status are shown in Table 4–3.

Maintaining Support Systems

Maintenance of support systems is crucial to the well-being of the elderly. Breakdown of family support due to death and relocation of family and friends may impair social support. Identification of appropriate social networks is of paramount importance. Day-care programs, respite care, and support groups for caregivers are often required to help an older individual.

The lives of older persons are often complicated by poverty due to diminishing income and inadequate pension, leading to poor housing conditions, poor nutrition, and the inability to afford health care. Home health care professionals, social workers, and community agencies making use of federal programs to provide Meals-on-Wheels and other resources can provide valuable assistance. Attendance at senior centers can help reduce isolation and loneliness and may give important respite time to other family members.

MEDICARE COVERAGE AND SETTING PREVENTION PRIORITIES

Under ideal circumstances, patients should be offered and given the opportunity to discuss the preventive interventions relevant to their needs, concerns, and preferences. Decisions should be made on the basis of the best medical evidence and the unique risks and circumstances of the individual. However, do not ignore Medicare reimbursement and other supplemental health insurance coverage (e.g., Medicare Part B), their limitations, and potential direct costs to the patient.

The number of screening procedures reimbursable through Medicare has increased recently. Screening mammography, Pap smears, pelvic examinations, and colorectal examinations are now often covered services. Secondary prevention tools such as diabetes self-management education and training, blood glucose monitors, and glucose testing strips may also be reimbursable.

Medicare still does not cover:

- Outpatient medication
- Routine preventive history and physical examination

TABLE 4–3. General Recommendations for Enhancing Functional Status

Function/Condition	Recommendation
Exercise	Encourage aerobic and resistance exercises as tolerated
Diet and malnutrition	Perform serial weight and serum albumin monitoring and dental evaluation
Cardiovascular condition	Suggest low-dose aspirin after age 50 for cardiovascular health and anticoagulation with warfarin in patients with atrial fibrillation
Smoking	Recommend smoking cessation*
Falls and accident prevention	Maintain physical activity; install alarm or Medi-alert bracelet; consider sedative medications, orthostasis, improper assistive devices, foot wear, and environmental hazards as possible risk factors
Ethical and legal issues	Explain end-of-life decision making and options (e.g., living wills and other advance directives)
Immunizations	Administer tetanus-diphtheria every 10 years, influenza annually after 65 years of age or if chronically ill, and pneumococcal vaccine at least once after 65 years of age
Sleep hygiene	Encourage regular times for sleep; suggest avoidance of stimulants and excessive drinking in the evening
Iatrogenic and adverse drug reactions	Minimize prescription medications, especially CNS-acting and anticholinergic drugs[†]
Driving	Note citations and accidents; advise to discontinue driving if increasing mental frailty or physical disability
Hypothermia and hyperthermia	Discuss symptoms and avoidance
Skin and foot care	Discuss how to assess for skin cancer in all patients and pressure ulcers in mobility restricted patients
Estrogen replacement	Discuss this option in postmenopausal period
Incontinence	Encourage frequent prompted voiding in cognitively impaired patients; suggest bladder training and pelvic floor (Kegel) exercises when appropriate

CNS = central nervous system.
*The benefits of smoking cessation persist late in life. However, smoking remains a risk factor for morbidity, although the risk lessens with age.
[†]Remember the saying, "starting low and going slow."

- Routine eye care and eyeglasses
- Dental care
- Preventive foot care (except for diabetes and peripheral vascular disease)
- Tetanus immunization (except postinjury)
- Mental health services (only covered at 50%)

PATIENT, FAMILY, AND CAREGIVER EDUCATION

As with all other age-groups, education of elderly patients and their families about the conditions that would most likely benefit from preventive care is extremely important for quantity and quality of life. The consequences of participating or not participating in a screening program, risks of developing a disease with or without the screening, and chances of false-positive and false-negative results should be discussed. Promoting physical activity, good nutrition, and environmental hazard surveillance is key to the health of seniors. The practitioner who learns to integrate those topics into routine office care through education, prevention screening, and encouragement can greatly enhance quality of life.

CHAPTER 5

Prevention and Screening Guidelines for Children and Adolescents

Jennifer Margolis • Susan Louisa Montauk

OBJECTIVES

- Be familiar with routine and preventive care for children and adolescents
- Explain the various aspects of anticipatory guidance and preventive care in children and adolescents
- List examples of screening guidelines for age-appropriate physical and developmental tasks in childhood and adolescence

INTRODUCTION

Preventive care begins before the birth of the child. Ideally, healthy childbearing should include preconception education, such as the recommendation that women of childbearing age who may become pregnant take folic acid to decrease the likelihood of neural tube defects. Family physicians who provide prenatal care generally discuss the expectations of the parents and offer anticipatory guidance regarding care of the newborn. However, because most family physicians do not provide obstetric care, many encourage expectant parents to schedule a prenatal consultation with them 6 to 8 weeks before the estimated delivery date. Other physicians do not begin the education process until the first newborn visit. The prenatal education model offered in this chapter is based on the one-time prenatal visit. Its content is meant to be adapted when other models of care are followed.

After the child is born, the well-child (or routine) visit provides regular opportunities throughout infancy, childhood, and adolescence for health maintenance, preventive care, and anticipatory guidance. It is important to focus on key age-appropriate health issues at every well-child visit. This chapter reviews some of the basic, more important health issues, but your preceptor may have others she finds to be particularly important.

Several organizations offer guidelines for the routine care of children and adolescents, and each physician should determine which recommendation he will follow. As with the other preventive chapters in this book, this chapter focuses on the guidelines of the United States Preventive Services Task Force (USPSTF). The USPSTF recommends seven well-child visits during the first 2 years of life. After 2 years of age, well-child visits are recommended at approximately 3, 5, and 11 to 16 years of age. During well-child visits, both the parent and child may be more relaxed than during a sick visit, providing an opportunity to get to know the child and the family.

> **NOTE**
>
> Children may be cared for and brought in by other caregivers in place of or in addition to parents. In this chapter, the term "parent" refers to the significant caregiver raising the child. A discussion of the medicolegal implications of custodial arrangements is beyond the scope of this book. Please confer with your preceptor if you have any questions.

GENERAL APPROACH TO CHILDREN

Medical students often express anxiety about dealing with young infants and small children. The child who is crying, uncooperative, or uncommunicative can heighten that anxiety even further. To help **put children at ease** you should:

- Be physically at the child's level
- Be gentle
- Speak softly
- Approach the child slowly
- Use toys to distract the child
- Wear bright colors
- Play games
- Talk about cartoon characters or pets

> **NOTE**
>
> Try to perform the physical examination of a small child while the parent is holding the child (i.e., on the lap or cuddling chest-to-chest).

Despite attempts to put children at ease, there are always going to be situations that are stressful and upsetting. It may be necessary to restrain a child for a procedure such as an ear examination. The child will often cry in response to being restrained, even when the procedure is not painful. Most children go through a normal period of development during which they are afraid of strangers and will cry no matter what is done. This can be distressing for the child, but it is usually transient and the child is often smiling by the end of the visit. Do not get discouraged or anxious. Remember that a gentle touch or hug can help the child to see you as a friend. For older children, a special treat at the end of the visit may work wonders. You should ask the parents before offering a treat. Some parents may allow their child to have stickers but not candy.

A distressed child can be a source of concern for parents. Parents may be reluctant to subject their children to what they perceive to be painful or frightening procedures. It is important to reassure parents that the pain is usually transient and there should be no long-term sequelae.

While an adolescent patient can provide his own history, an infant or young child "communicates" through his parents. However, it is still important to interact directly with the patient, even with very young infants. As children grow and can respond verbally, encourage them to participate in the interview. Some physicians encourage the parents of adolescents to leave the room for at least part of the office visit to encourage the confidential bond that may be the key to future care.

THE PRENATAL VISIT: ANTICIPATORY GUIDANCE AND HISTORY

Family Issues

Some **key questions to ask about the family** include:

- How do the parents feel about having a new baby?
- What are the medical histories and health habits of the family and household members? Is there any family history of congenital problems?
- Will there be any support from extended family and friends?
- Is either parent planning to stay home full or part time?
- Have plans been made for babysitters or day-care?

NOTE

Remind parents to attend to each other and their other children. Other family members may be overlooked with the excitement of a new baby on the way or in the household.

Safety

Following is a list of **safety tips** that parents should keep in mind when there is a new infant in the family:

- Make sure that **water heater thermostats** are set below 120°F to avoid the risk of scalding.
- Put an **approved rear-facing car seat** in the back seat of all cars for transporting infants up to 20 pounds.
- Put the baby in a **supine sleeping position,** which will decrease the risk of sudden infant death syndrome.

- Do not allow people to **smoke** around the baby. Exposure to tobacco smoke is associated with an increased risk of respiratory disease in infants and young children.

Nutrition

All mothers should be encouraged to breast-feed. To encourage breast-feeding, inform the expectant mother of the following facts:

> **NOTE**
>
> Breast milk provides ideal nutrition, protects infants against common respiratory and gastrointestinal infections, and decreases the incidence of allergic disease.

- Most mothers can successfully nurse their infants.
- There are few absolute contraindications to breast-feeding.
- Breast-feeding promotes bonding and provides psychological advantages for both mother and child.
- Studies suggest that breast milk intake produces long-term positive effects on health.
- Many mothers continue to nurse their infants even after returning to work. Milk expressed using a breast pump can be given to the infant by other caregivers.

Before a woman makes the final decision to breast-feed, make sure that she knows how her partner and other family members feel about breast-feeding. Determining whether family members are going to offer support, withhold support, or even undermine the process is an integral part of the decision. In addition, women who have had a previous distressing experience may need to be validated by the information that virtually all difficulties with breast-feeding are not a result of maternal inadequacy but of a lack of intensive instruction and support

Babies who do not breast-feed should receive iron-fortified formula.

THE NEWBORN: THE FIRST VISIT

In general, family physicians try to see all newborns immediately after birth (in the hospital) or within the first few days after birth (in the office). Many family physicians see all breast-feeding infants at 2 weeks of age to be sure that feeding is going well. This visit may be delayed until 4 weeks of age if the infant is receiving formula, particularly if the parents have had other children.

Anticipatory Guidance and History

Birth history

Review the pregnancy, labor, and delivery history and record APGAR scores, birth weight, length, and head circumference. Also document any problems that occurred in the newborn nursery or since going home.

Family issues

When a new baby arrives, family dynamics undergo change. Provide support to the primary caregivers and ask the following questions to determine how well the family is adjusting to the new member:

- How does the mother feel, both physically and emotionally, after giving birth? (Beware of postpartum depression.)
- How are the other adults and children in the home adjusting?
- Who lives at home and who participates in childcare?
- What role do other significant adults in the household (i.e., other than the primary caregiver) play in the infant's care and the household's day-to-day activities?
- Are there any health problems or significant changes in the family situation?

Nutrition

For mothers who breast-feed, review the frequency and duration of feeds, the mother's comfort level with breast-feeding, and any problems she has experienced. If the family is combining breast-feeding with bottle-feeding of breast milk, ask for specifics about both.

> **NOTE**
>
> Approximately 90% of the milk in each breast is suckled out within the first 10 minutes of nursing on that breast.

If a newborn is being fed formula, review the amount, frequency, and type of formula used. Make sure that the directions on any formula that must be reconstituted are being followed.

Inquire if the parents are supplementing with anything besides breast milk or formula.

> **NOTE**
>
> Do not prop bottles for infants in bed because of the potential for tooth decay and ear infections.

Immunizations

One immunization is given during the newborn period—hepatitis B. If the first dose of hepatitis B vaccine is not given in the hospital, it can be given at the first office visit.

Supplements

Iron

Most infants fed breast milk or iron-fortified formula do not need supplemental vitamins or iron for the first 6 months. Infants born before 36 weeks' gestation may have low iron stores and need supplements.

Vitamin D

Dark-skinned infants who are breast-fed during the winter in areas where they have no exposure to sunlight may need supplemental vitamin D. The actual vitamin D requirement in the absence of sunlight is unknown. Light-skinned infants receive sufficient vitamin D if they are exposed to sunlight for as little as 30 minutes per week unclothed or 2 hours per week fully clothed.

Physical Examination

> **NOTE**
>
> The coverage of periodic physical examinations in this chapter is not complete. Rather, this chapter is meant to cover key areas that will enhance the knowledge gained in courses that focus on physical diagnosis.

The first physical examination by the family physician should cover all organ systems. **The examination of a newborn infant or any baby new to the practice should not simply be focused; it should be complete.**

Vital signs

Newborn **temperatures** are taken rectally. This is a good time to ask if the parent is comfortable taking the newborn's temperature.

Weight can be an important indicator of health. Normal infants may lose up to 10% of their body weight during the first few days. Because a mother's breast milk usually starts to come in on the third or fourth day after delivery, breast-fed infants should stop losing weight by 1 week of age. By 2 weeks of age, breast-fed infants should be at birth weight or higher. Formula-fed infants tend to regain their birth weight more quickly.

Weight, length, and **head circumference** should be plotted on a growth chart.

HEENT

The **eyes** should be checked for a red reflex. Opacities may be indicative of congenital cataracts or glaucoma. A white retina may indicate a retinoblastoma. The **skull** should be checked to be sure the fontanelles are still open, and the **mouth** should be inspected for cleft palate.

Heart

Auscultate the heart for murmurs, but remember that murmurs may be difficult to hear with the typical pulse rate of 120 to 160 beats/min in a newborn.

Lungs

Auscultate the lungs for clarity of breath sounds.

Abdomen

Palpate the abdomen for masses that may result from polycystic kidneys. Assess for hepatomegaly and splenomegaly.

Skin and umbilical cord

Some skin lesions are normal (e.g., mongolian spots in dark-skinned infants, hemangiomas, erythema toxicum, milia, neonatal acne). Large congenital pigmented nevi and sebaceous nevi require referral to a dermatologist. Infants with defects in the subcutaneous tissues of the scalp should also be referred because of malignant potential in later years. Vesicular or pustular lesions with inflammation may indicate a serious viral or bacterial infection requiring immediate treatment.

The umbilical cord should dry up and fall off spontaneously between 3 days and 3 weeks of age. A small amount of drainage or bleeding during this time is normal. The cord should be kept dry and cleaned with alcohol until it has fallen off and there is no more drainage. A foul smell, purulent drainage, or erythema around the cord may indicate infection. Cord remnant erythema can result from too much or too aggressive cleaning with alcohol.

Screening Tests

Universal (i.e., throughout the United States) **newborn screening** is done for:

- Phenylketonuria
- Galactosemia
- Homocysteinuria
- Hypothyroidism
- Hemoglobinopathies

The tests for phenylketonuria and galactosemia are reliable only after the infant has been fed. Thus, for accuracy, blood samples should be obtained at least 48 hours after birth. Thyroid-stimulating hormone should be drawn after 24 hours of age. Infants are often discharged from the hospital earlier than 48 hours of age, in which case the tests for phenylketonuria and galactosemia must be repeated at home by a visiting nurse or at the first office visit.

INFANCY TO AGE FIVE

Anticipatory Guidance and History

Safety

Following are some safety tips to protect children from infancy through 5 years of age:

- **Car seats** are important for all children through 5 years of age and should be placed in the back seat.
- **Walkers** should not be used near stairs.
  - ☐ Always carefully discuss the safe use of walkers.
  - ☐ Many physicians discourage the use of walkers because of potential hazards; in fact, they are banned in Canada.
- **Tricycles** are great for motor development and fun but need to be carefully monitored to avoid accidents in the driveway or street.
- Medications and all other ingestible substances should be placed high up, far away from where small hands might get them, or otherwise locked away.
- **Ipecac** should be available in all homes, and parents need to be educated about its use.
  - ☐ The main contraindications to ipecac include ingestion of a corrosive chemical (e.g., drain cleaner) or a volatile substance that could be aspirated into the lungs.
  - ☐ Know your local poison control phone number and share it with parents.

Development

Developmental milestones are important. Parents enjoy learning about markers such as when to expect their child to smile, sit, walk, and talk. As visits progress, parents look for reassurance that their child is normal in development and physical health. Table 5–1 covers many different developmental, physical, and speech milestones. Always ask if parents have any concerns so you can specifically address those concerns.

When questions of developmental delay arise, the Denver Developmental Screening Test can be administered to evaluate gross motor function, fine motor function, social adaptiveness, and language development from birth through early childhood. Some family physicians administer this 30-minute screening tool in their office, while other physicians refer

TABLE 5–1. **Key Developmental Milestones: Infancy Through Preschool**

Age (Months)	Physical and Behavioral Milestones	Language Milestones
2	Smiles spontaneously	—
4	—	Coos
6	Rolls over*	Babbles
9	Sits alone, separation and stranger anxiety may begin	—
12	Pulls to a standing position and "cruises" (i.e., walks while holding onto things such as furniture)	Says "momma" or "dadda"
15	Walks well, stoops, climbs up stairs, drinks from a cup, feeds self with fingers, stacks two blocks, curious about and explores surroundings, tests limits, displays negativity and temper tantrums	Speaks 3–6 words, understands simple commands, listens to short stories, points to named body parts
18	Walks backward, pulls toy along, stacks three blocks	Speaks 15–20 words and a lot of jargon
24	Climbs down stairs, kicks ball, stacks five blocks, bowel and bladder control begin, helps with dressing and undressing	Uses two-word phrases, 65% of words are intelligible, follows two-step commands, imitates, matches animal pictures pictures and sounds
24–36	Jumps, rides tricycle, copies a circle and cross, interacts with peers, shares, starts to understand reasoning and discipline, practices daytime bladder and bowel control†, right- or left- handedness is manifested, some negativity or tantrums may persist	Speaks in sentences using verbs and adjectives, has a 200-word vocabulary, 80% of words are intelligible
36–48	Separates easily from parent; Speaks clearly; dresses without supervision; balances on one foot for 5 seconds; hops on one foot; picks longer of two lines; knows colors; counts to five; knows opposites and analogies; distinguishes right from wrong; knows name, address, and phone number; draws a person with head, body, arms, and legs	

*Many babies roll over earlier than 6 months of age, so watch carefully after 3 months of age if the infant is near the edge of a surface that is above the floor.
†A few "normal" children, most often boys, may not achieve full bowel and bladder control until the middle of the fourth year.

patients who appear to show delays to a physician who specializes in developmental disabilities.

> **NOTE**
>
> Any child who is not talking in full sentences with mostly intelligible speech by 3 years of age should be referred for speech and hearing evaluation.

Socialization

A playgroup or preschool may help with socialization and parent-child separation if the child is not in day-care or does not have siblings.

> **NOTE**
>
> Children who have learned to separate easily from their parents and take part in group activities before entering kindergarten make the adjustment to school more easily.

Discipline

There are many different approaches to discipline in our culture. Ask how the child is disciplined and discuss the importance and efficacy of using "time outs."

Intellectual skill building

Reading is the key to language and intellectual development. Encourage all parents to read to their children. **Music** may help build math skills and enhances play. In general, children love to learn singing games.

Immunizations

- Since the introduction of *Hemophilus influenzae* type B (HIB) vaccine in 1985, the incidence of invasive HIB infections in young children in the United States has fallen by 99%.
- Poliomyelitis has been eradicated from the western hemisphere since the vaccine was introduced in the 1950s.
- Measles, ubiquitous before 1965, is now rare in the United States.

Every year there are changes in immunization recommendations. An immunization schedule recommended by the Advisory Committee on Immunization Practices and endorsed by the American Academy of Family Physicians is published annually and can be found at the Centers for Disease Control and Prevention (CDC) web site (see Appendix III).

In addition to the standard childhood vaccines recommended by the Advisory Committee on Immunization Practices, others should be considered for certain high-risk children. These include influenza and respiratory syncytial virus vaccines. Lyme disease vaccines may be considered in high-risk geographic areas for individuals 15 years of age and older.

Supplements

Fluoride supplementation is indicated if there is an inadequate amount (i.e., less than 0.3–0.6 ppm) in the water supply.

Physical Examination

Vital signs

Blood pressure should be measured beginning when the child is 3 years old using an appropriate-sized cuff for the child. Weight should be recorded at each visit and plotted on a growth chart.

> **NOTE**
>
> Children usually double their birth weight by 4 months of age and triple it by 1 year of age.

HEENT

Check the **eyes** for a red reflex for the first 6 months after birth. Eyes often appear to "cross" in early infancy, which is generally a normal finding until 6 months of age. After 6 months of age, true eye crossing (strabismus) requires referral to an ophthalmologist. True strabismus can be detected by observing the reflection of a flashlight in the pupils; the reflections should be symmetrical. If the child is old enough to cooperate, the cover test can be used. One eye is covered while the other is focused on a fixed light. When one eye is alternately covered and uncovered, the contralateral pupil should not deviate medially or laterally.

Primary teeth start erupting as early as 4 months or as late as 12 months of age, and continue to erupt during the second year. The full set of 20 teeth is usually present by 24 to 36 months of age. Dental visits should begin at approximately 3 years of age, when the primary teeth are all erupted. Tooth brushing should begin as soon as the first tooth appears. Earlier referral to a dentist is indicated if there are signs of dental decay or abnormal dental development. Most experts recommend that children should be weaned from the bottle to the cup by 12 months of age to decrease the incidence of tooth decay.

Heart

Heart murmurs in infants are usually benign. If you think you hear a heart murmur, auscultate the heart through the back.

NOTE

A murmur heard through the back generally deserves expedient follow up.

Musculoskeletal system

The **hips** should be checked for dysplasia through the first year, until the child is walking well.

Skin

Check for diaper rash until toilet training is complete. Check for eczema, which is often first noted behind the ears.

Screening Tests

Hearing evaluations

Hearing evaluations of small children are usually done using gross assessment for the first few years. The child may need to be sent for quantifiable evaluation if there is a history of hearing-related problems (e.g., language delay). Pure-tone testing using an audiometer or similar device can be done in the office starting at 3 years of age. Tympanometry to detect middle ear fluid can be performed by 6 to 12 months of age.

Screening for iron deficiency

Iron deficiency is common in infants and young children and can have adverse effects on growth and intellectual development if untreated. Screening for iron deficiency is done at 9 to 12 months of age.

NOTE

Normal hemoglobin and hematocrit levels are lower in children than adults. Use a reference table of pediatric "norms" to evaluate results.

Screening for lead poisoning

Early treatment of lead poisoning prevents developmental and behavioral disorders. Screening should begin when the child begins to become mobile at 6 to 9 months of age. Questionnaires have been developed by the CDC to help identify those children who are at risk.

Screening for tuberculosis

Tuberculosis screening with the intradermal Mantoux test is required by some local health departments and schools for all children. It should be considered for all high-risk children.

AGES FIVE THROUGH ELEVEN

Anticipatory Guidance and History

School

The child's schooling should be evaluated at each well-child visit. Ask about attention span, academic achievement, behavior, and how the child interacts with peers. Ask about sports, music lessons, and other extracurricular activities. The child should be well-rounded but not overextended. Children need time for relaxing with friends and family. Quiet activities such as reading and an adequate amount of undisturbed sleep are important.

Limit setting and discipline

It is important to set limits for children. Encourage parents to limit the time their children spend watching television and help them make wise choices about the programs they watch. Ask about the forms of discipline the family uses and how they set rules. Age-appropriate, simple household chores can be assigned to each child to teach a sense of family and community responsibility and involvement.

Safety and hygiene

Discuss safety issues relevant to the home, the car, and public places (e.g., the street). Include the importance of bicycle helmets. Ask about supervision of the child before and after school. Most preteens need adult supervision, although some 11 to 12 year olds may be safe for short periods of time during daylight hours if they have shown sufficient maturity and know how to obtain prompt help. Make families aware of latchkey programs that may be available for children through sixth grade and community organizations (e.g., YMCA, Red Cross) that offer classes for preteens on first aid and babysitting.

Some age-appropriate topics to discuss include:

- Correct anatomical terms (use terms when discussing parts of the body, sexual characteristics, and body changes, but also ask the child and parents what terms they use) [4 year olds]
- Personal hygiene (5 year olds)
- Healthy diet (5 year olds)
- Stranger safety (6 year olds)
- The hazards of tobacco, drug, and alcohol abuse (8 year olds)

Nutrition

Following the **nutrition pyramid** (see Figure 20–1), although difficult (especially with picky eaters), should be encouraged. Discuss limiting refined sugars and fats.

Exercise

Encourage **daily exercise.** Electronic games and television should be treated as an addition to, not a replacement for, physical activity.

Intellectual skill building

Between the ages of 6 and 7 is a good time to get the child's first library card. Encourage parents to read age-appropriate stories, novels, and poetry to their children during the early school years. Suggest that children read out loud with their parents as well as read quietly alone. When feasible, children should be exposed to a wide variety of music.

Supplements

Fluoride supplementation is needed if there is an inadquate amount (i.e., < 0.6 ppm) in the water supply.

Physical Examination

Blood pressure should be measured at every well-child visit. Weight and height should continue to be plotted on growth charts.

Screening Tests

Test **vision** in all children over 4 years of age using a wall-mounted eye chart. Charts with pictures or the Snellen eye chart can be used for children who are unable to read. It is also important to assess **hearing.**

AGES TWELVE THROUGH SEVENTEEN

Anticipatory Guidance

Adolescents and confidentiality

In general, the more education you can provide adolescent patients, the more positive impact you have on their health. A careful, confidential, preventive approach to care can often convince adolescents to involve their parents even after initial reticence. At times, however, the adolescent's need for privacy and control or the sensitive nature of the health problem negate the adolescent's ability to give permission to involve the parents.

> **NOTE**
>
> Confidentiality between a physician and her adolescent patient may be the most important "tool" to promote prevention.

Most states allow physicians to treat adolescents 15 years of age and older, and often younger, for sexually transmitted diseases, substance abuse, birth control, and physical or sexual abuse without informing the parents. Many preceptors verbally assure both the patient and parents of patient confidentiality by the time the patient is 13 years of age.

Lifestyle concerns

You may feel uncomfortable speaking with an adolescent about issues such as condoms, drugs, or abuse, especially if you think that your patient may not be sexually active, likely to use drugs, or be abused. However, keep in mind that peers are the main educators of peers. Thus, by sharing information about controversial topics with an adolescent you may not only help to prevent future health concerns in that adolescent, but you may indirectly be responsible for positive lifestyle changes in your patient's peers.

> **NOTE**
>
> When discussing controversial issues with your adolescent patient, consider using the statement, "I realize you may not need the information yourself, but I talk with all teens your age about these things. With this knowledge you may be able to help, even save the life of, one of your friends or classmates."

Try to educate your adolescent patients before misconceptions have the chance to take root. For example, simple teaching about pubertal events (Table 5–2) should be initiated before the onset of puberty.

Sex

Interviews with high school students suggest that the peak time for learning about adult sexuality is during prepuberty and early puberty. If an adolescent is or may soon become sexually active, consider discussing both the health benefits of abstinence and those of contraception when abstinence is not followed. Over the last 5 years, the age until first intercourse and the use of birth control have increased while pregnancy rates and the number of abortions have decreased in adolescents. However, many young girls still become pregnant. An adolescent who is sexually active may not tell either a doctor or a parent for many reasons. Thus, many family physicians share the necessary and appropriate information with all adolescent patients.

> **NOTE**
>
> Check for possible pregnancy whenever necessary.

TABLE 5–2. **Timing of Pubertal Events**

Event	Girls	Boys
Growth spurt	Begins at about 11 years of age Peak height velocity is about 8 cm/year at 12 years of age By menarche, 90%–95% of height is reached	Begins at about 13 years of age Peak height velocity is about 9.5 cm/year at 14 years of age Often grow 2 cm after Tanner stage 5
Thelarche*	Full Tanner stage 5 breast development usually follows growth spurt May show uneven breast development initially	Breast and areolar development is common in early adolescence, but usually regresses within 1–2 years May show uneven breast development initially
Pubarche	Begins between 8 and 14 years of age (average of 11 years) Complete by about the end of the growth spurt	All normal boys have some genital maturation before pubarche
Menarche (girls), external genitalia (boys)	Usually begins at 10–16 years of age at about 47 kg (103 pounds) body weight Begins about 1 year after peak height velocity Begins 0.5–5.75 years after breast bud with average of 2.2 years 55%–90% of cycles are anovulatory for the first 20 months	Main Tanner stage for penile length increase is 4 Final penile length is about 15 cm
Facial and axillary hair	Often develop a small amount of facial hair during Tanner stages 4–5 Axillary hair appears in late puberty	Hair is found initially above the lip and on lower chin Hair is seldom found on upper chin until both genitalia and pubic hair are complete Axillary hair appears in late puberty
Orgasm, ejaculation	In studies, 30%–50% report having had an orgasm by 17 years of age	First ejaculation is usually 11–15 years of age, but the range is 8–21 years of age Ejaculatory ability is coincident with pubic hair development, about 1year before first wet dream

Adapted with permission from Montauk SL, Clasen ME: Sex education in primary care: infancy to puberty. *Med Aspects Human Sex* 23(1):22–36, 1989.
*Thelarche occurs before pubarche in 85% of adolescents.

Substance abuse

The average age for adolescents to begin using **tobacco** products is 13 to 14 years of age. Educate all adolescent patients about tobacco use, including cigarettes and chewing tobacco.

It is also important to discuss **alcohol** use and abuse with adolescent patients. Inform patients that one-third of adolescent deaths from motor vehicle accidents involve alcohol. Alcohol is also a significant factor in drowning and diving accidents.

Ask specifically about your patients' use of cigarettes, alcohol, and illicit drugs as well as about the habits of their peers and parents. Substance abuse by friends and parents increases the likelihood of current or future abuse.

> **NOTE**
>
> Children of alcoholics are four times more likely to have problems with alcohol.

Injury prevention

Ask about **guns** in the home. If guns are present, make sure the guns are locked up. Watch for **depression** and inappropriate expression of **anger.** Homicide and suicide account for approximately 40% of injury-related deaths in adolescents. Educate your patient about **seat belts** and **bicycle helmets,** because motor vehicle accidents account for the largest proportion of adolescent injuries.

> **NOTE**
>
> Injuries kill more adolescents than disease.

History

The adolescent history can provide indicators about the patient's mental health. School performance, involvement in sports and other extracurricular activities, after-school jobs, the family's spiritual belief system, and the family's health beliefs all provide important information.

> **NOTE**
>
> Normal development dictates a periodic disequilibrium between adolescents and their caregivers that can be very stress inducing for all involved.

A

Stage 1
Preadolescent. Nipple elevation

Stage 2

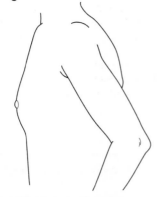

Breast bud stage. Elevation
as a small mound; enlargement
of areolar diameter

Stage 3

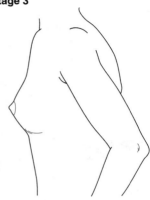

Further enlargement of elevation
of breast, nipple, and areola; all
one contour

Stage 4

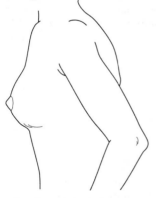

Areola and nipple form a
secondary mound projecting
from breast

Stage 5

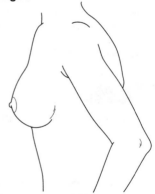

Mature stage; in most girls, areola
has receded and second mound
is breast only

FIGURE 5–1. Tanner stages of development. (A) Sex maturity ratings of breast changes in adolescent girls.

B

Stage 1

Preadolescent–no pubic hair except for fine vellus hair

Stage 2

Sparse, slightly pigmented, downy hair over the labia or base of the penis

Stage 3

Hair extends over the pubic symphysis and becomes darker, coarser, and curlier

Stage 4

Hair becomes adult-like, more coarse and curly.

Stage 5

Adult-like hair, increases in quantity and extends to medial thighs

FIGURE 5–1 (*Continued*). (*B*) Sex maturity ratings of pubic hair changes in adolescent girls and boys. (Adapted with permission from Tanner JM, Institute of Child Health, University of London, London.)

Development

Knowledge of **Tanner stages** (Figure 5–1), **pubertal stages** (see Table 5–2), and general information about anticipated normal adolescent **behavioral changes** often helps with differential diagnosis, education, and reassurance. Sexual maturation should be noted and should correspond with the child's age, somatic growth, and family history. A small child with delayed sexual development may become an average-sized adult, especially if a parent reports a similar growth pattern. On the other hand, a child who is growing faster than expected, with advanced sexual development, may reach a shorter than average adult height if she matures too quickly. Sexual precocity signs before 8 years of age in girls and 9 years of age in boys may require an evaluation for pathology.

NOTE

Remember that it is typical for adolescents to believe that they are invulnerable.

Common Office Problems

CHAPTER **6**

Acne Vulgaris

Charles Margolis

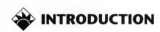 **INTRODUCTION**

> ### OBJECTIVES
> - Recognize the common presentation of acne
> - Understand the commonly used treatment modalities and the rationale for their use

Acne vulgaris, commonly referred to as simply "acne," is a disorder of the pilosebaceous units resulting in the formation of comedones, papules, pustules, and occasionally nodules. It occurs primarily on the face and upper back and is caused by overproduction of sebum within the pilosebaceous unit; increased "stickiness" of the squamous cells lining the duct, which blocks the pores; and the proliferation of a bacterium called *Propionibacterium acnes*.

Complex hormonal changes play a role in the development of acne lesions by regulating sebum production. In both genders, testosterone increases sebum production. Sebum also appears to be modulated by more than 12 other hormones, but their roles are not as well understood.

Acne is generally mild and significant scarring is uncommon, except in severe cases. However, because lesions can affect appearance and self-image, acne may have negative emotional consequences. Successful treatment of acne, particularly during adolescence, may be beneficial to the patient's emotional health and may enhance the patient–doctor relationship, which is often helpful when tackling more complex adolescent health issues.

TERMINOLOGY (ALSO SEE TERMINOLOGY IN CHAPTER 23)

Comedo, closed: a small follicular papule with inflammation (**red papule**) or without inflammation (**whitehead**)

Comedo, open: a dilated follicle with a central plug of sebaceous matter capped with dark epithelial debris (**blackhead**)

Cystic lesion: the lesion seen when a nodule fails to discharge its contents into the skin

Nodule: a firm, raised, localized skin lesion usually more than 1.5 cm in diameter

Nodulocystic acne: an advanced stage of acne that generally includes nodules, cystic lesions, and deep pustules and can lead to scarring

Papule: a raised lesion that is less than 1.5 cm in diameter

Pilosebaceous: relating to the hair follicles and sebaceous glands

Pustule: a lesion containing pus confined to a vesicle

Telangiectasia: dilated, superficial blood vessels that often appear "spider-like"

 BACKGROUND

Acne is the most common dermatologic problem seen by family physicians. The incidence of acne is similar in both genders, but it is often more severe in boys. Easily visible acne is very common in adolescent boys. For girls, menarche is associated with an increase in acne severity, and acne is often worse around menses. Pregnancy also can affect acne severity.

 PREVENTION

Primary Prevention

Sunlight improves acne in some patients but worsens it in others. Depending on the individual patient, sunlight may lead to the formation of more comedones or it may suppress the development of papules and pustules. Patients should be asked how sunlight affects their lesions and advised accordingly.

Secondary Prevention

To prevent new or advanced lesions, evaluate the patient's risk factors for acne. Some risk factors are alterable.

Iatrogenic risk factors include medications such as oral contraceptives, lithium, isoniazid, phenytoin, halogenated medications, and systemic steroids (both medically appropriate and illicit use for body building).

Environmental risk factors include external oils such as those in makeup (water-based makeup is better than oil-based makeup for some patients) and cooking oils (e.g., cooks laboring over grills).

Trauma from picking at comedones frequently leads to the formation of papules and pustules and should be discouraged. External compression (e.g., chin straps used by athletes) may also lead to inflammation of comedones.

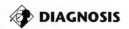 DIAGNOSIS

Presentation

Some patients may seek medical attention specifically for acne or present with a "complexion problem." Other patients may not mention acne as a problem but may be pleased to hear about treatment options.

History

History of present illness

- How long has acne been a problem?
  - □ In male patients, the onset of symptoms is usually in adolescence.
- In female patients, acne often begins in adolescence, but many experience its onset after 20 years of age.
- Does anything seem to make the acne worse or better (e.g., sunlight, stress)?
- Have you been exposed to iatrogenic or environmental risk factors (e.g., medications, external oils) [see secondary prevention; p 58]?
- What therapies have you tried in the past (e.g., over-the-counter preparations of benzoyl peroxide)?
  - □ If previous treatments were beneficial, they may be continued.
- If previous treatments were not beneficial, ascertain the patient's level of adherence to necessary regimens before excluding their use.
- What do you think causes your acne?
  - □ This is a good time to dispel myths.
- What bothers you most about your acne?
  - □ An assessment of the emotional impact on the patient is often warranted, particularly during adolescence when emotional lability is an issue.
- Many patients are despondent about their acne, in some cases because of the failure of previous treatments. Always project a positive attitude about treatment to encourage adherence to the medical regimen.
- Where are your acne lesions typically located?

Past medical history

- Is the patient taking a medication that is likely to induce or exacerbate acne (see secondary prevention; p 58)? If so, have alternative treatments been tried and with what effect?
- Would your female patient who is not on oral contraceptives benefit from being on oral contraceptives (see Oral Contraceptives; p 63)?

Family history

- Is there a history of nodulocystic acne in close relatives?

Social history

- What is the patient's occupation or hobby (see secondary prevention; p 58)?
  - □ Cooks exposed to cooking oils and athletes who wear chin straps are more at risk for acne.

> **NOTE**
>
> Many anecdotes refer to the effect of stress on the appearance of acne lesions; however, there is no evidence from controlled studies demonstrating a relationship between stress and acne.

Review of Systems

This means of diagnosis is not usually helpful for treatment decisions.

Physical Examination

Acne lesions are usually located on the face, upper back, and chest, in descending order of frequency. These are the locations with the greatest concentration of pilosebaceous units. The lesions include comedones (whiteheads and blackheads), papules, pustules, and nodules. Scars may also be present from previous lesions.

Laboratory Tests

Routine laboratory studies are not indicated unless severity or other physical findings suggest hormone abnormalities, such as virilization in a female patient.

DIFFERENTIAL DIAGNOSIS

Rosacea (also called **acne rosacea**) involves flushing, erythema, telangiectasia, and occasionally papules and pustules. It occurs in adults and increases in frequency with age. It appears on the nose, conjunctivae, and infraorbital areas. The cause is not yet known.

Perioral dermatitis is often associated with overuse of topical corticosteroids on the face, either in the present or recent past (i.e., rebound perioral dermatitis). It usually appears as papules and pustules on erythematous bases, most commonly around the mouth and in the nasolabial folds. It occurs in adults rather than teenagers.

Folliculitis appears as pustules surrounding a hair. Each of the pustules is surrounded by a reddish halo. It may occur in the beard distribution or on any hairy body part.

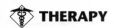 **THERAPY**

Treatment should be offered to all patients with acne. Acne is usually simple to treat. Therapy "failures" are often secondary to poor adherence to the required regimen, so carefully explore the patient's degree of adherence before abandoning a specific treatment.

Nonpharmacologic Therapy

Education about the factors that contribute to acne development is very important. It is also important to dispel myths about the factors that are likely to cause acne (e.g., chocolate, masturbation). Printed educational materials are widely available and should be used to supplement verbal advice.

Diet appears to have little, if any, effect on the frequency or type of acne lesions present.

Pharmacotherapy (Table 6–1)

Topical medications are often effective and should be tried before systemic medications, which may have greater side effects and risks. It is important to apply topical medication in a thin film and spread it over the entire area where acne lesions may occur, not just where the lesions are currently present. To minimize side effects, the initial applications may need to be less frequent than the usual daily or twice daily recommendations.

Topical benzoyl peroxide

Some patients use over-the-counter benzoyl peroxide before consulting with a physician, having heard from peers, family, the media, or pharmacists about its efficacy. Benzoyl peroxide gel, commonly used in a 5% or 10% over-the-counter concentration, is often quite effective in decreasing colony counts of *P. acnes* and works best for treatment of open comedones (i.e., blackheads). Thus, if your patient has not tried this fairly safe alternative, consider it as your first choice.

When used alone, benzoyl peroxide is commonly applied once daily to cleansed areas. If no negative irritation is present after several days to 1 week, applications can be increased to twice daily. Three applications daily is a safe regimen, but few patients tolerate three applications or can adhere to the schedule.

Some individuals are intolerant of benzoyl peroxide, developing contact or irritant dermatitis. Sometimes this is caused by using too much too soon.

Follow-up visits are commonly scheduled 6 or 8 weeks after beginning treatment to allow time for the therapeutic medication effects.

TABLE 6–1. **Acne Pharmacotherapy**

Medication	Comments	Side Effects
Benzoyl peroxide*	Available without a prescription, first-line treatment	Redness, irritation
Topical antibiotics	As effective as oral antibiotics, hard to apply to the back	Redness, irritation
Topical tretinoin	Especially effective for closed comedone	Redness, irritation, pregnancy complications[†]
Oral antibiotics	Convenient, use when topical treatments fail	Mild nausea, may affect oral contraceptive efficacy, sun sensitivity (tetracycline), pregnancy complications[†]
Oral contraceptives	May have other positive therapeutic effects, often as effective as other medications	Mild nausea, headaches
Oral isotretinoin	Highly effective, benefit often prolonged, use only with highly effective birth control if pregnancy is possible	Highly teratogenic[†], xerosis, epistaxis, arthralgia, elevated triglyceride and lipid levels (requiring frequent blood draws), pseudotumor cerebri

The side effects listed are the most common. There are many additional side effects that are rare.

*Some clinicians add topical antibiotics to the benzoyl peroxide regimen. Gels are available that include both a macrolide antibiotic and benzoyl peroxide (e.g., 3% erthyomycin and 5% benzoyl peroxide)

[†]Isotretinoin, tetracycline, and sulfa drugs are associated with fetal complications.

NOTE

When a follow-up visit is required, keep in mind that skin turnover takes approximately 1 month.

Topical antibiotics

Some topical antibiotics (e.g., clindamycin, erythromycin, metronidazole) also decrease colony counts of *P. acnes*. If benzoyl peroxide does not achieve appropriate results, many clinicians discontinue benzoyl peroxide and prescribe a topical antibiotic. It is generally recommended that topical antibiotics be used twice daily.

Tretinoin

Tretinoin, a vitamin A analog, is highly effective, especially against closed comedones (i.e., whiteheads). Tretinoin reduces squamous cell stickiness and proliferation. It may be used in combination with antibacterial agents; however, its use is often limited by skin irritation, particularly in fair-skinned individuals. Therefore, dosing starts slowly, with every other day use progressing to daily use and higher concentrations as tolerated. If skin irritation is a problem, consider using creams, which are less irritating than gels. Instruct the patient to apply tretinoin at night, and watch for hypersensitivity to the sun during warm months.

> **NOTE**
>
> Tretinoin prevents the formation of new lesions rather than clearing up old lesions; therefore, positive effects may not be seen for 3 to 4 weeks.

Oral antibiotics

Oral antibiotics are more convenient to use than topical medications, especially when acne is located on the back. Tetracycline is the most commonly used oral antibiotic. The most common dose is 500 mg twice daily, although daily doses can range from as low as 250 mg to as high as 2 g. Erythromycin, trimethoprim-sulfamethoxazole, and minocycline may be used as well.

> **NOTE**
>
> Tetracyclines may be teratogenic and will stain developing teeth; therefore, women of childbearing age should be carefully screened and educated about their use. Many clinicians only prescribe tetracyclines for men or women on adequate birth control. Unfortunately, tetracycline may interfere with oral contraceptive efficacy.

Oral contraceptives

Several studies have demonstrated that oral contraceptive formulations containing triphasic norgestimate are quite effective against acne. This is particularly important to keep in mind for patients already taking oral contraceptives. However, some clinicians recommend triphasic norgestimate–containing oral contraceptives for patients who are not already taking oral contraceptives if other areas of their health may benefit.

Isotretinoin

Isotretinoin, an oral medication related to tretinoin, is useful in severe (e.g., nodulocystic lesions that may lead to scarring if not adequately treated) or treatment-resistant cases of acne. Its exact mechanism of action is unknown. Because isotretinoin has a wide variety of side effects, it is advisable to exhaust other treatment options first.

> **NOTE**
>
> The potential fetal abnormalities associated with isotretinoin use are so severe that most physicians do not prescribe isotretinoin to women who are or may become sexually active, unless they are taking very reliable birth control.

 ## URGENCIES & EMERGENCIES

Highly inflamed lesions can be associated with emotional turmoil in some adolescents. When quick response to treatment is desired, as in the case of a teenager wishing to attend an important dance, it may be appropriate for experienced practitioners to use intralesional injections of corticosteroids.

 ## SPECIAL POPULATIONS

Children

"Neonatal" or "infantile" acne has been attributed to placental transfer of maternal androgens, relatively high androgen levels arising from the adrenal glands, and transient increases in end-organ response to androgenic hormones. This is a self-limiting condition that usually resolves spontaneously within several months. Thus, reassurance is usually the treatment of choice.

Seniors

The persistence of inflammatory acne after 50 years of age is unusual, although occasionally older patients will have comedones, often located on the temples. These respond well to tretinoin treatment.

Pregnancy

Acne is usually not affected in early pregnancy, improves during the second and third trimesters, and flares after delivery or weaning. Be sure to avoid medications that may cause complications (see Table 6–1).

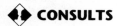 **CONSULTS**

Referrals to dermatologists for acne management are rarely necessary, although some family physicians less familiar with the treatment of difficult cases commonly refer acne patients to dermatologists. Patients also may request referral to a dermatologist, feeling that acne is a problem requiring a specialist. In most cases, an explanation of the simplicity of treatment is often helpful in continuing care by the family physician.

CHAPTER 7

Allergic Rhinitis

Bruce Gebhardt

 INTRODUCTION

The topic of allergic rhinitis is a model for understanding common allergic responses. Many of the principles discussed in this chapter relate to other manifestations of environmental allergies, such as sinus headaches, asthma, and allergic conjunctivitis.

OBJECTIVES

- Describe the common presentations of allergic rhinitis
- Explain preventive measures for allergic rhinitis
- Recognize the prevalence of allergic rhinitis and its potential complications
- Compare and contrast treatment options for allergic rhinitis
- Identify when it is appropriate to refer patients with allergic rhinitis

Allergic rhinitis is a common abnormal immune [i.e., immmunoglobulin E (IgE)] response to airborne environmental elements that results in increased mucous secretion, vasodilation, runny nose, nasal congestion, sneezing, watery eyes, and nasal pruritus. The associated response has two linked phases that are both mediated by an abnormal immune response to antigens. The phase of allergic rhinitis affects the clinical presentation and therapy choices.

Type I allergic response (i.e., **early-phase** overactive immune response in the nasal mucosa) involves the production of IgE antibodies and consequent degranulation of **mast cells.** The mast cells release **histamine** and other inflammatory compounds such as **prostaglandins** and **leukotrienes.**

Type II allergic response (i.e., **late-phase** overactive immune response in the nasal mucosa) involves the arrival of granulocytes, eosinophils, basophils, and mononuclear cells in response to the release of inflammatory products. The type II response leads to more inflammation 4 to 12 hours after exposure.

TERMINOLOGY

Allergic crease: a horizontal nasal crease that results from chronically performing the allergic salute (also called a nasal crease)

Allergic salute: frequent upward rubbing of the nose that often results in a nasal crease

Allergic shiners: black, dark halos around the eyes caused by midfacial venous congestion; most commonly seen in children

Atopic: relating to atopy

Atopy: a type I allergic reaction mediated by an abnormal IgE antibody response and caused by allergens such as dander, pollen, and food; associated with familial tendencies

Episodic allergy: an allergy caused by a time-limited, intermittent exposure to an allergen (e.g., allergic response to perfume in an elevator)

Perennial allergy: an allergy caused by one or more allergens that are plentiful throughout the year, thus generating symptoms year-round or close to year-round (e.g., an allergy to dust mites)

Rhinitis: inflammation of the nasal mucosa

Rhinitis medicamentosa: the rebound response of overuse of nasal decongestant spray

Seasonal allergy: an allergy caused by season-specific allergens (e.g., ragweed in "hayfever")

Vasomotor rhinitis: rhinitis caused by a nonallergen (e.g., a cool environment) and associated with rapid vasodilation and congestion; congestion is often provoked by a change in environmental humidity or temperature

⬦ BACKGROUND

Allergic rhinitis is very common and may affect as much as 20% to 25% of the population in the United States, making it the most common nasal problem. In high allergy areas (e.g., river valleys), allergic rhinitis may actually affect more than half of the population.

The onset of allergic rhinitis is usually before 30 years of age, with peak incidence in childhood and adolescence.

🛡 PREVENTION

Risk Factors

- Exposure to allergic triggers
- Presence of other atopic problems
- Family history

Prevention

Prevention is the first-line treatment for allergic rhinitis and consists of **avoidance of allergic triggers.** Offer patients suggestions to avoid exposure to molds, dander, and dust mites (see Chapter 8, Secondary Prevention; p 79).

Patients may not be able to avoid outdoor allergens, but some strategies may help to ameliorate exposure and symptoms.

- Wear a surgical mask when mowing the grass or weeding.
- Do not plant high pollen-producing plants, shrubs, or trees in the vicinity of the home.
- Stay inside as much as possible during "allergy season" and "high-count" days.

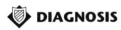 DIAGNOSIS

Allergic rhinitis is often one of several manifestations of the allergic response. Many atopic patients concurrently suffer with allergic conjunctivitis, asthma, and eczema.

Presentation

Some patients may call or visit the office to request a nonsedating antihistamine, well aware that they have allergic rhinitis. A large number of people self-diagnose, self-treat with over-the-counter (OTC) medications, and do not think to mention the problem unless asked specifically. Allergic rhinitis is often not identified until a patient presents with a chief complaint such as, "I have sinus problems," "My asthma is acting up again," or "I can't get rid of this cold."

There are multiple **clinical presentations** associated with allergic rhinitis.

- Allergy-mediated congestion can lead to eustachian tube dysfunction. This, in turn, may lead to serous otitis (otitis media with effusion), recurrent otitis media, a chronic sore throat, a chronic cough, and hearing impairment.
- Obstructed sinus drainage can lead to bacterial sinusitis and headache.
- Postnasal drip can lead to sore throat and hoarseness.
- Chronic mouth breathing in children can lead to orthodontic problems.
- Chronic exposure to allergens is associated with deviation of the nasal septum and chronically enlarged tonsils.

History

NOTE

The key to the diagnosis of allergic rhinitis is patient history.

History of present illness

- Are you experiencing symptoms such as congestion (sinus or nasal), clear nasal discharge, fatigue, pruritus of the nose or eyes, or sneezing?
- Are the symptoms episodic, seasonal, or constant?

- What triggers the occurrence of symptoms?
  - □ Common allergic triggers in and around the home include perfumes, pollen, pollution, grass, animal dander, cleaning chemicals, and cigarette smoke. All of these may have an exacerbated response when increased emotional stress is a cofactor.
- Are you experiencing fever, muscle aches, or yellow-green sputum or nasal discharge (may indicate infection)?
- What treatments have you tried (e.g., OTC medications, prescription medications, self-taught avoidance measures) and how effective were the treatments?

Past medical history

Ask the patient about:
- Otitis diagnoses
- Tympanostomy tubes
- Asthma
- Sinus headaches
- Seasonal problems with allergies
- Chronic cough
- Chronic sore throat
- Allergy shots

Family history

- Is there a family history of nasal allergies or sinus problems?
  - □ If one parent has had allergic rhinitis, the risk is 40%.
  - □ If both parents have had allergic rhinitis, the risk is 70%.

Social history

- Are you regularly exposed to allergens at home (e.g., smokers, pets, damp basement), work, or school?

Review of Systems

Focusing on individual systems, ask the patient about symptoms associated with allergy, upper respiratory infection, or both (Table 7–1).

Physical Examination (Table 7–2)

Laboratory Tests

The **radioallergosorbent test (RAST)** measures IgE levels for a range of possible allergens. It is not very specific; patients may test positive to an allergen but not be truly allergic to that allergen. Although RAST is not as

TABLE 7–1. **Review of Systems: A Comparison of Allergic Rhinitis and URI**

System	Signs and Symptoms	Likelihood of Positive Finding* Allergic Rhinitis	URI
Dermatologic	Exzema (itchy, red to pearly rash commonly seen in flexor creases or behind the ears)	+++	+
	Viral exanthem (red maculopapular rash commonly noted on trunk and extremities)	—	+++
HEENT			
Eyes	Pain	+	++
	Itchy sclera	+++	+
	Injected sclera	++++	++
	Yellow conjunctival discharge	—	++
	White or translucent conjunctival discharge	+++	+
	Unilateral eye involvement	+	++
	Bilateral eye involvement	++++	+
Ears	Pain	+	++++
	Itchy auditory canal	++++	+
	Perceived internal pressure	++	++
Nose	Rhinorrhea	+++	+++
	Sneezing	+++	+++
	Congestion	+++	+++
	Yellow discharge	—	++
	White or translucent discharge	+++	+
Throat/neck	Pain	—	+++
	Itchy pharynx	+++	+
	Hoarseness	+	+++
	Cervical lymph node enlargement	—	++
Respiratory	Asthma symptoms (wheezing, dry cough, shortness of breath)	++	+
	Bronchitis symptoms (productive cough, yellow-green sputum)	—	+++

URI = upper respiratory infection.
*The plus signs represent the approximate likelihood of a positive finding in the review of systems if the specified system (organ) is involved. However, a patient can have either allergic rhinitis or a URI without perceiving that any of the above systems (organs), other than the nose, are affected.

TABLE 7–2. Physical Examination Findings in Allergic Rhinitis

System	Findings
HEENT	Chronic nasal congestion; mouth breathing; injected conjunctiva; infection or effusion of the tympanic membranes; boggy, pale or bluish nasal mucosa with clear nasal discharge; postnasal drip; allergic shiners or nasal crease; nasal polyps; enlarged oral pharynx or tonsils; halitosis
Dermatologic	Eczema in flexor creases (e.g., elbow, knee)
Lymphatic	Enlargement or tenderness of the lymph nodes (especially in the neck)
Respiratory	Wheezing (may indicate an asthmatic exacerbation)

specific as skin testing, it may be helpful if the patient has skin disease, is unable to discontinue medications that may interfere with skin testing (e.g., histamine blockers, steroids), or has a history of anaphylaxis.

Nasal smear evaluation (i.e., examination of nasal secretion for eosinophils) is noted as a test to consider for allergic rhinitis in many texts. Unfortunately, it is not very sensitive; a negative smear does not rule out allergic rhinitis.

Imaging Studies

Radiographs do not play a role in the diagnosis of allergic rhinitis unless a secondary complication (e.g., sinusitis) is suspected.

Additional Studies

Skin testing is the gold standard for allergen identification. Skin testing is highly sensitive and specific for allergens; however, it does not always identify the cause of symptoms, and negative skin tests do not rule out allergic rhinitis. Although patients may request testing to identify the specific allergen responsible for their symptoms, skin testing is usually not necessary to identify appropriate therapy.

Skin testing should be considered if a patient does not respond to empiric treatments, needs medication on a chronic or nearly chronic basis, or is insistent. Skin testing should not be done if there is a rash or other skin disease over the area that needs to be tested. Patients who do require skin testing should not take antihistamines for at least 1 week before the test.

⬧ DIFFERENTIAL DIAGNOSIS

Common differential diagnoses of allergic rhinitis include:
- Bacterial sinusitis (indicated by yellow or green mucous, fever, facial and tooth pain, headache)

- Nonallergic rhinitis eosinophilia syndrome
- Obstruction (e.g., foreign body, polyp, tumor, deviated septum)
- Rhinitis medicamentosa
- Vasomotor rhinitis
- Viral upper respiratory infection

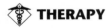 **THERAPY**

Nonpharmacologic Therapy

Avoidance of allergens should be incorporated into all treatment programs (see prevention; p 67).

Pharmacotherapy

Allergic rhinitis may be mild and successfully self-treated with OTC oral allergy medication or cromolyn nasal spray. If the allergen exposure is expected to be less than 3 days, or the role of a mild infection is unclear, OTC nasal decongestant sprays can be used.

Allergic rhinitis that is moderate to severe and disruptive to patient functioning may benefit from prescription medication. This can be divided into two subgroups: medications that modify the pathophysiology (e.g., antihistamines, steroids, mast cell stabilizers, immunotherapy) and medications that directly modify symptoms (e.g., decongestants, anticholinergics).

Antihistamines

Antihistamines block histamine release from mast cells and can alleviate sneezing, rhinorrhea, and pruritus, but not congestion. Antihistamines are systemic drugs that may not be appropriate for treating a local problem. This may be an advantage if other symptoms (e.g., allergic conjunctivitis) are present or if the patient's allergy season is only a few weeks out of the year.

There are two broad categories of antihistamines: **sedating** and **nonsedating.** Sedating antihistamines (e.g., diphenhydramine, chlorpheniramine) are usually OTC medications. Nonsedating antihistamines (e.g., cetirizine, fexofenadine, loratadine) usually require a prescription. The nonsedating antihistamines have a better side-effect profile and longer duration of action than the sedating antihistamines, but may be more expensive. There is one antihistamine nasal spray formulation (i.e., azelastine) available.

Decongestant–antihistamine combinations are also available and are advantageous for certain presentations. Taking a combination of decongestant and antihistamine means exposure to the possible negative side effects from two different drugs, when only one of the medications (i.e., antihistamine or decongestant) may be indicated.

Steroids

Steroids can be delivered systemically or intranasally. While systemic steroids are used infrequently for allergic rhinitis, **intranasal steroids are the single most effective treatment for chronic allergic rhinitis.** As many as 90% of patients experience relief with intranasal steroids. Intranasal steroids are generally safe, are very effective, treat local disorders locally, and can be used year-round for perennial rhinitis.

When steroids are administered, the side effect of major concern is systemic absorption and disruption of the hypothalamic-pituitary-adrenal axis. This side effect is especially worrisome in children; however, it occurs so rarely that most intranasal steroid products are approved for children 6 years of age and older.

Sprays vary in delivery systems, odor, and taste. Be sure to educate patients about the proper use of the available nasal sprays. Relief usually takes approximately 1 week to occur; therefore, for seasonal allergic rhinitis, it is best to start intranasal steroids before the patient's allergy season begins.

> **NOTE**
>
> Inform all patients using steroid sprays that they will not experience immediate relief of symptoms.

Mast cell stabilizers—cromolyn

Cromolyn is available as an OTC nasal spray. It is a first-line treatment option for children because of its safety profile. It is not as effective as intranasal steroids, but may be a reasonable alternative. An oral form, though available, is not used for allergic rhinitis. Like intranasal steroids, cromolyn does not immediately reduce symptoms; rather, it is administered to prevent symptoms from occurring.

Immunotherapy

Immunotherapy is effective in 85% of patients and may reduce or eliminate the need for other medications. Approximately 60% of patients experience long-lasting symptom reduction after injections are discontinued.

> **NOTE**
>
> Although the side effects of immunotherapy are usually minor (e.g., local reaction at injection site), anaphylaxis is possible.

Family physicians often administer immunotherapy injections ("allergy shots") prescribed by an allergist. Observe the patient for anaphylaxis for 30 minutes after giving the injection. Some patients may avoid immunotherapy because of dislike of needles, time constraints, or expense.

> **NOTE**
>
> Before administering an immunotherapy injection, screen the patient for evidence of uncontrolled asthma, which increases the risk of anaphylaxis.

Decongestants

Decongestants are available in nasal (topical) and oral formulations. The nasal sprays (e.g., oxymetazoline) work well, but can only be used for a few days continuously. If used longer than 3 to 4 days, rebound congestion may occur. Patients who use topical decongestant nasal sprays chronically often refer to them as "addictive" and may use the sprays for years, even to the point of perforation of the nasal septum. Discontinuing nasal decongestants after long-term use can be difficult.

> **NOTE**
>
> Chronic sympathomimetic stimulation can lead to rebound congestion (i.e., rhinitis medicamentosa) and a vicious cycle of medication use followed by rebound congestion.

Oral decongestants are available as OTC medications or by prescription. Because they are sympathomimetics, side effects such as palpitations and increased blood pressure are possible. Oral decongestants may not be suitable for patients with hypertension, coronary artery disease, or an uncontrolled anxiety disorder. Men with prostatic hypertrophy may experience urinary retention.

Anticholinergics—ipratropium

Ipratropium nasal spray is indicated for the treatment of rhinorrhea. It is a prescription drug that should be considered when other medications are ineffective or when vasomotor rhinitis is a possible diagnosis.

Leukotriene inhibitors

Leukotriene inhibitors are oral prescription medications for asthma that have shown benefit for the treatment of allergic rhinitis. They are not currently FDA approved for allergic rhinitis but may be considered for patients with both asthma and allergic rhinitis.

URGENCIES & EMERGENCIES

Allergic rhinitis can cause severe nasal congestion and secondary problems such as headache. When patients are miserable, immediate relief with an oral steroid burst is useful. When used with more traditional therapies, a steroid burst will relieve symptoms within 24 hours and allow time for intranasal steroids to work.

Anaphylaxis is a life-threatening condition. In regard to allergic rhinitis, it is mainly of concern when using immunotherapy. If your preceptor's office is giving allergy shots, they will carefully screen patients with coexisting asthma. Peak flows should be greater than 70% of the patient's best before giving the shot. A crash cart is essential office equipment if allergy shots are being given. Epinephrine is the therapy of choice for anaphylaxis.

SPECIAL POPULATIONS

Children

Cromolyn is an OTC medication and is the first-line treatment for allergic rhinitis in children. One nonsedating antihistamine, cetirizine, is FDA approved for children 2 years of age and older. Sedating antihistamines are available in many OTC formulations (e.g., diphenhydramine) that are appropriate for children.

> **NOTE**
>
> In children, asthma and allergic rhinitis occur concurrently in a large percentage of patients. This concurrence decreases with age.

Seniors

Antihistamines with anticholinergic properties should be used cautiously in older patients. They may cause side effects such as confusion, sedation, hypotension, urinary retention, and worsening glaucoma. Because seniors have an increased rate of hypertension and coronary artery disease, decongestants are less suitable in this population.

Pregnancy

Cromolyn is the drug of choice for pregnant patients with allergic rhinitis. Some antihistamines (e.g., tripelennamine, chlorpheniramine, diphenhydramine) have also been used safely. Inhaled steroids (e.g., beclomethasone) are used for the treatment of asthma during pregnancy and should be safe when used intranasally for allergic rhinitis. Pseudoephedrine, a decongestant, has also been used safely in pregnant patients.

Immunotherapy is generally not started in pregnancy, but may be continued in pregnancy if already begun. If immunotherapy is to continue after a pregnancy is verified and the family physician will not be responsible for prenatal care, the health care provider who will be providing prenatal care should be notified. The allergist should also be informed.

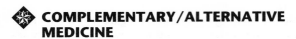 COMPLEMENTARY/ALTERNATIVE MEDICINE

The evidence for homeopathy is conflicting. There are studies showing benefit in the treatment of allergic rhinitis. These studies compared placebo, not conventional medicines, to homeopathy.

◆▶ CONSULTS

Consider referral to an **allergist** when a patient does not respond to your treatments or when a patient's allergy and treatment history suggests that allergy shots may be a better alternative than chronic medication use. Allergists may also have the expertise and staff to provide more thorough patient education. Most family physicians do not perform skin testing or prescribe immunotherapy.

Otolaryngologists may be consulted to help with surgically correctable complications of allergic rhinitis (e.g., frequent otitis media).

CHAPTER 8

Asthma

Jeff Kirschman

STUDENT OBJECTIVES

- Define "asthma"
- Describe both primary and secondary prevention of asthmatic symptoms
- Obtain an appropriate history for both new onset asthma and for poorly controlled chronic asthma
- Explain pharmacologic and non-pharmacologic treatment modalities and therapeutic interventions for chronic asthma

 INTRODUCTION

Simply stated, asthma is a chronic inflammatory disorder of the airways characterized by reversible airflow obstruction and airway hyperresponsiveness. In susceptible individuals, inflammation of the airways causes recurrent episodes of wheezing, breathlessness, chest tightness, and coughing, particularly at night and in the early morning. These episodes are usually associated with widespread but variable airflow obstruction that often reverses spontaneously or with treatment. Inflammation also causes an associated increase in the existing bronchial hyperresponsiveness to a variety of stimuli.

TERMINOLOGY

Cor pulmonale: right ventricular hypertrophy induced by lung disease

FEV_1/FVC: a ratio of the two indices (i.e., forced expiratory volume in 1 second and forced vital capacity) used to determine the presence of obstructive or restrictive lung disease by providing a measure of the amount of air that can be exhaled in the first second to the total amount of exhaled air; generally, this ratio is 75% or higher in healthy individuals and may be decreased in patients with obstructive lung diseases [e.g., asthma, chronic obstructive pulmonary disease (COPD)]

Forced expiratory volume in 1 second (FEV_1): the volume of air expired in the first second after a full inspiration; the FEV_1 usually is decreased in patients with obstructive lung disease

Forced vital capacity (FVC): the total volume of air forcibly expired from the lungs after a maximum inspiration

Lung compliance: the ability of the lungs to rebound (i.e., the elastic properties of the lungs); decreased in patients with emphysema

Pack year: the equivalent of one pack per day for 1 year with 20 cigarettes per pack

Peak expiratory flow rate (PEFR): measurement of the maximum rate of airflow attained during a single forced expiration

Spirometry: measurement of the volume of air inhaled or exhaled

Status asthmaticus: a severe asthma exacerbation with extreme intractable bronchospasm

Tachypnea: a rapid respiratory rate

Vital capacity (VC): the maximum volume of air that can be expelled slowly and completely after a full inspiratory effort

Wheeze: a breath sound often described as "whistling" or "squeaking" that is produced by a rush of air passing through constricted bronchioles

◆ BACKGROUND

It is estimated that asthma occurrences are experienced by 4% to 6% of the population in the United States. Approximately 50% of persons with asthma experience onset before 10 years of age, though less than half of these cases continue into adulthood. Despite scientific advances in understanding its pathophysiology and treatment, asthma is one of a few diseases of increasing prevalence in the United States. Over the past 20 years, from 1980 to 1994, the self-reported prevalence rate increased by 75%. Approximately 13.4 million people reported having asthma in 1994.

In the United States, the number of deaths with asthma as the underlying cause increased from 8.2 per 1,000,000 population in 1975 to 1978 to 17.9 per 1,000,000 population in 1993 to 1995.

The average rate of office visits associated with asthma complaints increased from 25 per 1000 population in 1980 to 1981 to 39 per 1000 population in 1993 to 1995. In contrast, the estimated annual hospitalization rates in which asthma was the primary diagnosis remained relatively stable, from 17.6 per 10,000 population in 1979 to 1980 to 18.1 per 10,000 population in 1993 to 1994.

Relative to caucasians, **African Americans** are seen for asthma in emergency rooms five times more often, are hospitalized for asthma at a rate three times higher, have a higher rate of self-reported asthma (57.8 versus 50.8 per 1000), and have a 2.5 times higher annual death rate associated with asthma (38.5 versus 15.1 per 1,000,000). African-American males between the ages of 18 and 34 have a death rate associated with asthma that is five times higher than that of white males of the same age.

Although males are twice as likely as females to experience childhood-onset asthma, this ratio equilibrates in the adult years. In 1993 to 1995, adult females had a higher rate of hospitalizations, emergency room visits, office visits, and self-reported asthma than males. Since the late 1960s, adult females have also had a consistently higher rate of death associated with asthma.

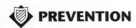 **PREVENTION**

Primary Prevention

Primary prevention of adult-onset asthma involves never smoking or smoking cessation, because cigarette smoke enhances the risk of sensitization to allergens. It is also important to control exposure to allergens in the workplace, which are estimated to be responsible for 2% to 15% of cases of adult-onset asthma.

Secondary Prevention

Identification of specific allergens provides direction for intervention and environmental control; however, control of environmental triggers should be individualized for the patient. Keep in mind that controlling the environment to minimize exposure to the identified allergen can be expensive and time-consuming for the patient.

Contact with problematic nonallergenic triggers (e.g., environmental tobacco smoke, irritant gases, dust, chemical fumes) should be limited by avoidance. Wall-to-wall carpeting may also be problematic for persons with environmental allergies because it harbors dust, dust mites, pet dander, and other airborne elements.

Allergies related to **furry pets** (e.g., cats) are most effectively dealt with by removing the animal. After removal of the animal, it may take up to 6 months for animal dander to fade away from the environment. If the animal cannot be removed from the household, it should be confined to noncarpeted areas and should not be permitted in the patient's room.

Mold growth in the home may be reduced by maintaining a low humidity (i.e., less than 50%) and changing furnace filters yearly.

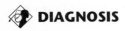 **DIAGNOSIS**

The presumptive diagnosis of asthma can be made based on history and physical examination. Further pulmonary function testing can help confirm and quantify your original assessment.

Presentation

The prominent clinical symptoms of asthma include a persistent, episodic cough; chest tightness; wheezing; and shortness of breath. Bronchospasm induced by exercise often presents with cough or shortness of breath during or after increased physical activity.

History

History of present illness

Questions to consider asking include:

- Are you awakened at night by coughing, wheezing, or shortness of breath?
- Do you experience coughing, wheezing, or unexpected shortness of breath during or after exercise?
- Are there certain times of the day or certain locations (e.g., work, home) that you notice more coughing, wheezing, or shortness of breath?
- Does this problem get better if you go away on vacation?
- Do cigarette smoke, perfumes, chemical fumes, or strong cooking odors bother you or cause you to wheeze?
- Is there anything at work or home that makes your symptoms worse?
- Do you have pets or wall-to-wall carpeting?

NOTE

In asthma, exposure precedes symptoms. Symptoms may not occur until 8 to 12 hours after exposure.

TABLE 8–1. **Asthma Severity Classifications**

		Asthma Severity		
Findings	**Intermittent**	**Mild Persistent**	**Moderate Persistent**	**Severe Persistent**
Presence of symptoms	≤ 2 times per week	3–6 times per week	Daily	Continuous
Exacerbation	Brief (few hours to a few days)	May affect activity and sleep	Affects activity and sleep >2 times per week, may last days	Frequent, affects all activity and sleep
Nocturnal symptoms	≤ 2 times per months	3–4 times per month	≥ 5 times per month	Frequent
PEF or FEV$_1$ (predicted)	≥ 80%	≥ 80%	> 60% and < 80%	≤ 60%
PEF variability*	< 20%	20%–30%	> 30%	> 30%

Adapted from *Expert Panel Report 2: Guideline for the Diagnosis and Management of Asthma.* Bethesda, MD: National Institutes of Health, National Heart, Lung, and Blood Institute; 1997. No. 97–4051.
FEV$_1$ = forced expiratory volume in 1 second; PEF = peak expiratory flow.
*Variability refers to values obtained throughout the day.

The history can also be used to determine the severity of the disease. In addition to the guidelines outlined in Table 8-1, severity can be assessed by:

- The number and type of inhalers used each month
- The number of times the patient needed oral steroid therapy in the last year
- The number of emergency room visits, hospitalizations, and intensive care unit admissions related to asthma

Past medical history

Ask adults about seasonal or chronic allergies, atopy, atopic dermatitis, frequent attacks of acute bronchitis, sinusitis, and gastroesophageal reflux disease.

Ask children about frequent respiratory infections.

Family history

A history of allergies, atopy, and asthma in first-degree relatives is associated with an increased incidence of asthma.

Social history

Exposure history forms the basis of prevention in asthmatic patients. Assess occupational setting, home environment, and tobacco use for possible continual aggravation of asthmatic symptoms.

Review of Systems (Table 8–2)

TABLE 8–2. Review of Systems in the Diagnosis of Asthma

System	Common Patient Complaints
Vital signs	Elevated respiratory rate
Constitutional	Fatigue and weakness during acute attacks, vague symptoms (e.g., insomnia secondary to nocturnal cough, overall fatigue) when stable
Dermatologic	Cyanosis
HEENT	Dry mouth secondary to mouth breathing
Cardiovascular	Palpitations or tachycardia
Respiratory	Wheezing, increased cough, dyspnea even at rest, difficulty "catching" breath
Musculoskeletal	Tremors secondary to overuse of β_2-agonist bronchodilator, abdominal muscle pain secondary to overuse during acute attacks
Psychologic	Increased anxious state related to breathing problem

Physical Examination

Vital signs

The patient's vital signs may show tachypnea, tachycardia, and pulsus paradoxus.

General appearance

During acute attacks, the patient may appear to be in respiratory distress with declining mental clarity and increasing fatigue. If the attack continues, the patient may talk in shorter sentences or prefer to sit up instead of lying down. When stable and resting, the patient may appear to be comfortable.

Dermatologic

Cyanosis may be present in patients with asthma.

HEENT

Examination may reveal flared nares, mouth breathing, and use of accessory muscles around the neck to assist in breathing. The patient may appear to be gasping for breath.

Cardiovascular

Examination of the cardiovascular system may reveal tachycardia.

Respiratory

> **NOTE**
>
> If a patient uses an inhaler immediately before coming to your preceptor's office, you may not get a true sense of the initial extent of respiratory compromise.

Tachypnea is usually seen in asthma. In mild asthma, fine, scattered expiratory wheezes may be appreciated. However, in many instances, no wheeze is heard. As the severity of asthma increases, both inspiratory and expiratory wheezes scattered through both lungs can be appreciated along with a prolonged expiratory phase.

> **NOTE**
>
> Airway noise may decrease in patients with very severe asthma when air is unable to flow through many of the bronchial tubes.

Musculoskeletal

Abdominal muscles may be retracting vigorously with respirations. The patient may also experience tremors.

> **NOTE**
>
> Accessory muscle use, retractions of the abdominal walls, and nasal flaring are all associated with increasing severity of an acute asthmatic attack.

Psychologic

The patient may present with an anxious affect.

Laboratory Tests

An **arterial blood gas** is only necessary in acute, severe disease when severe hypoxemia is suspected.

> **NOTE**
>
> High carbon dioxide levels require careful evaluation and observation for impending respiratory failure.

A **complete blood count** may demonstrate leukocytosis or eosinophilia, but is not necessary unless there is the suggestion of other medical problems.

Imaging Studies

Chest radiographs are not necessary as part of the routine diagnostic work-up. However, a chest radiograph is required if there is the suggestion of infection (e.g., pneumonia), localized disease, or a foreign body (e.g., toys, coins, fish bones).

Abnormalities are rarely noted on a chest radiograph even when asthma is present. The most common abnormal findings are bronchial wall thickening and hyperinflation.

Additional Studies

Spirometry is the accepted diagnostic standard to show airway reversibility. It can be used in conjunction with a short-acting bronchodilator to document the presence and severity of significant reversible airway obstruction (Table 8–3). If spirometry with a bronchodilator is negative but asthma is still important to rule in or out, consider a methacholine challenge test. If a patient has a negative methacholine challenge test, consider a different diagnosis.

TABLE 8–3. **Spirometry Challenge Tests**

FEV$_1$	Required Test	Procedure	Results
< 80%	Bronchodilator test	Give a short-acting bronchodilator and repeat spirometry 15–20 minutes after administration	Airway reversibility is confirmed if the FEV$_1$ improves by 12% or 200 ml
>80%	Methacholine challenge test*	Administer an increasingly higher controlled dose of methacholine with repeated FEV$_1$ measurements	A 20% drop in FEV$_1$ with a dose no higher than 8 mg/ml of methacholine is considered a positive test

FEV$_1$ = forced expiratory volume in 1 second.

*Do not perform a methacholine challenge test if there is severe airflow obstruction (i.e., FEV$_1$/FVC ≤ 70%) or in any setting that is not prepared to deal with respiratory distress, because this is a provocative test.

Peak expiratory flow rates (PEFR) can be used in the office setting to demonstrate airway reversibility after bronchodilator administration. PEFR should not be used to replace confirmation by formal spirometry.

Pulse oximetry can be used to assess oxygenation. **Allergy testing** and **immunotherapy** may benefit patients with asthma who have year-round or seasonal allergies.

DIFFERENTIAL DIAGNOSIS

Chronic obstructive pulmonary disease (COPD) can be differentiated from asthma using spirometry to assess the forced expiratory volume in 1 second (**FEV$_1$**). The airway reversibility of asthma will appear as a substantial increase (i.e., 12% to 20%) in the FEV$_1$ after the use of inhaled β$_2$ agonist. If the FEV$_1$ does not substantially increase, spirometry should be repeated after a 2-week trial of oral corticosteroid therapy (40 to 60 mg of prednisone daily). The corticosteroid trial should reduce inflammation, resulting in less bronchospasm and increased airflow.

If a focal wheeze is appreciated, consider other lung diseases such as a **foreign body, infection,** or **tumor.** Tables 8–4 and 8–5 provide the differential diagnoses of cough and dyspnea respectively.

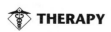 THERAPY

The treatment of asthma is approached either as long-term management to maintain lung function or acute management of asthma exacerbations.

TABLE 8–4. Differential Diagnosis of Cough

Pathology	Notable Features	History	Physical Exam	Diagnostic Procedures or Methods
Acute bronchitis	Viral syndrome may precede cough	7–10 day cough is common	Wheezing may be present	None
Aspiration pneumonitis	Acute onset	Precipitating event	Focal consolidation on lung exam	Chest radiograph shows pneumonia
Asthma	Lack of viral syndrome before cough	Recurrent episodes of cough or wheezing, worse at night	Diffuse wheezing may be heard	Spirometry shows reversible airway disease, provocation testing may be required
COPD	Smoker's hack on awakening, patient is generally older	Smoker with 20+ pack/year history	Prolonged expiratory phase on auscultation	Spirometry, chest radiograph
CHF	Dependent edema, shortness of breath	Dyspnea on exertion	Abnormal cardiac exam	EKG, chest radiograph, echocardiogram
Environmental allergies	Cough related to exposure, clears with removal	Symptoms usually long-standing	May show evidence of allergic rhinitis or atopic disorder	Provocation testing with suspected allergen or avoidance
Foreign body	Foul breath	Chronic tickle in throat, difficulty swallowing	Foul smell, purulent drainage may be present, upper respiratory wheeze may be heard	Chest radiograph, laryngoscopy for possible radiolucent objects
GERD	No associated respiratory features	Heartburn that is worse at night, cough after meals and spicy foods	Tender over epigastric region, symptoms reproduced with deep palpation	Trial of histamine blockers or proton pump inhibitors
Medication side effect	Slight cough, usually non-productive, without fever	Recent start of new drug (β-blocker, ACE inhibitors)	Lungs usually clear, wheezing may be appreciated	Trial of medication discontinuance, then possible rechallenge

(*continued*)

TABLE 8–4. **Differential Diagnosis of Cough (*Continued*)**

Pathology	Notable Features	History	Physical Exam	Diagnostic Procedures or Methods
Occupational exposure	Exposure precedes cough, cough may follow up to 24 hours after exposure	Exposure to respiratory irritant	Lungs may be clear	Removal from source results in improvement, spirometry with provocation testing to verify
Pneumonia	Spiking fevers, chills, dyspnea	Short onset (1–2 days)	Lungs reveal focal consolidation	Chest radiograph
TB, pulmonary	Hemoptysis	—	Rales may be heard	Chest radiograph, positive PPD 6 weeks after exposure
Tumor	Recurrent pneumonia, hemoptysis, weight loss	Smoker, recurrent pulmonary problems	Focal consolidation may be heard	Chest radiograph, chest CT
URI (common cold)	Postnasal drainage	Patient says cough comes from their throat, tickle in the throat	Nasal congestion	None, diagnosed by history and clinical presentation

ACE = angiotensin-converting enzyme; CHF = congestive heart failure; COPD = chronic obstructive pulmonary disease; CT = computed tomography; EKG = electrocardiogram; GERD = gastroesophageal reflux disease; LRI = lower respiratory infection; PPD = purified protein derivative; TB = tuberculosis; URI = upper respiratory infection; VRI = viral respiratory infection.

Long-term management focuses on avoiding exacerbations and allowing the patient to maintain normal activity levels with normal or near-normal lung function. **Acute exacerbation management** relies on the clinician educating the patient to recognize problems early and institute appropriate intervention in a timely manner.

Nonpharmacologic Therapy

Massage therapy and other stress reduction techniques (see COMPLEMENTARY/ALTERNATIVE MEDICINE; p 92) have been shown to decrease the rate of asthma attacks. Current recommendations focus on treatment of the underlying lung tissue inflammation.

TABLE 8–5. **Differential Diagnosis of Dyspnea**

Onset of Dyspnea	Differential Diagnosis
Acute onset	Asthma
	Acute bronchitis
	Endocarditis or pericarditis
	Hyperventilation
	Pulmonary embolus
	Pulmonary infarct
Chronic progressive onset	Bronchiectasis
	Chronic bronchitis
	Cor pulmonale
	Emphysema
	Eosinophilic lung disease
	Interstitial lung disease
	Pleural effusion
	Pneumonia
	Pneumothorax
	Pulmonary fibrosis
Acute or chronic progressive onset	Arteriovenous malformations or fistula
	Lung cancer
	Congestive heart failure
	Foreign body
	Sleep apnea (primary hypoventilation)
	Valvular heart disease

Pharmacotherapy

Long-term management

Long-term pharmacologic therapy is initiated in a stepwise manner based on the level of severity as assessed by the physician, with intensive therapy from the beginning (Tables 8–6 and 8–7).

Once control is achieved, follow-up visits every 1 to 6 months are essential for monitoring therapy. The gradual reduction of medications (using the "last-on, first-off" policy) can start after achieving several weeks to months of control. Because steroid inhalers currently provide the most effective long-term control for persistent asthma symptoms, they should be the last daily medication to be lowered. Steroid inhalers may be tapered 25% every 2 to 3 months until achieving the lowest dose required to maintain control.

Acute exacerbation management

The management of acute asthma exacerbations concentrates on the quick relief of the patient's bronchoconstriction through the repeated, rapid use of

TABLE 8–6. Daily Medication Recommendations for the Long-Term Management of Asthma for Patients Older Than 5 Years

Step	Symptoms	Treatment Guidelines
1	Intermittent (one intermittent pharmaceutical)	No daily medications, treat acute exacerbations with inhaled short-acting β_2-agonist bronchodilators
2	Mild persistent (one pharmaceutical)	Inhaled corticosteroid (200–500 µg)
		OR
		Cromolyn or nedocromil
		OR
		Leukotriene receptor antagonists (e.g., montelukast, zafirlukast, zileuton) in age-appropriate patients with mild disease
		OR
		Sustained-release theophylline* titrated to serum concentrations of 5–15 µg/ml
3	Moderate persistent (two pharmaceuticals)	Inhaled corticosteroid (800–2000 µg)
		AND
		A long-acting bronchodilator (especially for nighttime symptoms):
		■ Long-acting inhaled β_2 agonist
		OR
		■ Sustained-release theophylline
		OR
		■ Long-acting β_2-agonist tablets or syrup
4	Severe persistent (three pharmaceuticals)	Inhaled corticosteroid (800–2000 µg or more)
		AND
		A long-acting bronchodilator (especially for nighttime symptoms):
		■ Long-acting inhaled β_2 agonist
		OR
		■ Sustained-release theophylline
		OR
		■ Long-acting β_2-agonist tablets or syrup
		AND
		Corticosteroid tablets or syrup long-term, as needed, with reduction to lowest possible daily dosing

Adapted from *Expert Panel Report 2: Guidelines for the Diagnosis and Management of Asthma.* Bethesda, MD: National Institutes of Health, National Heart, Lung, and Blood Institute; 1997. No. 97–4051.

*Sustained-release theophylline is used as an alternative; it is not the preferred therapy.

TABLE 8–7. **Daily Medication Recommendations for the Long-Term Management of Asthma for Patients Younger Than 5 Years**

Step	Symptoms	Treatment Guidelines
1	Intermittent (one intermittent pharmaceutical)	No daily medications, treat acute exacerbations with inhaled short-acting β_2-agonist bronchodilators
2	Mild persistent (one pharmaceutical)	Inhaled corticosteroid (200–400 μg) OR
		Cromolyn (MDI or nebulizer) or nedocromil (MDI only)*
3	Moderate persistent (one or two pharmaceuticals)	Inhaled corticosteroid via MDI with spacer and face mask (400–800 μg/day) OR
		Nebulized budesonide ($<$ 1 mg twice daily)
		Once control is established:
		Medium-dose inhaled corticosteroid plus nedocromil OR
		Medium-dose inhaled corticosteroid plus long-acting bronchodilator (e.g., theophylline†)
4	Severe persistent (three pharmaceuticals)	Inhaled corticosteroid via MDI with spacer and face mask ($>$ 1 mg every day) OR
		Nebulized budesonide ($>$ 1 mg twice daily)
		If needed, add oral steroids at 2 mg/kg/day and reduce to the lowest possible dose on an alternate-day, early morning schedule.

Adapted from *Expert Panel Report 2: Guidelines for the Diagnosis and Management of Asthma.* Bethesda, MD: National Institutes of Health, National Heart, Lung, and Blood Institute; 1997. No. 97–4051
MDI = metered dose inhaler.
*Use the MDI with a spacer and face mask.
†Theophylline is not the preferred therapy.

short-acting β_2 agonists and reduction of pulmonary inflammation with an oral corticosteroid (i.e., prednisone). Intravenous steroid therapy should be limited to patients who cannot tolerate oral dosing of prednisone, because studies have shown equal efficacy and time of onset with intravenous and oral prednisone. Although intramuscular steroids may help some patients, they are generally not as helpful because of uneven absorption.

Patients in respiratory distress (i.e., severe wheezing, cyanosis, inability to walk or talk) should be seen immediately in the office or sent to the emergency department by ambulance depending on their severity.

URGENCIES AND EMERGENCIES

Asthma attacks need to be treated aggressively and early to prevent further pulmonary function degradation. Acute asthma exacerbations that do not respond to home therapy should be seen in the office as soon as possible. If the asthma attack has been ongoing for an extended period and there is use of accessory muscles without a good response to office therapy, consider ambulance transport to a hospital for further treatment, because respiratory arrest is a possibility.

In very severe asthma (e.g., status asthmaticus), wheezing may not be appreciated because the high degree of bronchoconstriction does not permit further air passage. In such instances, the patient will usually appear to be in severe respiratory distress. Intensive medical care is indicated.

 SPECIAL POPULATIONS

Children

Prevention

Asthma is more closely associated with allergies in children than in adults. *In utero* exposure to the blood products of tobacco smoke is an important predictor of wheezing within the first year of life. Although wheezing does not always represent asthma, it suggests an environmental risk factor.

Exclusive breast-feeding for the first 4 months of life is associated with a statistically significant decrease in the risk of asthma and wheezing until 6 years of age.

History

When taking the history, include questions about parental occupations (e.g., possible chemical exposures brought home), exposures at day-care and school, smokers in the home or day-care facility.

Diagnosis

Although spirometry is useful in children over the age of 4, some children may not be able to cooperate with the test until they are at least 7 years of age.

Therapy

All children with asthma and their parents should be taught how to use a spacer device in conjunction with a metered dose inhaler (MDI) to deliver inhaled medications. Studies have shown that when used correctly, MDI–spacer combinations have efficacy and treatment results similar to that of nebulized inhalation therapy, even during acute exacerbations. Use a mask with the spacer and MDI to deliver inhaled medications for infants and other individuals who are unable to use the MDI–spacer combination alone. Long-term management for children older than 5 years of age is similar to adults (see Table 8–6).

Seniors

Presentation

In elderly persons, asthma symptoms are commonly attributed to other disorders such as emphysema, congestive heart failure, and lower respiratory infections. Whereas wheezing is the predominant complaint in younger patients, cough tends to be the predominant symptom in the elderly and may manifest itself at night.

Diagnosis

Spirometry may be performed. The methacholine challenge test and other general inhalation challenge tests are not used in elderly patients because of the fear of adverse effects from the challenge agents or the reversal agents.

Therapy

Inhaled β_2 agonists remain the mainstay of therapy for the immediate relief of asthma symptoms in elderly patients, though caution should be used because of the increased risk of cardiac arrhythmias. The use of anticholinergic agents (e.g., ipratropium bromide) should be limited to those patients who have an element of COPD or are intolerant of inhaled β_2 agonists.

Elderly patients do not respond as well as younger patients to mast cell antagonists (e.g., cromolyn and nedocromil), though therapy should be attempted if the patient requires oral corticosteroid maintenance therapy. Theophylline should be used cautiously because of its narrow therapeutic window, though many suggest the use of single nighttime dosing for control of nocturnal symptoms.

Acute asthma attacks without other complicating factors are infrequent in the elderly. However, when acute attacks occur, the complexity of stepwise asthma therapy can easily lead to problems related to polypharmacy. More extensive monitoring and education than is needed by younger adults may be indicated.

Pregnancy

The treatment of asthma remains basically the same during pregnancy. The hypoxemia of poorly controlled asthma during pregnancy can result in increased perinatal mortality and morbidity caused by premature birth and low birthweight. In addition, most of the medications used in the treatment of asthma pose little risk to the fetus.

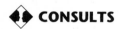 **COMPLEMENTARY/ALTERNATIVE MEDICINE**

- **Echinacea** is often used to help decrease the likelihood that a respiratory infection will become worse (e.g., a viral infection becoming bacterial). It may strengthen the immune system and has few contraindications.
- Gingko may reduce bronchial hypersensitivity.
- **Saiboku-to** was studied in steroid-dependent asthmatics over 6 to 24 months and was found to be helpful, although more detailed clinical trials are indicated.
- **Coleus forkholii,** an Ayurvedic herb, showed a bronchodilating effect in two studies.

There are no current well-done studies to suggest that **chiropractic care** can assist in the management of patients with acute respiratory disorders.

Homeopathy has been reported to be helpful in patients with asthma; however, studies have only been done on a few patients and they lack objective measures.

Some studies have suggested that **acupuncture** can decrease breathlessness in patients with asthma; however, other studies have been inconclusive. Thus far, acupuncture does not have an important role in respiratory therapy.

Massage is often used to help loosen mucus trapped in the bronchioles. It can be ordered in most hospitals.

CONSULTS

A **pulmonary consult** should be considered if the patient demonstrates severe (moderate to severe in children) airway obstruction on spirometry and does not respond well to initial therapy. Also consider **case managers** and **asthma education programs** offered by some insurance programs.

Bronchitis

Jeff Kirschman

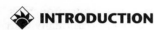

STUDENT OBJECTIVES

- Define acute bronchitis
- Describe the progression of acute bronchitis with and without intervention
- Characterize treatment modalities and therapeutic interventions for acute bronchitis

INTRODUCTION

Bronchitis is inflammation of the mucous membranes of the bronchial tree. Acute bronchitis is most commonly caused by infection and chemical irritation. Viral infections represent as many as 95% of all cases in healthy, nonsmoking patients. This chapter discusses acute bronchitis. See Chapter 10 (Chronic Obstructive Pulmonary Disease) for a discussion of chronic bronchitis.

TERMINOLOGY (See Chapter 8)

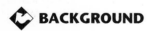

BACKGROUND

Respiratory diseases remain one of the leading reasons for visits to physician's offices. Data concerning the true prevalence and incidence of acute bronchitis in the ambulatory setting are scant. Partly because of poor diagnostic criteria, the diagnosis of "acute bronchitis" is frequently assigned to a variety of acute upper and lower respiratory tract infections.

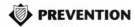

PREVENTION

Primary Prevention

Patients should be urged to avoid respiratory irritant exposures, especially cigarette smoke.

Secondary Prevention

Patients with a recurrent diagnosis of acute bronchitis should be evaluated for other respiratory diseases and systemic illnesses.

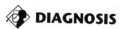 **DIAGNOSIS**

The clinical diagnosis of acute bronchitis is vague because of the absence of clear signs and symptoms and the lack of definitive laboratory tests. "Acute bronchitis" is a clinical diagnosis based purely on the clinician's evaluation of a persistent cough, usually with sputum production that develops rapidly and concurrently.

Presentation

Cough is the most frequent complaint associated with acute bronchitis. Patients may describe "constant" or "frequent" cough, occasionally with "coughing jags" or "coughing fits" that are not controlled with over-the-counter cough suppressants. The cough may be productive of purulent sputum for up to 10 days.

NOTE

Even in a healthy nonsmoker, the cough associated with bronchitis can persist for up to 6 months after the upper respiratory infection.

History

History of present illness

- Do you have head cold symptoms, tiredness, chills, or muscle aches?
- Are you experiencing any shortness of breath or wheezing? When does the wheezing occur?
- Have you had a temperature higher than 100°F?

Past medical history

- Have you had many chest or lung infections?

Family history

- Does anyone in your family have asthma, allergies, or eczema?

Social history

- Do you smoke?

Review of Systems (Table 9–1)

Physical Examination

No specific findings on physical examination are pathognomonic for acute bronchitis.

Vital signs

The patient's **temperature** may help you decide whether antibiotics are needed. Cough from congestive heart failure may be associated with weight gain, elevated blood pressure, or both.

HEENT

Examination of the nasal and oral cavities may reveal other causes for the patient's cough (e.g., purulent postnasal drainage, foreign body, throat infection).

Cardiovascular

Auscultate the heart for murmurs, irregular rhythm, or cardiomegaly, all of which are suggestive of a cardiac cause for the cough.

Respiratory

Lung findings are usually diffuse, not focal. Auscultation of the lungs may reveal intermittent, scattered high- or low-pitched rhonchi, or wheezing.

Gastrointestinal

Examination of the abdomen may reveal midepigastric pain that is consistent with reflux esophagitis.

TABLE 9–1. **Review of Systems in the Diagnosis of Acute Bronchitis**

System	Associated Signs and Symptoms
Constitutional	Myalgias, fever, chills, dyspnea
HEENT	Sinus pain and pressure, nasal drainage, nasal congestion (URI), ear pain (otitis)
Cardiovascular	Palpitations, chest pain (cardiac disease)
Respiratory	Wheezing, shortness of breath, dyspnea on exertion, cough, sputum, pain with deep breath
Gastrointestinal	Reflux esophagitis* (gastroesophageal reflux)

URI = upper respiratory infection.
*Reflux esophagitis is a nonbronchitis source of cough.

Laboratory Tests

Laboratory tests are rarely indicated if the patient presents with the typical signs and symptoms of acute bronchitis. Cultures and microscopic examination of the sputum are usually not helpful because the most common pathogens are viral. Even for the few cases that are the result of bacterial pathogens, the bacteria will most likely be *Mycoplasma pneumoniae* or *Chlamydia pneumoniae*, neither of which are seen with routine sputum cultures.

Cases of acute bronchitis that are associated with wheezing or have lasted more than 1 month suggest airway obstruction. Thus, pre- and postbronchodilator peak-flow testing in the office may help determine the most appropriate next step for further work-up. A low peak flow may suggest that a trial of a bronchodilator is indicated.

Imaging Studies

Imaging studies are rarely indicated. However, if the diagnosis is unclear, imaging studies are used to differentiate between pneumonia, tumor, foreign body, tuberculosis, and probable bronchitis.

DIFFERENTIAL DIAGNOSIS OF COUGH
(See Table 8–4, p 86)

THERAPY

Therapy is mainly supportive (e.g., hydration or therapy to help an acute, cough-induced insomnia).

Nonpharmacologic Therapy

Instruct the patient to rest until afebrile and to increase fluid intake, particularly during febrile episodes. Some patients feel that a vaporizer helps. Unfortunately, it also increases mold counts and may worsen the problem.

Pharmacotherapy

Acute bronchitis commonly requires antipyretics and analgesics for fever and pain and medication for cough suppression. If over-the-counter medications (e.g., guaifenesin for mucolysis and dextromethorphan for cough suppression) have failed, consider using benzonatate or compounds that contain codeine or hydrocodone.

For **smokers who have moderate to severe or unresolving acute bronchitis,** the selective use of antibiotics may be beneficial. Antibiotic coverage in smokers should be directed against *C. pneumoniae*, *M. pneumoniae*, and *Bordetella* species. Such antibiotics include erythromycin and tetracycline as well as the newer macrolides (e.g., azithromycin, clarithromycin), the 'floxacins, doxycycline, and trimethoprim/sulfamethoxazole (TMP/SMX).

In most cases of *C. pneumoniae* and *M. pneumoniae,* young nonsmoking patients spontaneously recover from the illness, though a few require further intervention if they develop more serious symptoms. Treatment of *C. pneumoniae* and *M. pneumoniae* in special populations of individuals living in close quarters (e.g., college, military installations, nursing homes) requires early intervention to prevent an epidemic.

Some clinicians treat patients with inhaled β-agonists if they present with more severe symptoms, particularly those suggestive of obstructive lung disease. Patients with moderate to severe bronchitis, using β-agonist inhalers at a rate of two puffs three or four times daily, tend to experience less coughing and an improved sense of well-being within 1 week after initiation. In addition, these patients tend to return to work sooner.

 ## URGENCIES & EMERGENCIES

In some patients with underlying chronic conditions, acute bronchitis may lead to acute respiratory failure; however, this is rare. Patients should be reminded to call the physician if their symptoms become worse.

 ## SPECIAL POPULATIONS

Children

The microbiology of acute bronchitis in children differs from that in adults. Adenovirus is most prevalent in children younger than 2 years, while respiratory syncytial virus (RSV) and parainfluenza viruses are seen in children 2 to 5 years of age. Treatment remains symptomatic, except for children with underlying lung disease (e.g., asthma, bronchial dysplasia secondary to prematurity).

Seniors

Elderly patients are even more susceptible to other sources of cough and shortness of breath, including congestive heart failure, exacerbation of chronic obstructive pulmonary disease, bronchogenic tumors, and gastroesophageal reflux disease. Oxygenation status is a more frequent concern. Respiratory rate determination and judicious use of a pulse oximeter are warranted. Seniors may deserve early intervention because they have an associated mortality rate of 5% to 10% with *C. pneumoniae.*

Pregnancy

Pregnancy alters immune status; therefore, symptoms associated with acute bronchitis may persist for several weeks or longer in the pregnant patient. All pharmacotherapeutic choices should reflect concerns for fetal effects.

COMPLEMENTARY/ALTERNATIVE MEDICINE (See Chapter 8; Complementary/Alternative Medicine, p 92)

- Lemon balm is said to have mild sedative and carminative (spasmolytic, antibacterial, antiviral) effects. The average daily dose is 8 to 10 g of the drug per day, made into two to five cups of tea.
- Marshmallow, mullein, or licorice teas are said to initiate soothing action on mucous membranes.
- Steam inhalations with the addition of eucalyptus leaves, camphor oil, or both may help open bronchial tubes.

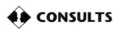 **CONSULTS**

Acute bronchitis in the healthy adult normally does not require referral to a consultant.

CHAPTER 10

Chronic Obstructive Pulmonary Disease— Chronic Bronchitis and Emphysema

Jeff Kirschman

OBJECTIVES

- List the diagnostic criteria for chronic bronchitis and emphysema
- Describe the progression of chronic obstructive pulmonary disease with and without intervention
- Elucidate treatment modalities and therapeutic interventions for chronic obstructive pulmonary disease

 INTRODUCTION

Chronic obstructive pulmonary disease (COPD) is a disease state represented by airflow obstruction that is generally progressive and may be partially reversible. COPD is caused by emphysema or chronic bronchitis and is a major cause of death and disability in the elderly.

Chronic bronchitis is diagnosed when a productive cough has been present for 3 months in each of 2 successive years and other causes of chronic cough have been excluded.

Emphysema is the abnormal, permanent enlargement of the air spaces distal to the terminal bronchioles. These spaces result from destruction of the walls of the bronchioles without obvious fibrosis.

TERMINOLOGY (See Chapter 8)

 BACKGROUND

COPD was the fourth leading cause of death in the United States in 1996. In 1994, there were 14 million cases of chronic bronchitis and 2 million

99

cases of emphysema. Approximately 10.7 million of the cases of chronic bronchitis were in Americans older than 45 years of age.

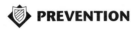 PREVENTION

Risk Factors

Cigarette smoking is the leading cause of COPD, with active smoking accounting for 80% to 90% of cases. Continued smoking leads to a rapid decline in pulmonary function. Other major risk factors include being white, male, and in a low socioeconomic group, as well as pollutants (domestic and occupational), atopy, and a family history of COPD.

> **NOTE**
>
> Approximately 10% to 15% of all smokers develop clinical evidence of COPD.

Primary Prevention

Primary prevention measures include never smoking cigarettes and avoiding exposure to respiratory pollutants.

Secondary Prevention

Secondary prevention consists of smoking cessation and minimization of exposure to inhaled irritants (e.g., second-hand cigarette smoke, aerosolized products, organic dusts, noxious gases).

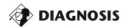 DIAGNOSIS

COPD is a diagnosis of exclusion; therefore, patients require a complete work-up to rule out other possible causes of their pulmonary symptoms.

Presentation

Patients with COPD initially present with a chronic cough and breathlessness. Early in the course of the disease, patients may complain of a "chest cold." The history often reveals that the cough has been present for several months; is sometimes associated with clear, white, or purulent sputum; and has recently become worse.

As COPD progresses, patients may also complain of dyspnea on exertion, wheezing, and panic-like attacks when they are hypoxic. Patients with COPD frequently find that they are extremely limited in their activities and feel trapped by the disease. They may complain of feelings of isolation and depression.

History

History of present illness

Questions to consider asking include:

- Do you have coughing, wheezing, or shortness of breath? If so, is it usually worse at night? Does it ever awaken you? Does exercise make it a little or a lot worse?
- Do you now or have you ever smoked? If so, how much do you smoke and for how long have you smoked?
  - □ Patients with COPD usually give a smoking history of at least 20 pack years
- Are there certain times during the day or certain locations (e.g., home, work) that you notice more coughing, wheezing, or shortness of breath? If so, does the coughing improve when you leave the location?
- Does cigarette smoke, chemical fumes, or smells make breathing more difficult for you?
- Have you ever had pulmonary function tests? If so, when and what were the results?
- Do you always have sputum and a cough?

Severity can be assessed by:

- The number and type of inhalers used per month
- The number of times the patient needed oral steroid therapy in the last year
- The carbon dioxide level on an arterial blood gas
- The extent of fingertip clubbing
- The patient's ability to perform activities of daily living (e.g., meal preparation, household cleaning, dressing, personal hygiene) over the last 3 months
- The number of emergency room visits, hospitalizations due to COPD exacerbations, intensive care unit admissions
- The number of times the patient has needed intubation

NOTE

Dyspnea on exertion that is chronic and progressive is suggestive of COPD, while intermittent breathlessness is suggestive of asthma.

Family history

- Is there a family history of COPD?
  - □ Some studies have indicated that a family history of COPD may increase the risk of developing COPD if exposed to respiratory irritants (e.g., cigarette smoke).

TABLE 10–1. Review of Systems in the Diagnosis of Chronic Obstructive Pulmonary Disease

System	Common Patient Complaints
Constitutional	Fevers (bronchitis)
Cardiovascular	Angina (oxygen starvation), right-sided heart failure, orthopnea
Respiratory	Dyspnea on exertion (early), dyspnea even at rest (late) nonproductive cough, wheezing, pain with deep breath, symptoms reversible with β agonists (bronchitis)
Musculoskeletal	Ankle edema, clubbing of finger tips
Neurologic	Depression*

*Depression can be related to functional limitations or physical illness secondary to neurologic changes with chronic hypoxia.

Review of Systems (Table 10–1)

Physical Examination (Table 10–2)

No specific findings on physical examination are pathognomonic for COPD. Often, a combination of findings suggests the presence of lung disease and requires further work-up.

Laboratory Tests (Figure 10–1)

Arterial blood gases (ABGs) should be drawn periodically to document the degree of hypoxemia and concomitant hypercapnea.

TABLE 10–2. Physical Examination Findings in Chronic Obstructive Pulmonary Disease

System	Findings
General appearance	Shallow, lethargic, movement requires great effort; "pink puffer" refers to thin individuals breathing through pursed lips; "blue bloater" refers to obese individuals with a bluish hue resulting from hypoxia
HEENT	Use of pursed lips during breathing
Cardiovascular	Distant heart sounds, jugular venous distention, ankle edema
Respiratory	Wheezing and a prolonged forced expiratory phase, restricted movement of the chest (especially the diaphragm) during inspiration, increased use of abdominal muscles during inspiration, increased anteroposterior diameter
Musculoskeletal	Clubbing of the fingertips

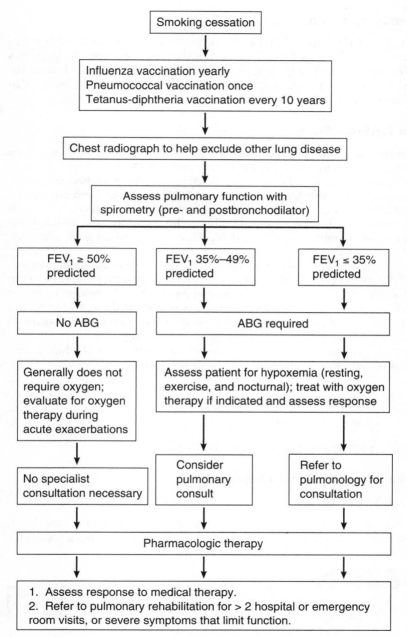

FIGURE 10–1. An overview of the evaluation and treatment of adults with chronic obstructive pulmonary disease. ABG = arterial blood gas; FEV_1 = forced expiratory volume in 1 second

Imaging Studies (see Figure 10–1)

A **chest radiograph** of a patient with COPD correlates poorly with symptoms, though it is useful in documenting the presence of other lung diseases (e.g., tumors, focal infections). Commonly seen nonspecific findings in patients with COPD include hyperinflation, bullae, blebs, diaphragmatic flattening, elongated cardiac silhouette, and peribronchial markings.

Additional Studies (see Figure 10–1)

Pulmonary function tests, particularly spirometry and pulse oximetry are the most important studies in the diagnosis of COPD.

Spirometry should be performed before and after bronchodilator treatment to assess the degree of airway reversibility. If there is no evidence of reversibility with a bronchodilator, a 2-week trial of oral corticosteriods may be considered with repeat testing at the end of the trial period. If the presence of obstructive airway disease is documented on spirometry, further testing should follow.

Pulse oximetry can be performed in the office and in the patient's home. If the patient complains of dyspnea on exertion, perform pulse oximetry in the office by walking the patient around the room while measuring oxygen saturation levels. If the patient complains of nocturnal breathlessness and awakenings, overnight pulse oximetry may be used to document nocturnal desaturation and the need for oxygen therapy during sleep.

An **electrocardiogram** may reveal supraventricular rhythm disturbances; however, these disturbances are not specific to COPD.

 DIFFERENTIAL DIAGNOSIS
(See Table 8–5, p 87)

 THERAPY (See Figure 10–1)

Nonpharmacologic Therapy

Smoking cessation

Smoking cessation is the mainstay of therapy to prevent further lung deterioration. See Chapter 25 for specific information about smoking cessation.

> **NOTE**
>
> More than 90% of patients with COPD had previously or are currently smoking cigarettes.

Pulmonary rehabilitation

Pulmonary rehabilitation, usually administered by ancillary health providers (e.g., respiratory therapists), provides the motivated patient with a set of therapies designed to maximize independence and functioning. These therapies must be tailored for the individual patient and should focus on increasing the patient's exercise tolerance, smoking cessation, and providing a support mechanism.

Nutrition

Patients with COPD may experience progressive weight loss without evidence of protein malnutrition, maintaining a normal serum albumin and lean body mass. Nutritional therapy should be directed toward maintaining adequate caloric intake. L-carnitine supplementation (2 g three times a day) may result in improved exercise capability.

Pharmacotherapy

Pharmacologic therapy for COPD is mainly directed at providing symptomatic relief. The treatment of bronchospasm is outlined in Table 10–3.

> **NOTE**
>
> All metered dose inhalers (MDIs) should be used with a spacer. Patients should demonstrate the use of their MDI with a spacer during the office visit.

Oxygen

The use of supplemental oxygen to correct hypoxemia associated with COPD has been shown to increase survival and quality of life. The American Thoracic Society suggests that long-term oxygen therapy be used for patients whose partial pressure of oxygen (PaO_2) is

- 55 mm Hg or less
- 59 mm Hg with cor pulmonale
- 60 mm Hg within specific conditions such as sleep apnea (if continuous positive airway pressure is not being used)

Oxygen supplementation should be limited to the minimum flow rate necessary to achieve a PaO_2 greater than 60 mm Hg or oxygen saturation greater than 90%.

Mucus and cough suppressants

The use of expectorant and mucolytic therapy should generally be limited to acute exacerbations. Most experts agree that cough suppressants should be avoided with COPD because they may serve as respiratory depressants and further increase hypoxia. As an alternative, increased mobilization of secretions can be accomplished by increasing oral hydration.

TABLE 10–3. **Pharmacotherapy for Bronchospasm in Chronic Obstructive Pulmonary Disease**

Classification	Treatment Guidelines
Step 1 (variable symptoms	Selective β_2-agonist MDI, 1–2 puffs every 2–6 hours as needed; do not exceed 8–12 puffs in 24 hours
Step 2 (mild to moderate continuing symptoms)	Ipratropium MDI, 2–6 puffs every 6–8 hours AND Selective β_2-agonist MDI, 1–4 puffs as needed up to four times daily (for rapid relief or as a regular supplement) CONSIDER Ipratropium and albuterol combination MDI if patient requires both agents daily OR Long-acting selective β_2-agonist MDI (e.g., salmeterol), 1–2 puffs every 12 hours if a significant reversible airway obstruction is present
Step 3* (mild to moderate increase in symptoms)	Sustained-release theophylline, 200–400 mg twice daily OR Sustained-release theophylline, 400–800 mg at bedtime for nocturnal bronchospasm AND/OR Sustained-release oral albuterol, 4–8 mg twice daily or at night for control of nocturnal bronchospasm AND/OR Mucokinetic agent (e.g., acetylcysteine, nebulized)[†]
Step 4* (still suboptimal control of symptoms)	Trial course of oral corticosteroids (e.g., prednisone), up to 40 mg daily for 10–14 days IF IMPROVEMENT Wean to lowest daily or alternate-day oral dose CONSIDER High-dose inhaled corticosteroid therapy as an alternative to oral corticosteroid
Step 5* (severe exacerbations)[‡]	Increased selective β_2-agonist MDI use or subcutaneous administration of epinephrine or terbutaline; exercise extreme caution when using these drugs in patients with concurrent cardiac disease and the elderly AND/OR Increase ipratropium dosage to 6–8 puffs every 3–4 hours AND Intravenous theophylline to bring serum theophylline level to 10–12 μg/ml (requires hospitalization) AND Intravenous methylprednisolone, 50–100 mg every 6–8 hours, tapering as soon as possible AND Antibiotics, if indicated

MDI = metered dose inhaler.
*These treatment regimens should be added to those for step 2.
†Minimal evidence exists concerning the efficacy of mucokinetic agents in bronchospasm.
‡For severe exacerbations, consider hospitalization, pulmonology referral, and oxygen therapy.

Vaccines

COPD patients should be encouraged to have annual influenza immunizations, at least one pneumococcal vaccination, and up-to-date diphtheria-tetanus vaccinations.

Antibiotics

Studies of acutely symptomatic patients with COPD have failed to demonstrate definite organisms in more than 50% of the patients. When bacterial pathogens are isolated in the lower respiratory tracts of adult patients with chronic bronchitis, the most common are *Streptococcus pneumoniae,* *Haemophilus influenzae,* and *Moraxella catarrhalis.* Antibiotic use should be limited to short courses during acute exacerbations, with therapy directed against these common bacterial pathogens.

NOTE

There is no well-defined role for antibiotic prophylaxis in the nonimmunocompromised COPD patient.

 URGENCIES & EMERGENCIES

COPD exacerbations require prompt intervention. Patients with increasing hypoxemia or hypercapnia should be evaluated for inpatient management.

 SPECIAL POPULATIONS

Children

Children who develop symptoms similar to those seen with COPD should be evaluated for the presence of α_1-antitrypsin deficiency.

Seniors

β-Agonist bronchodilators (e.g., albuterol) should be used with caution in the elderly because of possible cardiac complications.

Pregnancy

COPD is generally not seen in pregnant women. Pregnant patients with early-onset COPD should be referred to a pulmonologist for further management.

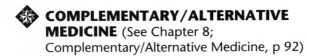

COMPLEMENTARY/ALTERNATIVE
MEDICINE (See Chapter 8;
Complementary/Alternative Medicine, p 92)

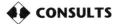

CONSULTS

Patients found to have moderate to severe COPD or COPD unresponsive to conservative therapy may benefit from an evaluation by a pulmonologist.

Coronary Artery Disease

Edward Onusko

OBJECTIVES

- Describe the impact of coronary artery disease in a primary care practice
- Prepare history questions that help define the risk and current problems related to coronary artery disease
- Explain how to use physical findings and in-office diagnostic studies to obtain objective evidence of cardiac disease
- Compile the pertinent components of the history, physical examination, and laboratory findings into an individual risk factor profile for coronary artery disease
- Recognize indications for further diagnostic studies and referral for treatment of cardiac disease
- Differentiate between the classes of drugs used to treat cardiac disease
- Explain key information about coronary artery disease and interventions that can alter cardiac risk factors using patient-appropriate terms

 INTRODUCTION

Coronary artery disease (CAD) may be defined as narrowing of the lumen of the coronary arteries secondary to the deposition of cholesterol plaque. CAD is associated with a wide variety of problems commonly seen in primary care offices, including ischemic heart disease [e.g., angina, myocardial infarction (MI)], congestive heart failure (CHF), arrhythmias, and valvular heart disease.

TERMINOLOGY

Acute coronary syndrome: acute MI or unstable angina

Angina pectoris: chest discomfort (i.e., pain, pressure, squeezing) caused by an ischemic myocardium

Angina, stable: a generally predictable pattern of angina pectoris that has not distinctly worsened over time

Angina, unstable: angina pectoris that is new or clearly increasing in frequency within the past 2 months, or is present at rest

Anginal equivalent: an atypical symptom (e.g., dizziness) that corresponds to myocardial ischemia

Angioplasty, balloon: a procedure involving dilation of the coronary arteries at the site of obstruction by inflation and then deflation of a balloon-tipped catheter

Atherosclerosis: narrowing of large and medium-sized arteries caused by the deposition of lipids in the intima of the vessel wall

Atypical chest pain: chest discomfort that does not have the typical characteristics of angina and may or may not be caused by myocardial ischemia

Central obesity: pattern of truncal fat deposition more typically seen in men (apple-shaped pattern) than in women

Diastolic dysfunction: impaired filling of the left ventricle prior to contraction resulting from increased stiffness of the myocardium

Dyslipidemia: abnormal blood lipids (i.e., high total cholesterol, high low-density lipoproteins, low high-density lipoproteins, or high triglycerides)

Hypertension: usually quantitatively defined as elevation of the systolic blood pressure above 140 mm Hg or the diastolic blood pressure above 90 mm Hg

Plaque, arterial: an area of lipid deposition on the inner surface of an artery

Stent, arterial: a spring-like device placed in the coronary artery after angioplasty to maintain patency of the vessel

Systolic dysfunction: depressed myocardial contractility

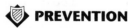 BACKGROUND

CAD is the most common cause of morbidity and mortality in the United States, affecting more than 10 million people. Along with other atherosclerotic diseases, it is one of the top 10 diagnoses seen in a family practice office.

PREVENTION

Risk Factors

Risk factors for CAD include:

- Cigarette smoking
- Older than 40 years of age
- Dyslipidemia
- Diabetes mellitus types 1 and 2
- Obesity (i.e., more than 20% over desired body weight), particularly if central obesity
- Emotional or physical stress
- Sedentary lifestyle
- Hypertension
- Excessive alcohol intake
- Family history of premature cardiac disease, particularly if onset was

younger than 55 years in a male family member or younger than 65 years in a female family member
- Male sex or postmenopausal female

Primary Prevention
Risk factor modification

Risk factor modification is the major form of primary CAD prevention. Diet, exercise, and smoking cessation are three key ingredients (see NON-PHARMACOLOGIC THERAPY; p 119).

> **NOTE**
>
> The average woman has a risk of death from CAD approximately equal to that of a man 10 years her junior. However, because women are likely to live longer than men, the number of actual deaths from CAD is similar in both sexes.

Screening

Many patients with risk factors for cardiac disease visit their family physicians for unrelated medical concerns. When treating a patient for a problem such as acute gastrointestinal disease, recurrent bronchitis, or depression, note all of the patient's health risk factors. These risk factors do not have to be addressed thoroughly at an acute visit but should receive attention in a timely manner. Sometimes the best approach is to ask the patient to return for a "prevention review" visit after pointing out key reasons why this type of visit is important for the patient's long-term health.

Physical examination findings that suggest atherosclerosis (e.g., a carotid or renal bruit), other cardiac disease (e.g., a murmur or irregular heart rhythm), or the presence of cardiac risk factors (e.g., fundoscopic changes of diabetes mellitus) necessitate further evaluation for CAD.

The significance of screening during a routine physical is emphasized and explored in Chapter 3. In addition, see Chapters 12, 13, and 16 for recommendations on who should be screened and how often.

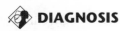 **DIAGNOSIS**

The tremendous impact of CAD in the United States dictates that it is essential for the general public to be educated about the signs and symptoms of heart disease that warrant evaluation by a health care provider. The greatest "clot buster" drugs will not be effective if the patient with angina does not recognize the urgent need to seek medical evaluation. Delay in the diagnosis of cardiac disease can result in significant morbidity and mortality; therefore, a healthy level of caution is indicated. The diagnostic information that follows is for suspected CAD, not for the urgent care of a suspected MI in progress.

Presentation

Patients with symptomatic CAD may present with a large variety of complaints, including:

- Discomfort in the chest, arm, neck, shoulder, or abdomen
- Shortness of breath or exercise intolerance
- Dizziness or syncope
- "Heartburn"
- Palpitations

NOTE

Women are less likely than men to present with classic symptoms of CAD, but more likely to present with nonspecific complaints (e.g., fatigue).

History

A careful history is the primary tool to explore a clinical suspicion of CAD. Physical examination and diagnostic studies may then provide more objective evidence that can help define treatment options, including the appropriate time for specialty referral.

History of present illness

Chest discomfort is the most common presentation for CAD in the outpatient setting. Use the following mnemonic (**P/PQRST**) to focus history taking on this important symptom.

- Provocation
  - What brings the symptom on or makes it worse (e.g., physical exertion, emotional stress)?
  - What were you doing the first time (or the most recent time) you experienced the symptom?
- Palliation
  - What relieves the symptom (e.g., rest, sublingual nitroglycerin)?
- Quality
  - What words best describe the pain (e.g., pressure, tightness, crushing, squeezing, heaviness)?
- Radiation
  - Where does the pain start and, if it moves, to where does it move (e.g., over the precordium radiating to the jaw, neck, arms, or abdomen)?

- □ What other symptoms accompany the chest discomfort (e.g., diaphoresis, nausea, palpitations, shortness of breath)?
- ■ Severity
  - □ How prominent is the symptom (rated on a scale of 1 to 10)?
  - □ What were you able to do or not able to do when the pain was present?
- ■ Temporal
  - □ When did the pain first start?
  - □ How long does the pain last?
  - □ How often does the pain occur?
  - □ Have you ever had the pain before?
  - □ How long after the onset of exertion does the pain begin?
  - □ Does the pain occur in the early morning hours (common in acute MI)?

In addition to the symptom of chest discomfort, ask the patient about **risk factors for cardiac disease** (see RISK FACTORS; p 110).

Obtain the patient's current **medication history,** including:

- ■ Current cardiovascular medications
- ■ Medications that may impact on coagulopathies (e.g., daily aspirin)
- ■ Medications that could cause or exacerbate the current symptoms (e.g., nonsteroidal anti-inflammatory drugs can increase gastrointestinal-related chest pain, herbal preparations may contain caffeine or sympathomimetics such as ephedra)
- ■ Adherence for all prescribed medication

Past medical history

- ■ Have you had previous evaluations for cardiac disease?
- ■ Do you have diabetes, blood pressure problems, or any other major medical problems?

Family history

Ask the patient about family members with:

- ■ CAD
- ■ Diabetes
- ■ Lipid abnormalities
- ■ High blood pressure
- ■ Cerebrovascular disease (e.g., stroke, transient ischemic attacks)
- ■ Peripheral vascular disease (e.g., surgical limb, foot, or digit loss; claudication)

Social history

Ask the patient about:

- ■ Use of tobacco products and alcohol
- ■ Exercise and diet

- Current major stressors
- Support systems (e.g., who lives at home)
- Job history (e.g., significant source of stress, sedentary work duties)

Review of Systems

All systems need to be carefully reviewed early on to establish a baseline; Table 11–1 highlights some important findings in selected systems that help to differentiate acute MI and CAD.

Angina deserves special mention in the review of systems because patients with it may present with what first appear to be noncardiac symptoms including gastrointestinal, pulmonary, musculoskeletal, or psychogenic symptoms. When you are uncertain as to whether a stable patient has angina, ask yourself the following questions before suggesting further work-up:

TABLE 11–1. Focused Review of Systems in the Diagnosis of Coronary Artery Disease

	Pertinent Findings	
System	**Pertinent Positives Indicating CAD**	**Pertinent Negatives Regarding Acute MI**
Constitutional	Sweating*, rapid weight gain (fluid retention)	Fever
Cardiovascular	Chest discomfort (with or without exertion*), palpitations	—
Respiratory	Shortness of breath with or without exertion, PND, orthopnea, nonproductive cough	Pain with deep breaths, productive cough
Gastrointestinal	Abdominal or mid-epigastric pain, nausea*	—
Musculoskeletal	Calf pain (due to claudication), neck or arm pain	Pain associated with recent trauma or strain to chest, arm, neck, or calf muscles
Neurologic	Dizziness or lightheadedness*, headache (due to urgently high blood pressure)	Circumoral or fingertip numbness or tingling (due to hyperventilation), dizziness with sensation of spinning (due to vestibular disorder)
Psychologic	Unusual anxiety*, panic with feeling of doom*	Multiple complaints consistent with somatization disorder

CAD = coronary artery disease; MI = myocardial infarction; PND = paroxysmal nocturnal dyspnea.
*These findings are common in patients with acute MI.

- How typical are this patient's symptoms and history for angina?
- How likely is it that this patient's atypical symptoms are from ischemia? What else is in the differential diagnosis?
- What are the patient's risk factors?
- What has the physical examination revealed?
- What does the patient think is happening?
- Is an electrocardiogram (EKG) or chest radiograph necessary?

NOTE

All that pains the chest is not angina. A work-up without thought may needlessly waste time and money and produce avoidable patient and family anxiety.

Physical Examination (Table 11–2)

Laboratory Tests

EKG

The EKG should be immediately available in any adult primary care setting. A 12-lead tracing should be evaluated for rate, rhythm, axis, hypertrophy, signs of ischemia (i.e., ST segment, T wave, or Q wave abnormalities), and signs of metabolic abnormalities (e.g., hypokalemia). Treatment of an acute coronary syndrome should not be delayed while waiting for other diagnostic tests.

TABLE 11–2. **Physical Examination Findings in Coronary Artery Disease**

System	Findings
Vital signs	Hypertension, hypotension, tachycardia, bradycardia, irregular pulse, tachypnea
General appearance	Comfort versus distress, pallor or cyanosis, obesity, diaphoresis
HEENT	Signs of diabetes or hypertension on fundoscopic examination
Cardiovascular	Gallops, murmurs, rubs, displaced cardiac impulse (by palpation), decreased peripheral pulses, jugular venous distention, bruits
Respiratory	Abnormal breath sounds (e.g., rales, wheezes, rhonchi), increased respiratory effort
Gastrointestinal	Organomegaly
Musculoskeletal	Peripheral edema

Blood

Cardiac enzymes [e.g., total creatine phosphokinase (CPK) and CPK-MB band, troponin I] are evaluated if acute MI is suspected. This evaluation is usually done in the emergency department or inpatient care setting. A complete blood count, fasting lipid profile, renal profile, glucose, and clotting studies (prothrombin time and partial thromboplastin time) are also done.

Urine

A **urinalysis** may reveal proteinuria (indicating hypertension or renal disease) or glucosuria (indicating diabetes).

Imaging Studies

Obtain **posteroanterior** and **lateral chest films.** Chest radiographs are helpful in assessing cardiac enlargement, pulmonary vascular congestion, and pulmonary pathology (e.g., pneumonia) that may be causing symptoms or affecting cardiac status.

Additional studies

Oximetry

Oxygen saturation by pulse oximetry can be helpful in assessing possible respiratory compromise.

Cardiac stress tests

Cardiac stress tests can be very useful in the nonurgent diagnosis of CAD. These tests consist of two parts:

1. **A mechanism to stress the cardiovascular system.** Exercise (e.g., treadmill, bicycle, arm ergometer) or the administration of pharmacologic agents (e.g., adenosine, dobutamine, dipyridamole) can result in increased myocardial oxygen requirements or alteration of cardiac perfusion.
2. **A means to measure the heart's response to stress.** When inadequate coronary blood supply is unable to provide sufficient perfusion to the stressed heart, ischemia may be evidenced by:
   - A drop in ST segments on the EKG
   - Abnormal distribution of radioisotope (thallium) perfusion to the myocardium
   - Ventricular wall motion abnormalities seen on echocardiography (dobutamine stress echocardiography)

The individual patient needs to be matched with the appropriate type of stress test (Table 11–3).

TABLE 11–3. **Cardiac Stress Tests**

Test	Description	Indications	Contraindications
Exercise EKG	Most commonly done on a treadmill; continuous EKG tracing is monitored for ST segment depression; least expensive stress test; less helpful if baseline ST segment abnormalities are present at rest (e.g., LBBB, ventricular pacemaker, digitalis effect)	For men or postmenopausal women with a moderate risk of CAD (or for risk stratification in patients considered high risk)	Not for patients with unstable angina, critical aortic stenosis, left ventricular outflow tract obstruction, a recent thrombotic event, or cerebral ischemia, or for those who have had a large MI within the past 3 days
Exercise EKG with thallium	Same as exercise EKG, but thallium (or another radiopharmaceutical) is injected immediately postexercise and its distribution by the cardiac circulation is imaged; may demonstrate fixed (suggesting previous MI) or reversible (suggesting compromised circulation worsened by stress) areas of myocardial ischemia	See indications for exercise EKG, except this test is better for patients with baseline ST abnormalities on EKG	See contraindications for exercise EKG
Pharmacologic stress EKG	Administration of adenosine or dipyridamole results in alteration of coronary artery blood flow; effect may then be assessed by thallium studies	For patients who are unable to do exercise because of physical limitations (e.g., severe emphysema, morbid obesity) or who have a high probability of a false–positive result (e.g., valvular disease, left ventricular hypertrophy).	Not for patients with active bronchospasm, high-grade heart block without pacemaker, or hypotension, or for those who are taking theophylline or caffeine

(continued)

TABLE 11–3. Cardiac Stress Tests (*Continued*)

Test	Description	Indications	Contraindications
Stress echocardiogram	IV dobutamine is the stressor; an echocardiogram detects the degree of wall motion abnormalities and measures the response; stress echocardiograms may have superior specificity and sensitivity to other forms of stress testing	For patients who are unable to tolerate physical exertion or other nuclear perfusion isotopes, or if information on ventricular wall thickness or valvular structure and function is also needed	Not for patients with symptomatic aortic aneurysm, those with uncontrolled ventricular tachycardia, and those who are difficult to image with echocardiography (e.g., because of morbid obesity, severe lung disease)

CAD = coronary artery disease; EKG = electrocardiogram; IV = intravenous; LBBB = left bundle branch block; MI = myocardial infarction.

Echocardiography

An echocardiogram may be useful in assessing systolic heart failure (poor contractility may be secondary to ischemia), diastolic dysfunction, valvular heart disease, and ejection fraction. However, an echocardiogram may not be helpful for CAD that is not associated with these other pathologies, except to rule them out. Echocardiography has the advantages of being noninvasive (as opposed to cardiac catheterization), nonprovocative (as opposed to a stress test), and relatively inexpensive.

> **NOTE**
>
> Do not delay indicated stress testing or cardiac catheterization while waiting for echocardiogram results.

Cardiac catheterization

Cardiac catheterization is invasive and more expensive than stress testing but gives a definitive picture of the coronary artery anatomy. It has the added advantage of allowing for immediate interventional therapy (e.g., angioplasty).

> **NOTE**
>
> Computed tomography (CT) scanning and magnetic resonance angiography of the coronary arteries are in development as screening tools.

 DIFFERENTIAL DIAGNOSIS (Table 11–4)

 THERAPY

Nonpharmacologic Therapy

Exercise prescriptions

> **NOTE**
>
> A stress test may be needed before undertaking an exercise program to evaluate the safety of stressing the heart and to determine what level of exercise the patient should be prescribed. Ask your preceptor before prescribing exercise for any patient with CAD.

TABLE 11–4. **Differential Diagnosis of Chest Pain**

Differential Diagnosis	Description of Chest Pain
Aortic dissection	Associated with severe hypertension
Esophageal rupture	Worse with emesis or swallowing
Gastroesophageal reflux	Worse when lying down; radiates to the back
Musculoskeletal pain	Worse with cough, deep breathing, palpation, or movement
Pancreatitis	Radiates to the back and is coincident with abdominal pain
Panic attack	Coincident with palpitations, severe anxiety, a feeling of doom, hyperventilation symptoms
Pericarditis	Worse with cough, deep breathing, or when lying down; radiates to the neck, shoulder, or back
Pneumomediastinum	Worse with cough, deep breathing, emesis, or swallowing; radiates to the jaw or neck
Pneumonia	Coincident with dyspnea and cough; worse with cough or deep breathing
Pneumothorax	Coincident with dyspnea; radiates to the back or shoulder
Pulmonary embolus	Coincident with dyspnea; worse with cough or deep breathing

Exercise is an important aspect of the patient treatment plan to achieve the goals of weight loss, blood pressure control, improved cardiovascular fitness, and correction of dyslipidemias. Twenty minutes of aerobic activity at least three times a week is usually recommended. Shorter, more frequent exercise (e.g., taking the stairs instead of the elevator, parking at the far corner of the lot and walking) is also beneficial.

NOTE

Choosing an activity that is enjoyable to the patient is important in ensuring adherence to the exercise regimen. Any activity is better than none at all.

Dietary recommendations

Dietary specifics suggested by most authorities include **salt restriction** for control of blood pressure and CHF, **saturated fat restriction** for dyslipidemias, plenty of fresh **fruits and vegetables,** and **caloric restriction** for obesity.

NOTE

As little as 10 pounds of weight loss may have a significant cardiovascular benefit.

Moderate alcohol use (i.e., 1 oz of ethanol per day for men and 0.5 oz for women) has been shown to be associated with a decreased risk of CAD; however, recommendations for regular alcohol use should be made with caution. Alcohol is an addictive substance that may have adverse effects on hypertension, obesity, diabetes mellitus, triglycerides, liver, and the upper gastrointestinal tract when consumed in excess.

Smoking cessation

Efforts by physicians have been shown to significantly impact on a patient's ability to quit smoking. See Chapter 25 for a discussion of smoking cessation.

Stress reduction

Relaxation techniques and lifestyle modifications that decrease psychological stress have been shown to be helpful in managing CAD, particularly when combined with other lifestyle changes.

Pharmacotherapy

Cholesterol plaque–induced fixed narrowing of the coronary arteries usually causes exercise-sensitive stable angina. Pharmaceuticals for stable angina are generally targeted at decreasing ischemia, providing anticoagulation, and modifying risk factors.

Ischemia

Ischemia can be decreased with **β-blockers, nitrates,** or **calcium channel blockers.** β-Blockers and calcium channel blockers appear to have similar clinical outcomes; however, β-blockers are preferred because they appear to have fewer adverse effects when treating stable angina. Recent studies have suggested that β-blockers may be better for anginal symptoms. Thus far, trials comparing nitrates to β-blockers and calcium channel blockers for antianginal treatment have been inconclusive.

NOTE

The American College of Cardiology and the American Heart Association recommend β-blockers as the first-line agents for chronic, stable angina unless their use is contraindicated.

Anticoagulation

Prophylaxis with one **aspirin** daily is usually indicated because of its antithrombotic (i.e., antiplatelet) effect. Prophylaxis with daily aspirin should also be considered for high-risk, asymptomatic patients.

Risk factor modification

Risk factors can be altered with **antihypertensives, lipid-lowering agents,** and **smoking cessation.** See Chapters 13, 16, and 25 for more information.

Procedures

The decision about whether to suggest coronary artery bypass grafting (CABG), angioplasty, or management with antianginal medications alone is often preceded by defining the coronary artery anatomy with a cardiac catheterization. At times the catheterization can proceed to include correction of certain structural abnormalities (e.g., coronary artery stenosis, valvular stenosis) using balloon angioplasty, stent placement in the coronary arteries, or laser or mechanical ablation (to minimize obstructing plaques).

CABG is an effective therapy for the treatment of CAD and may provide more effective symptomatic relief than medical management. It improves survival rates in patients with left main artery disease, three-vessel disease, or significant CAD with left ventricular dysfunction.

URGENCIES & EMERGENCIES—ACUTE CORONARY SYNDROMES

Unstable angina and **acute MI** are likely to be sudden, thrombotic, platelet-mediated events caused by acute rupture of plaque in the endothelium of the coronary arteries. The patient and the clinician must be able to recognize the presentation of an acute coronary syndrome and act accordingly. Actively instruct patients with known CAD in the management of patterns of unstable angina.

> **NOTE**
>
> When treating a patient with a possible MI, follow the mantra, "Time is Muscle." The sooner an acute coronary occlusion is treated with therapies such as thrombolytics, the greater the benefit to the endangered myocardium.

Many therapies for unstable angina and acute MI (Table 11–5) can be administered in the outpatient setting. These therapies may decrease clot

TABLE 11–5. Urgent Outpatient Therapy for a Suspected Myocardial Infarction

- Administer **CPR** if needed.
- Call **911** or your local emergency system activation number.
- Administer **oxygen.**
- Administer **nitroglycerin** sublingually for chest pain.
- Administer **aspirin** for antiplatelet therapy.
- Use a cardiac **monitor** to assess for arrhythmias.

CPR = cardiopulmonary resuscitation.

formation, ischemia, and pain as well as improve outcomes. Life-threatening delays in therapy may result from waiting for nonessential laboratory tests to return, trying to contact other health care providers, or misdiagnosing nontypical complaints as being noncardiac in origin.

NOTE

Because thrombolytics or urgent angioplasty may be a highly effective treatment alternative in acute coronary syndromes, patients should get to the hospital as soon as possible.

Coagulation can be decreased with **aspirin, heparin** and **glycoprotein IIb/IIIa inhibitors.** Aspirin's antiplatelet effects have been shown to be highly efficacious in acute coronary syndromes. Heparin anticoagulation has been a mainstay of therapy. Glycoprotein IIb/IIIa inhibitors are some of the newer drugs being used for their antiplatelet activity in this setting.

Ischemia and pain can be reduced with **oxygen, nitroglycerin,** and **morphine.** Oxygen should be administered by nasal cannula. Patients with chronic obstructive pulmonary disease should be monitored carefully because they may retain carbon dioxide. Nitroglycerin should be given sublingually, topically, or intravenously to decrease vasoconstriction and pain. Morphine should be given intravenously for sedation, to enhance vasodilation, and to decrease pain not relieved by nitrates.

NOTE

The mnemonic "MONA" (**m**orphine, **o**xygen, **n**itrates, **a**spirin) has been used for treatment of acute ischemia.

Outcomes may improve with **β-blockers** and **angiotensin-converting enzyme (ACE) inhibitors.** β-Blockers improve outcome when used in acute MI and chronically in the postinfarct patient and are probably underused for these indications. ACE inhibitors may enhance the remodeling process that begins soon after ischemic injury of the myocardium.

SPECIAL POPULATIONS

Children

Cardiac disease in children is usually not secondary to CAD. Some forms of vasculitis (e.g., Kawasaki's disease) may result in nonatherosclerotic aneurysmal abnormalities of the coronary arteries, with a risk of sudden death.

Because cardiac risk factors are well defined in the adult population and effective treatment of these factors (e.g., hypertension, dyslipidemia) has been demonstrated to decrease morbidity and mortality, it is tempting to define certain children as being at high risk for CAD. Is the first grader with the highest cholesterol in his class at risk for heart disease? Is the tenth grader on the basketball team with blood pressure in the 95th percentile at higher risk of experiencing an MI on the court? Or are these children normal?

Whether such definitions of risk are appropriate and whether treatment of the risk factor does more harm than good is the subject of continued debate and research. However, it is known that education of school-aged children about the health effects of tobacco use, exercise, diet, and other aspects of a healthy lifestyle is beneficial.

Seniors

Normal physiologic changes associated with aging may complicate or worsen cardiac disease processes. These changes include:

- **Blunting of heart rate response to exercise** (secondary to diminished β-adrenergic receptor responsiveness)
- **Decreased compliance of the arteries** (results in hypertension and increased cardiac workload)
- **Decreased compliance of the ventricles** (results in increased end-diastolic pressures)

For example, seniors are more dependent on atrial contraction to adequately fill the relatively stiff ventricles, thus making atrial fibrillation a more symptomatic problem than it might be in a younger person. In addition, β-blocker therapy for hypertension is less effective in seniors because of decreased baseline β-adrenergic receptor responsiveness.

Because CAD is usually a lifelong, progressive process, the prevalence increases with advancing age and is very common in the elderly. Frequent comorbidities, increased propensity for adverse drug reactions, and adherence problems all complicate the evaluation and treatment of cardiac risk factors, management of adverse cardiac events, and postevent monitoring and treatment in the elderly patient.

Pregnancy

Normal pregnancy is a hyperdynamic cardiovascular state. Heart rate, cardiac output, and blood volume are increased. Normal women have enough cardiac reserves to respond to the increased demands without problems. However, women with significant baseline cardiac disease may find pregnancy to be a stressor that compromises their cardiovascular well-being. These women must be followed carefully during pregnancy, labor, and delivery.

 ## COMPLEMENTARY/ALTERNATIVE MEDICINE

The following therapies have only some scientific, but much anecdotal acceptance.

- **Vitamin E** has known antioxidant effects that are postulated to help prevent the endothelial damage that occurs with the atherosclerotic process.
- **Chelation therapy** has been advocated as a means of reversing plaque buildup, but is generally not accepted by cardiologists for this purpose.
- **Garlic** has purported benefits in the treatment of CAD, but proof of efficacy from controlled trials is lacking.
- **Fish oil** and other omega-3 fatty acid supplements may be effective treatments for hyperlipidemia.
- **Adjunctive therapies** (e.g., hypnotherapy, acupuncture, guided imagery, yoga, biofeedback) may aid traditional treatment of cardiac risk factors (e.g., cigarette smoking, hypertension).

CONSULTS

Specialty consultation is indicated for highly technical diagnostic evaluation (e.g., cardiac catheterization) or when therapies are needed that are beyond the usual scope of the family physician. As with all diagnoses, your preceptor may refer sooner or later than one of his colleagues because of variable comfort levels with the evaluation and treatment of CAD.

CHAPTER **12**

Diabetes Mellitus

Philip Diller • Rick E. Ricer

 INTRODUCTION

Diabetes mellitus is the name given to a group of metabolic disorders that all result in a common biochemical abnormality—elevated blood glucose levels. The rise in blood glucose levels is the result of dysfunction in insulin sensitivity, insulin secretion, or both.

Diabetes mellitus is classified as type 1, type 2, or gestational. Type 1 and type 2 are very different diseases. Although this chapter concentrates on type 2 diabetes, the characteristics of type 1 diabetes are also outlined to enhance your ability to differentiate between the two.

OBJECTIVES

■ Describe the impact of diabetes mellitus in the United States and in individual family practice settings

■ Explain the American Diabetes Association criteria for diagnosing diabetes mellitus

■ Compare and contrast the major forms of diabetes mellitus

■ Understand the concept of syndrome X and its relationship to the evaluation and management of type 2 diabetes mellitus

■ Recognize the long-term complications of type 2 diabetes mellitus

■ Outline the components of an individualized approach to the management of type 2 diabetes mellitus

Type 1 Diabetes Mellitus

Type 1 diabetes is an autoimmune disease, possibly initiated by a viral infection, which causes beta cell destruction in the pancreas leading to an **absolute insulin deficiency.** Type 1 diabetes may also be secondary to other processes that destroy the beta cells of the pancreas (e.g., chronic pancreatitis, trauma to the pancreas).

Patients with type 1 diabetes:

■ require exogenous insulin to maintain glucose homeostasis
■ have a propensity toward ketoacidosis
■ are usually younger at onset than those with other types of diabetes
■ are commonly at or below ideal body weight

- have very low levels of C-peptide (a marker of endogenous insulin production)

Type 2 Diabetes Mellitus

Type 2 diabetes accounts for 90% to 95% of all cases of diabetes in the United States. The process that usually causes type 2 diabetes is **resistance to circulating insulin at the cellular level.**

The expression of genetically determined insulin resistance appears to be modulated by environmental factors; most notably, obesity and lack of exercise (Figure 12–1). A person who is obese but has no genetic predisposition may never develop type 2 diabetes. Likewise, a person who is genetically predisposed to insulin resistance may never develop type 2 diabetes if his weight remains controlled throughout life, particularly if he exercises regularly. The weight at which a genetically predisposed individual will develop type 2 diabetes appears to vary; some individuals have normal blood glucose levels at 20% over ideal weight while others may have abnormal levels at or below ideal body weight.

Type 2 diabetes is often part of a constellation of signs, symptoms, physical findings, and disease processes referred to in the medical literature by several different names: **syndrome X,** metabolic syndrome, and insulin-resistance syndrome. We shall use the term "syndrome X." Syndrome X predisposes a person to accelerated atherosclerosis (see Figure 12–1). One current theory is that hyperinsulinemia causes hypertension,

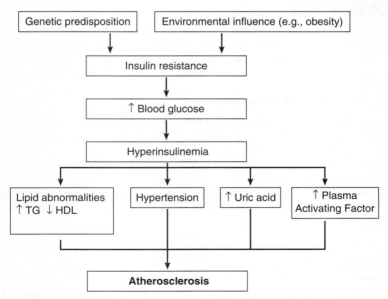

FIGURE 12–1. The path to atherosclerosis in syndrome X. *HDL* = high-density lipoproteins; *TG* = triglycerides.

a low level of high-density lipoprotein (HDL) cholesterol, and elevated triglycerides, all of which lead to atherosclerosis. It is also possible that the **decrease in intracellular glucose** associated with insulin resistance leads either directly or indirectly to atherosclerosis.

Although most persons with type 2 diabetes have syndrome X, other processes can cause what is currently classified as type 2 diabetes. These processes include:

- chronic use of glucocorticosteroids
- Cushing's disease
- a combination of an abnormally high insulin resistance and inadequate insulin secretion

NOTE

Insulin resistance and poor insulin secretion are likely to be the causes of type 2 diabetes in people who are not obese.

It is important to determine whether type 2 diabetes is or is not associated with syndrome X because the approach to treatment for each subset differs. However, because type 2 diabetes associated with syndrome X is more common, this chapter focuses on the prevention, evaluation, and treatment of patients with syndrome X.

NOTE

Knowledge of syndrome X is becoming increasingly more important to the understanding of the cause and treatment of type 2 diabetes and the implementation of appropriate patient education.

Gestational Diabetes Mellitus

Gestational diabetes is the result of abnormal glucose metabolism during pregnancy. Hyperglycemia appears to be caused by a combination of the hormonal changes of pregnancy and individual predisposition. Blood glucose must be tightly controlled throughout pregnancy to help avoid complications such as stillbirth, preterm labor, and large-for-gestational-age babies.

The development of gestational diabetes mellitus indicates an increased risk of developing type 2 diabetes in the future (estimated risk of 50% to 70%).

TERMINOLOGY

C-peptide: byproduct of insulin production by the pancreatic beta cells; normal levels imply the pancreas is producing appropriate amounts of insulin, low levels imply the pancreas is producing too little (e.g., diabetes), and high levels imply the pancreas is producing too much (e.g., an islet cell tumor)

Classic diabetes mellitus symptom triad: polyuria, polydipsia, and polyphagia

Diabetes: diseases having in common the symptom of polyuria; usually implies diabetes mellitus, but can also refer to diabetes insipidus (rare)

> ### NOTE
> The polyuria and resulting polydipsia of diabetes insipidus is caused by an abnormality in antidiuretic hormone, not hyperglycemia.

Diabetic neuropathy: changes in the nerves resulting from microvascular abnormalities; this disorder can lead to autonomic dysfunction (e.g., orthostatic hypotension, tachycardia, gastroparesis) and peripheral neuropathy

Diabetic retinopathy: changes in the retina characterized by exudates, hemorrhages, microaneurysms, and neovascularization

Fasting blood glucose: the glucose reading on blood drawn at least 8, but preferably 12, hours after no oral intake except water

Hemoglobin A_{1C} (HbA$_{1C}$, glycosylated hemoglobin): a lab value used to estimate average blood glucose concentrations over the past 3 months

Macrovascular changes: atherosclerotic changes of the larger vessels that can lead to coronary artery disease (CAD) and peripheral vascular disease (PVD)

Microvascular changes: changes of the smaller vessels that can lead to retinopathy, microscopic renal disease, and neuropathy

Peripheral neuropathy: a complication of diabetes that results from compromised blood flow through the microvascular pathways; characterized by anesthesia, paresthesia, hyperesthesia, neuralgia, or loss of proprioception or vibratory sense in the extremities

Silent myocardial infarction: evidence of a heart attack without angina or other symptoms (e.g., Q waves on electrocardiogram)

Target organs of diabetes mellitus: the major organ systems harmed by diabetes mellitus, including the brain, heart, eyes, and kidneys

◈ BACKGROUND

Diabetes mellitus is one of the top 10 diagnoses seen in family practice. The vast majority of cases are type 2 diabetes. The American Diabetes Association (ADA) estimates that 15.7 million people (i.e., 5.9% of the population in the United States) have diabetes, about one-third of whom are not aware that they have the disease. Prevalence is projected to increase to 22 million people by the year 2025 because of an aging population.

African Americans, Hispanic Americans, and especially Native Americans have a higher risk of developing diabetes than Caucasians do. Type 2 diabetes is the number one cause of new cases of blindness, end-stage renal disease, and nontraumatic lower limb amputations. Persons with type 2 diabetes are two to four times more likely to have coronary artery disease (CAD) or a cerebrovascular accident (CVA).

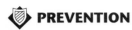 **PREVENTION**

Primary Prevention

Type 1 diabetes mellitus

Because type 1 diabetes appears to be triggered by an undetermined viral illness, no information on its primary prevention is known.

Type 2 diabetes mellitus

Maintenance of appropriate body weight and exercise may delay or prevent the appearance of type 2 diabetes in genetically susceptible individuals.

Secondary Prevention

The focus of secondary prevention is to decrease the likelihood of target organ disease. This includes attempting to normalize blood glucose levels and maintain an appropriate weight, the use of angiotensin-converting enzyme (ACE) inhibitors to help prevent renal damage, and the control of lipid abnormalities and hypertension.

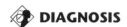 **DIAGNOSIS**

Screening

Type 1 diabetes mellitus

Screening is not routinely done for type 1 diabetes.

Type 2 diabetes mellitus

The **United States Preventive Services Task Force** found insufficient evidence for or against screening asymptomatic adults for type 2 diabetes.

The ADA recommends screening persons or populations with the following characteristics for type 2 diabetes:

- 45 years of age and older (screen every 3 years)
- History of delivery of a baby over 9 pounds
- Family history of diabetes in parents or siblings
- History of gestational diabetes
- Obesity greater than 20% over ideal body weight

- Sedentary lifestyle
- Recurrent candidal infections
- Past problems with glucose tolerance
- Components of syndrome X, such as hypertension or specific dys-lipidemias (i.e., HDL < 35 or triglycerides > 250)

Presentation

Type 1 and type 2 diabetes mellitus often initially present with symptoms related to hyperglycemia; commonly, unexplained rapid weight loss and lethargy. The classic triad of polyuria, polydipsia, and polyphagia is a presentation seen in only a minority of patients. Patients may report blurred vision, rapid changes in visual acuity, injuries that are slow to heal, nocturia, paresthesia, and recurrent bacterial or fungal infections. Since fasting blood glucose levels greater than 150 mg/dl tend to diminish a patient's sense of well-being, new or exacerbated depression or a sense of "feeling bad" may be reported.

Unlike type 2 diabetes, type 1 sometimes presents with an acute metabolic dysfunction or even as ketoacidosis.

History

History of present illness

When diabetes mellitus is suspected, ask about the symptoms of the disease (see PRESENTATION, above).

When diabetes mellitus has already been diagnosed, consider asking the following questions:

- How was your diabetes mellitus previously diagnosed?
- What laboratory tests have been ordered?
- What have been your recent blood sugar readings? How often do you check your blood sugar levels?
- What is your usual blood pressure?
- What is your current treatment plan?
- Do you check your feet regularly?
- What type of diet are you following?
- Have you ever visited a dietitian? When was the last time?
- What type of exercise program are you following?
- Has your weight changed over the past 6 to 12 months? What is your goal weight?
- How has diabetes affected your life?
- Have you ever received special diabetes education?

Past medical history

- Do you have a history of recurrent infections, gout, high blood pressure, lipid abnormalities, heart attacks, renal problems, CVAs, peripheral vascular disease (PVD), transient ischemic attacks (TIAs), angina, or gestational diabetes?

- Have you ever been hospitalized because of problems related to diabetes?
- When did you last visit the eye doctor or podiatrist, and what were their findings?
- What medications are you currently taking (including, over-the-counter medications, supplements, herbs, and vitamins)?
- Have you ever had negative reactions to medications?

NOTE

The complications of syndrome X (e.g., atherosclerotic changes, the macrovascular and microvascular complications associated with type 2 diabetes) may begin or even significantly advance before blood glucose levels diagnostic for type 2 diabetes are reached.

Family history

Ask the patient about family history of:

- diabetes (including age of onset and associated weight if subtype is not yet known)
- obesity
- dyslipidemias
- hypertension
- stroke
- myocardial infarction (MI)

TABLE 12–1. **Review of Systems in the Diagnosis and Management of Diabetes Mellitus**

System	Common Patient Complaints
Dermatologic	Ulcers of the lower extremities, fungal infections*
HEENT	Thrush*
Cardiovascular	Chest pain (angina)
Respiratory	Shortness of breath
Gastrointestinal	Abdominal pain, nausea (gastroparesis), pain with swallowing (esophageal candidiasis*), constipation (neuropathy or dehydration), diarrhea (neuropathy), chest pain or heart burn (gastroesophageal reflux)
Urogenital	Vaginal candidiasis*, urinary tract infections*, impotence
Musculoskeletal	Intermittent claudication (peripheral vascular disease), lower extremity edema (congestive heart failure)
Neurologic	Peripheral neuropathy symptoms, visual changes
Psychologic	Lethargy, depression, poor concentration

*These conditions are related to glucose level or immunodeficiency.

- TIAs
- PVD
- amputations
- kidney and eye problems

Social history

- Do you use alcohol or tobacco products? Ask the patient to quantify.
- What are your support systems?
- What is your occupation?

Review of Systems (Table 12–1)

Physical Examination (Table 12–2)

Physical examination helps to screen for end-organ damage that can be caused or exacerbated by complications and to rule out other causes of symptoms.

TABLE 12–2. **Possible Physical Examination Findings in Diabetes Mellitus**

System	Findings
Vital signs	Tachycardia, orthostatic changes (autonomic dysfunction), elevated blood pressure, change in weight
Dermatologic	Ulcerations of the lower extremities, fungal infections (especially of the feet), abnormal toenails, evidence of foot or lower leg trauma that patient is unaware of (peripheral neuropathy)*
HEENT	Thrush, extraoccular muscle movement[†], decreased vision[‡], fundoscopic abnormalities (retinopathy)
Cardiovascular	S_3, jugular venous distention (CHF), aortic sclerosis murmur, carotid bruit, femoral bruit, decreased peripheral pulses (arteriosclerotic disease)
Respiratory	Rales (CHF)
Gastrointestinal	Enlarged abdominal aorta, renal bruits (arteriosclerotic disease), central obesity, striae
Musculoskeletal	Asymptomatic foot sores*
Neurologic	Decreased sensation in the feet[§], decreased reflexes, orthostatic hypotension, steady heart rate despite the Valsava maneuver, deep breathing, Horner's syndrome, palsies in the third, fourth, and sixth cranial nerves, decreased ankle jerk

CHF = congestive heart failure; S_3 = third heart sound.
*Evidence of pressure-related problems should prompt a check for malfitting shoes.
[†]Diabetes mellitus is the most common cause of sixth-nerve palsy and a common cause of third-nerve palsy.
[‡]Acuity can change depending on the level of the blood glucose and the changes of the lens secondary to high blood glucose levels.
[§]Early in the course of disease there may only be decreased proprioception or decreased vibratory sense.

> **NOTE**
>
> Periodic, dilated funduscopic examinations are important. Many family physicians refer this to an optometrist or ophthalmologist.

Laboratory Tests

Laboratory tests that should be obtained include:

- lipid profile (for dyslipidemias, including the elevated triglycerides and decreased HDL of syndrome X)
- renal function tests (for increased creatinine)
- urinalysis (for proteinuria), including tests for microalbuminuria
- blood glucose
- Hemoglobin A_{1C} (HbA_{1C})

> **NOTE**
>
> Serum and plasma glucose are 15% greater than whole blood glucose. Because capillary blood resembles arterial blood more than venous blood does, capillary blood glucose (e.g., from a fingerstick) is 7% greater than venous blood.

The ADA criteria for the diagnosis of diabetes mellitus are based on blood glucose levels and are currently the accepted standard of care (Table 12–3). The oral glucose tolerance test, once a common outpatient diagnostic technique, is rarely used except with prenatal patients. HbA_{1C} is a method used to estimate average blood glucose concentrations over a 3- to 4-month period. Although the HbA_{1C} is a useful laboratory tool for following patients with the diagnosis of diabetes mellitus, it has poor diagnostic sensitivity.

Additional Studies

Liver function tests should be done if the patient is likely to start medications such as metformin.

An electrocardiogram can be used to screen for evidence of a silent MI.

On rare occasions, it is difficult to identify if a patient has type 1 or type 2 diabetes without the use of blood tests. Type 1 diabetes is strongly suggested by the presence of islet cells and anti-insulin autoantibodies. However, because these signs fade within the first 6 months of diabetes onset, a negative test does not exclude type 1 diabetes. Because functional islet cells generally disappear 2 years after the onset of type 1 diabetes, type 2 diabetes is strongly suggested if it has been 2 years since the diagnosis and the patient's fasting C-peptide value is greater than 1.0 ng/dl.

TABLE 12–3. **American Diabetes Association Criteria for the Diagnosis of Diabetes Mellitus**

One random blood glucose value > 200 mg/dl **plus** symptoms of diabetes
OR
Two fasting blood glucose values > 126 mg/dl
OR
Two 2-hour postprandial blood glucose values > 200 mg/dl
OR
Any combination of two of the blood glucose values above

 DIFFERENTIAL DIAGNOSIS

The differential diagnoses of hyperglycemia include other endocrine disorders, tumors, alcoholic ketoacidosis, hepatic disease, central nervous system pathologies, and pharmaceutical side-effects (resulting from oral, intravenous, or intramuscular steroids; intravenous pentamidine; adrenocorticotropic hormone; thyroxine; epinephrine).

 THERAPY

Successful control of diabetes mellitus is directly related to the patient's capacity and motivation to practice self-care and the health system's capacity and commitment to educate the patient. Each treatment regimen needs to be individualized according to the patient's education level, prior experience, health beliefs, physical limitations, financial barriers, and psychosocial conditions. Patient and family education need to continue throughout the patient's lifetime.

Type 1 Diabetes Mellitus

The cornerstone of management of type 1 diabetes is exogenous insulin given in such a way as to mimic the body's normal production pattern. Insulin can simplistically be viewed as the key that opens the door to the cell (e.g., muscle cell, nerve cell, organ cell) so that glucose can enter and be metabolized for energy. Because persons with type 1 diabetes do not produce insulin, they are dependent on insulin given exogenously.

The use of specific types of insulin (e.g., short-acting, intermediate-acting, or long-acting insulin), the required dosages, and the frequency and types of administration are beyond the scope of this chapter.

Type 2 Diabetes Mellitus

General goals for the management of type 2 diabetes are explained in Tables 12–4 and 12–5.

Nonpharmacologic therapy

Because most cases of type 2 diabetes are part of syndrome X, the major initial goal of therapy is weight loss. If the patient can maintain an appropriate weight, hypertension, lipid abnormalities, high uric acid levels, and elevated blood glucose levels can often all return to normal without the use of medication. **Diet and exercise are the mainstays of treatment** even when medications are needed to control diabetes.

Diet

Although there is not one "diabetic diet" that works for everyone, the ADA recommends a diet that consists of 1500 to 1800 calories per day as a good starting point. Caloric restriction may be necessary for weight loss. When indicated, caloric restriction should be moderate (i.e., 500 calories less per day than the average calculated from a food history, since 3500 calories = 1 pound). All else being equal, this allows for an average weight loss of one pound per week. General dietary guidelines can be found in Table 12–6.

A dietitian or diabetes educator can provide significant expertise, explaining the diet in terms relevant to the individual patient. Other household members should be included in the educational process, especially the person who most commonly prepares the meals.

Exercise

Exercise equivalent to brisk walking for 30 minutes three times a week has been shown to decrease insulin resistance. Exercise programs should be tailored to the needs and specifications of each individual patient.

TABLE 12–4. **General Management Goals for Type 2 Diabetes**

- Determine the extent of blood glucose control by a record of home sugars or periodic HbA_{1C} levels.
- Assess for complications, comorbid conditions that may lead to complications (particularly target-organ disease), and the current state of other syndrome X pathologies.
- Assess the patient's capacity for self-management and social support systems.
- Determine which members of the diabetic care team are involved or need to be involved for general education and diet and exercise planning.
- Discuss and help set achievable goals for blood glucose control and control of complications.
- Check for adherence to diet, exercise, and medication regimens.
- Reassess goals systematically and alter the plan if necessary.
- Continue patient education at every opportunity.

TABLE 12–5. Suggested Goals for Glycemic Control of Diabetes Mellitus

Biochemical Index	Nondiabetic Patient	Goal for Diabetic Patient	When Action is Suggested*
Preprandial glucose	< 100 mg/dl	80–120 mg/dl	< 80 or > 140 mg/dl
Bedtime glucose	< 120 mg/dl	100–140 mg/dl	< 100 or > 160 mg/dl
HbA$_{1C}$	< 6%	< 6%	> 8%

*Action refers to lifestyle adjustments, pharmacotherapy, or both.

Consider a cardiac stress test before initiating an exercise regimen in a patient at risk for cardiovascular disease (see Table 11–3). Many clinicians consider a stress test to be imperative if evidence of microvascular disease already exists. Patients who have microvascular disease should avoid strenuous aerobic exercise or exercise that involves straining, jarring, or Valsalva-like maneuvers. Low-impact cardiovascular conditioning such as swimming, walking, and stationary cycling is acceptable for these patients.

Pharmacotherapy

Oral therapy

Recent studies suggest that intensive control of blood pressure and blood glucose levels may be beneficial in the treatment of both type 1 and type 2 diabetes, especially for the prevention and treatment of microvascular complications. If the target blood glucose level (see Table 12–5) has not been maintained after an adequate trial of weight loss and exercise, oral therapy is indicated.

TABLE 12–6. General Dietary Guidelines for Type 2 Diabetes

Dietary Elements	Amounts
Protein	10%–20% of total calories*
Carbohydrates	55%–70% of total calories
Fat	30%–35% of total calories†
Dietary fiber	25–30 g of both soluble and insoluble fiber‡
Alcohol	Two drinks or fewer per day
Sodium	2400–3000 mg per day

*Patients with nephropathy may benefit from further protein restriction.
†Less than 10% of the total fat intake should be saturated fats. Monosaturated fats should be encouraged.
‡The soluble and insoluble fiber should come from a variety of sources.

There are several classes of oral medications from which to choose when treating type 2 diabetes (Table 12–7). Because the biguanides and thiazolidinediones decrease insulin resistance, and insulin resistance is the basic cause of increased blood glucose, drugs in these classes have become common first-line agents.

TABLE 12–7. **Notable Aspects of the Oral Diabetic Medications**

Biguanides (metformin)
- Do not increase insulin; therefore, no hypoglycemia or weight gain results
- Appear to decrease insulin resistance, mildly decrease hepatic glucose neogenesis, and increase cellular glucose reuptake
- Stimulate lactate production from the intestines, which can lead to lactic acidosis in patients with renal insufficiency, liver disease, congestive heart failure, or hypoxia
- Should be discontinued a few days before studies that use contrast dye that is filtered through the kidneys
- Can be combined with other treatments for type 2 diabetes

Thiazolidinediones (pioglitazone and rosiglitazone)
- Increase the number of insulin receptors and decrease insulin resistance
- Can be combined with other treatments for type 2 diabetes
- Can cause liver problems; therefore, liver function tests need to be drawn before beginning treatment and periodically thereafter

Sulfonylureas (chlorpropamide, tolbutamide, tolazamide, glipizide, glyburide, gynase, glimepiride)*
- Stimulate pancreatic insulin secretion, making patients more hyperinsulinemic
- May slightly decrease insulin resistance
- May lead to hypoglycemia
- Tend to increase patient's weight

Meglitinides (repaglinide)
- Mechanism of action similar to that of sulfonylureas
- Rapid onset of action
- Given just before a meal so that insulin stimulated from the pancreas corresponds with increased glucose load of the meal

α-Glucosidase inhibitors (acarbose and miglitol)
- Inhibit break down of complex carbohydrates to simple sugars, delaying their absorption
- Inhibit a-glucosidase on the intestinal brush border
- Do not decrease calorie load because carbohydrates are still absorbed
- Increase gas formation (via fermentation of complex carbohydrates in the intestines) that can lead to flatulence, gas, distention, and diarrhea

*Chlorpropamide, tolbutamide, and tolazamide are older, longer-acting agents. Glipizide, glyburide, gynase, and glimepiride represent newer, shorter-acting members of this class.

As long as the body is able to produce insulin, treatment with oral agents is effective at decreasing blood glucose levels. Monotherapy studies suggest that metformin, the sulfonylureas, or repaglinide can decrease HbA_{1C} by 1.5% to 2%, thiazolidinediones, by 1% to 1.2%, and acarbose by 0.72% to 1%. These drugs can also be used in combination.

Comorbidities and current pathologies associated with syndrome X should be considered when choosing a diabetic medication. For example, metformin may decrease body weight. Metformin and the thiazolidinediones may decrease triglyceride levels and increase HDL levels, although only slightly. Other oral medications appear to have no effect on these parameters. Unfortunately, none of the oral hypoglycemics appears to decrease blood pressure.

NOTE

Some of the medications used for hypertension (e.g., β-blockers, hydrochlorothiazide) may reduce blood pressure while simultaneously worsening blood glucose levels and the lipid profile.

Insulin

Patients with type 2 diabetes often produce an overabundance of insulin in the early disease process. With increasing age and progression of the disease, the ability of the pancreas to produce insulin may decrease, making insulin therapy necessary. It may also be necessary earlier in the disease process for patients who have difficulty complying with diet, exercise, weight loss, and oral medication regimens.

As important as exogenous insulin can be, it has drawbacks. Administration of insulin controls blood sugars, but does not stop the process of atherogenesis. Insulin stimulates appetite, which can lead to weight gain, which leads to increased insulin resistance, which requires the use of higher doses of insulin. All patients need to be carefully educated about the complexities of insulin administration and its benefits and potential adverse effects. Inexperienced patients generally have a great fear of the idea of administering insulin shots.

When initiating insulin administration, patients must be instructed in dose calculations. An initial dose of insulin can be calculated using one of the following formulas:

- Divide the average fasting blood glucose (ml/dl) by 18
- Divide body weight (kg) by 10

It is common to initially use only long-acting insulin preparations. The dosage can be increased in 2- to 5-unit increments every 3 to 4 days until the target blood glucose level is reached. Some reduction in the oral agents may be necessary. If poor control of blood glucose persists, twice-a-day dosing or split dosing of different types of insulin may be necessary. This level of treatment requires more frequent monitoring of blood glucose levels, usually through home monitoring several times each day.

Follow-up Care

Follow up of a patient who appears to have good control of the diabetes is typically every 3 to 4 months. Patients having difficulty controlling blood glucose levels need more frequent appointments. During each follow-up visit, a review of medication problems, adherence issues, and home monitoring results is appropriate. Performing a review of systems (see Table 12–1) and a physical examination (see Table 12–2) at regular follow-up visits can help to identify the complications of diabetes early. At a minimum, most clinicians suggest a weight check, blood pressure check, and a foot examination to assess whether any signs of diabetic neuropathy are present.

Blood glucose and HbA$_{1c}$ monitoring

Encourage home blood glucose monitoring. The frequency should be based on the severity of the disease process, complications encountered, comorbid conditions, and treatment protocols. Office-based random or fasting blood glucose levels, usually by finger stick, can be helpful in checking adherence and accuracy of home monitoring.

The ADA suggests that the HbA$_{1c}$ be monitored every 3 months for all diabetic patients.

Complications

> **NOTE**
>
> The complications of diabetes mellitus usually take years to develop; therefore, continual follow up is necessary to establish an effective plan for lifelong treatment.

The types of complications and number of patients who develop complications appear to vary depending on many factors, including the type of diabetes. For example, the percentage of patients in a primary care practice with nephropathy or neuropathy appears to be fairly similar for types 1 and 2. Patients with type 1 diabetes are more likely to have retinopathy than their type 2 counterparts, while it is the opposite for the macrovascular (i.e., cardiovascular, cerebrovascular, peripheral vascular) complications.

> **NOTE**
>
> All patients with diabetes mellitus are in a higher risk group for infection and should be considered for a pneumococcal vaccination and a yearly influenza vaccination.

Renal disease and retinopathy

Tight control of blood pressure and blood glucose levels can retard progression of retinopathy and nephropathy. A urine dipstick test to check for the presence of microalbuminuria and a serum creatinine test should be done at least yearly. If any abnormality in renal function is identified (Table 12–8), treatment with an ACE inhibitor is indicated. Some clinicians treat patients with normotensive diabetes who have no laboratory evidence of renal disease prophylactically with a low dose of an ACE inhibitor.

Patients with diabetes should have a dilated retinal examination on a yearly basis to assess the presence of retinopathy or to monitor the progression of retinopathy.

NOTE

Early laser therapy of proliferative retinopathy may be vision saving.

Neuropathic pain, paresthesias, and foot problems

The feet should be examined for dorsalis pedis and posterior tibialis pulses, pain sensation, light touch sensation, proprioception, vibratory sensation, and lesions. Patients should be educated about home foot care in preventing foot problems, especially as the patient loses sensation in his feet.

Improvement in peripheral neuropathy is best accomplished by aggressively controlling blood glucose levels. Treatment for neuropathic pain syndromes can include certain seizure medications (e.g., carbamazepine), low doses of tricyclic antidepressants (e.g., amitriptyline), or capsaicin cream.

Polyuria and polydipsia

Achieving a fasting blood glucose level of less than 200 mg/dl will usually alleviate polyuria and polydipsia.

CAD

Because many diabetics have asymptomatic CAD, the practitioner may choose to do noninvasive screening such as a cardiac stress test or echocardiogram (see Chapter 11).

TABLE 12–8. **Quantified Definitions of Abnormalities in Creatinine**

Findings	24-Hour Collection	Timed Collection	Spot Collection
Normal creatinine	< 30 mg/24 hr	< 20 μg/min	< 30 μg/mg
Microalubminuria	30–300 mg/24 hr	20–200 μg/min	30–300 μg/mg
Clinical albuminuria	> 300 mg/24 hr	> 200 μg/min	> 300 μg/mg

Blood pressure should be taken at each visit and aggressively controlled whenever possible. The blood pressure goal for persons with diabetes should be less than 130/85 mm Hg, and ideally less than 120/80 mm Hg. Many clinicians consider ACE inhibitors to be the agents of choice because they can also retard nephropathy.

NOTE

Women with diabetes who are on estrogen replacement therapy do not appear to benefit from an estrogenic cardioprotective effect and have the same MI risk as men of comparable age.

Aggressive lipid control is indicated in patients with diabetes to reduce the risk of accelerated atherosclerosis. Most articles suggest following lipids annually; target goals are shown in Table 12–9. Tight diabetic control will help decrease lipid abnormalities and is the treatment of choice before beginning a lipid-lowering medication. Since poorly controlled diabetes increases lipids, HbA_{1c} should be less than 8 before starting lipid-lowering medications. If a patient has persistent difficulty controlling blood glucose levels, a lipid-lowering medication may be indicated with an HbA_{1c} greater than 8.

 URGENCIES & EMERGENCIES

Hyperosmotic states or coma and ketoacidosis can occur in patients with diabetes. Ketoacidosis is rare in type 2 diabetes. Aggressive intravascular hydration and insulin therapy are usually necessary.

The decision for further evaluation or admission to the hospital should be based on the severity of the patient's symptoms or the acute problems that are causing the blood glucose level to increase, not on the numerical value of the glucose alone.

TABLE 12–9. **Lipid Target Goals for Patients with Diabetes Mellitus**

	Total Cholesterol (mg/dl)	Triglycerides (mg/dl)	HDL (mg/dl)	LDL (mg/dl)
With CVD	< 170	< 150	> 35	< 100
Without CVD	< 200	< 150	> 35	< 130

CVD = cardiovascular disease; HDL = high-density lipoprotein; LDL = low-density lipoprotein.

SPECIAL POPULATIONS

Children

Children with diabetes usually have type 1. However, with the trend of increasing obesity in the United States, type 2 is being diagnosed more frequently, especially in older children and adolescents.

Seniors

The prevalence of type 2 diabetes increases with age. Seniors are more likely to have decreased production of insulin from the pancreas and develop a total absence of insulin secretion. Seniors are also more likely to have comorbid conditions that contraindicate the use of certain oral medications.

Pregnancy

Patients with type 1 diabetes who become pregnant are at higher risk for complications in pregnancy and are usually followed by a maternal–fetal medicine specialist.

Pregnancy is a diabetogenic state. Human placental lactogen and other pregnancy hormones act to oppose the effects of insulin. Therefore, gestational diabetes can occur during pregnancy in a patient who has never had problems with glucose control. Women with gestational diabetes usually have little or no notable symptoms and rarely develop ketoacidosis. They need to be tightly controlled throughout pregnancy to avoid complications such as large-for-gestational-age babies, fetal demise, preterm labor, and babies with hypoglycemia or respiratory distress syndrome. In the United States, pregnant women are screened with a 1-hour glucose tolerance test at 24 to 28 weeks' gestation. If the screening test is abnormal, a 3-hour glucose tolerance test is indicated.

Oral diabetic medications are contraindicated in pregnancy; therefore, treatment consists of tight glucose control with diet and insulin. Fasting blood glucose levels should be less than 90 mg/dl, and 2-hour postprandial sugars should be less than 120 mg/dl. If blood glucose levels can not be tightly controlled, a consultation with or referral to a maternal–fetal medicine specialist is indicated.

 COMPLEMENTARY/ALTERNATIVE MEDICINE

Biofeedback has been shown to increase peripheral temperature (from 9% to 31% in one study), and is therefore surmised by some clinicians to help alleviate peripheral circulation abnormalities in patients with diabetes. Biofeedback may also have a role in controlling incontinence, which is a complication of autonomic neuropathy.

Chili peppers have long been used topically to decrease pain, and recently have been incorporated into a pharmaceutical preparation (i.e., capsaicin cream). Some patients with diabetes have found the use of capsaicin cream helpful in reducing painful peripheral neuropathy.

◆▶ CONSULTS

Many family physicians refer children with type 1 diabetes to an **endocrinologist** because of the intense ancillary needs of these patients and their families. Patients who have poorly controlled diabetes despite compliance with therapy may also be referred to an endocrinologist.

Foot care is important to the secondary prevention of infection in patients with diabetes. Many family physicians refer patients who show signs of peripheral neuropathy, PVD, foot infection, or complicated toenail care to a **podiatrist** yearly.

Patients with signs of even minimal microvascular disease should see an **ophthalmologist** or **optometrist** at least yearly for a dilated retinal examination.

Patients who have been recently diagnosed with diabetes and have poor control of their blood glucose levels should meet with a **diabetes education specialist** or **dietitian** to review diet specifications and other aspects of care.

CHAPTER **13**

Dyslipidemias

Philip M. Diller • Susan Louisa Montauk

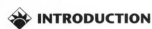

♦ INTRODUCTION

Cholesterol and triglycerides (TGs) are lipids, and blood is mostly water. Because oil and water do not mix well, lipids need a transport mechanism to circulate throughout the bloodstream. The apolipoproteins accomplish this by coating the "oily" lipids, allowing the lipoprotein particles to travel within the "watery" blood.

> ### OBJECTIVES
> ■ Learn a clinical classification scheme for dyslipidemias that guides goal setting and medication selection
> ■ Characterize an approach to the diagnosis, treatment, and follow up of dyslipidemias

Dyslipidemias are a group of metabolic diseases characterized by abnormal elevations or reductions in TGs or one or more of the serum lipoproteins [i.e., very-low-density lipoproteins (VLDL), low-density lipoproteins (LDL), high-density lipoproteins (HDL), and chylomicrons]. Although an elevated total cholesterol (currently defined as greater than 200 mg/dl) is usually associated with dyslipidemia, it is not always.

The second consensus report of the National Cholesterol Education Program (NCEP II) uses current knowledge about components of the lipid profile in vivo to set patient target levels. This classification scheme recognizes abnormalities in the lipid profile and recognizes two major types of dyslipidemia—isolated and combined (Table 13–1).

TERMINOLOGY

Amaurosis fugax: a symptom of retinal artery occlusion that is often described as "a shade coming down over the eye"
Apolipoprotein: the protein component of serum lipoproteins
Arcus senilis: an opaque ring around the iris, most commonly associated with aging but also associated with hyperlipidemia
Bile acid sequestrants: drugs that bind bile acids in the gut (e.g., cholestyramine, colestipol)

Dyslipidemia: concentrations of plasma lipids that are statistically associated with an increased risk for arteriosclerosis

Fibric acids: drugs that enhance metabolism of triglyceride particles (e.g., gemfibrozil, fenofibrate)

Hypercholesterolemia: an abnormally high concentration of cholesterol in the bloodstream (usually quantified as greater than 200 mg/dl)

Hyperlipidemia: an elevated concentration of any or all of the plasma lipids (e.g., cholesterol, TGs, LDL) that leads to an increased risk for arteriosclerosis

Lipid profile: a set of blood tests that usually includes the total cholesterol, HDL cholesterol, TGs, and the calculated LDL cholesterol

Lipoprotein: a class of serum proteins that are important for the transport of lipids

Rhabdomyolysis: an acute, potentially fatal disease of the skeletal muscle that involves muscle destruction and leads to both myoglobinemia and myoglobinuria

Statins: drugs that block 3-hydroxy-3-methylglutaryl coenzyme A (HMG CoA) reductase

Triglyceridemia: elevated concentrations of TGs in the plasma (usually quantified as a fasting value greater than 250)

Xanthelasma: xanthoma on the eyelid

Xanthoma: a benign yellow subdermal lesion composed of lipid-laden foam cells that are histiocytes containing cytoplasmic lipid material

◆ BACKGROUND

The epidemiologic data concerning dyslipidemias are a function of the specific cutoff points used to define a targeted value. The level of LDL,

TABLE 13–1. **The NCEP II Classification of Dyslipidemias**

Dyslipidemia Type	Lipid Abnormalities
Isolated	■ High LDL ■ Low HDL ■ High TGs
Combined	■ High TGs and low HDL ■ High LDL and high TGs ■ High LDL and low HDL ■ High TGs, high LDL, and low HDL

The values considered *high* for LDL and TGs vary based on the patient's risk factors (see Table 13–6).
HDL = high-density lipoproteins; LDL = low-density lipoproteins; TGs = triglycerides.

HDL, or TG that is targeted for clinical intervention varies somewhat among patients and depends on:

- the presence of other coronary artery disease (CAD) risk factors
- the presence or absence of CAD
- the age of the patient

Data from the third National Health and Nutrition Examination Survey (NHANES III) and the NCEP II suggest that 1 in 5 adults (20 to 74 years of age) have total cholesterol levels greater than 240 mg/dl and 1 in 3 adults have total cholesterol levels between 200 and 239 mg/dl. Assuming that a "healthy" total cholesterol level is less than 200 mg/dl, approximately 52 million people qualify for lipid-lowering intervention.

PREVENTION

Screening

The United States Preventive Services Task Force (USPSTF) recommends periodic screening for high cholesterol in all men between the ages of 35 and 65 years and women between the ages of 45 and 65 years. Screening in healthy individuals between the ages of 65 and 75 years, adolescents, and young adults may be recommended when they have other risk factors for coronary disease. Screening may include total cholesterol, TGs, HDL, and LDL.

> **NOTE**
>
> Physicians must individualize screening based on age, gender, and risk factors for CAD (see Chapter 11, risk factors; p 110).

Most physicians agree that patients of all ages should be screened if there is evidence of or a family history of an inherited lipid disorder of considerable severity (e.g., familial hypercholesterolemia); a strong family history of problematic dyslipidemias, early cardiac death, or occlusive cardiovascular disease [e.g., angina, myocardial infarction (MI), cerebrovascular accident, claudication]; or multiple risk factors for CAD.

Dietary Interventions

To assess a patient's diet, instruct the patient to complete a 3- to 7-day diet record before coming to the office. Review the diet record with the patient, pointing out all high-fat and high-cholesterol foods, as well as any other dietary concerns. Dietary interventions may lower LDC levels by as much as 5%–15%.

TABLE 13–2. **Levels of Dietary Intervention Recommended in the NCEP II**

Level	Cholesterol	Total Fat	Saturated Fat
Step 1	< 300 mg/day	< 30% of total calories	< 10% of total calories
Step 2	< 200 mg/day	< 30% of total calories	< 7% of total calories

NCEP II = second consensus report of the National Cholesterol Education Program.

NCEP II levels of dietary intervention

The NCEP II suggests two levels of dietary intervention (Table 13–2). The step 1 diet provides a healthy dietary regimen and can be advocated for all patients, irrespective of the presence of dyslipidemia. Food groups are demonstrated in Figure 20–1.

The step 2 diet is more stringent and should be advocated for those patients who have met with a dietitian and have followed a step 1 diet, but whose lipid levels are still unacceptable.

Vegetarian diet

Vegetarian diets that included approximately 10% of total calories from fat have been studied as part of an overall lifestyle program in a highly motivated population. The program demonstrated actual plaque regression; therefore, patients should be aware of the potential benefits of a nutritionally complete vegetarian diet. Encourage interested individuals to explore this diet as an alternative or adjunctive treatment option.

Oils

Vegetable oils contain no cholesterol. However, there are some (e.g., palm oil, coconut oil) that can accelerate atherosclerosis because they are largely saturated and can accelerate cholesterol synthesis.

NOTE

"No cholesterol" on a food label does not necessarily mean that the food is a good choice for people with high cholesterol levels.

Secondary Prevention

Secondary prevention efforts are imperative for patients with arteriosclerotic disease and dyslipidemia. These patients need to be treated aggressively to help reduce the likelihood of disease progression and future cardiovascular events.

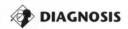 **DIAGNOSIS**

The diagnosis of dyslipidemia is made via a blood test (see LABORATORY TESTS, below).

Presentation

Dyslipidemia has a long latent period before most related signs and symptoms, such as those associated with CAD, appear. Most patients are asymptomatic and are identified through screening.

History

The protocol for history taking is similar to that for CAD (see Chapter 11; p 112).

Review of Systems (Table 13–3)

Physical Examination

The physical examination seeks to identify signs indicating CAD, occult vascular disease, or dyslipidemia (Table 13–4).

Laboratory Tests

Dyslipidemia is identified with a **lipid profile,** which includes total cholesterol and its subsets: TGs, HDL, and LDL. Their relationship is based on the Friedewald equation: **total cholesterol = TGs/5 + LDL + HDL**. With current laboratory techniques, total cholesterol, TGs, and HDL are measured directly; LDL is calculated. VLDL can be calculated from TGs (VLDL = TGs/5, as long as TGs are less than 400 mg/dl).

Physiologic variation and laboratory error dictate that it is often best to perform a second lipid profile at least 1 week after the first profile. The average of the two results should be used as the patient's baseline. For the best accuracy, blood samples for a lipid profile should be collected from

TABLE 13–3. **Focused Review of Systems in the Diagnosis of Dyslipidemia**

System	Associated Signs and Symptoms
Dermatologic	Hair loss on legs (PVD); yellow lesions below the skin (i.e., xanthomas) on trunk, buttocks, arms, elbows, or thighs
HEENT	Thyromegaly (hyperthyroid), new buffalo hump (Cushing's disease)
Cardiovascular	Chest pain, palpitations, orthopnea, PND, dyspnea on exertion, dizziness (CAD)
Respiratory	Shortness of breath, PND, orthopnea (CAD)
Gastrointestinal	Upper abdominal pain (atypical angina, pancreatitis)
Musculoskeletal	Claudication (PVD), arm pain coincident with chest pain (CAD), Achilles tendonitis, previous gout attacks
Neurologic	Vision abnormalities (amaurosis fugax), transient weakness or inability to use muscles (TIA)
Psychologic	Depression (hypothyroidism)

CAD = coronary artery disease; PND = paroxysmal nocturnal dyspnea; PVD = peripheral vascular disease; TIA = transient ischemic attack.

TABLE 13–4. **Physical Examination Findings in Dyslipidemia**

System	Findings
Vital signs	Blood pressure or obesity
General appearance	Apple-shaped
Dermatologic	Palmar striae on the hands (i.e., yellowish discoloration of the palmar crease; associated with type III hyperlipoproteinemia); thickened tendons (hands, feet, pretibial, Achilles), xanthomas (elbows, trunk, knees, buttocks), hair loss above the ankles (PVD)
HEENT	Xanthelasma (50% associated with high cholesterol), arcus senilis*, shimmering retina†, thyromegaly (hypothyroidism)
Cardiovascular	Bruits, absent or reduced lower extremity pulses, aortic murmurs, calf pain (DVT)
Respiratory	Shortness of breath (heart failure)
Gastrointestinal	Renal artery bruit, aortic enlargement, splenomegaly, hepatomegaly
Musculoskeletal	Poor muscle tone, buffalo hump (Cushing's disease)

DVT = deep venous thrombosis; PVD = peripheral vascular disease.
*Arcus senilis is abnormal if found in individuals younger than 50 years.
†Shimmering retina occurs when triglycerides are greater than 1000 mg/dl.

patients who have fasted for 10 hours. In practice, a nonfasting lipid profile is often adequate because, if within normal limits, neither a fasting
lipid profile nor a second specimen is required.

NOTE

Although a nonfasting specimen rarely changes the total cholesterol
by more than 15 points, TGs can be significantly elevated.

The common acquired causes of dyslipidemia and relevant laboratory
findings are shown in Table 13–5.

⬦DD⬦ DIFFERENTIAL DIAGNOSIS

The differential diagnoses of a secondary dyslipidemia include:

- Pregnancy
- Systemic lupus erythematous
- Pancreatitis
- Medication side effect (e.g., from estrogen, androgens, cortico-
  steroids, β-blockers, thiazide diuretics)
- Metabolic disorder (e.g., hepatic disease, renal disease)
- Endocrine disorder (e.g., diabetes, hypothyroidism, Cushing's syn-
  drome, Addison's disease)

**TABLE 13–5. Laboratory Assessment of Common Acquired Causes
of Dyslipidemia**

Acquired Causes	Laboratory Testing	Dyslipidemia on Lipid Profile
Hypothyroidism	TSH	↑ LDL with or without ↑ TGs
Nephrotic syndrome	Urinalysis	↑ LDL and TGs
Chronic renal failure	Renal profile	↑ TGs
Diabetes	Glucose	↑ TGs, ↓ HDL and LDL
OCPs, thiazides, or corticosteroids	None (history only)	↑ TGs and LDL, ↓ (mild) HDL
Alcohol	None (history only)	↑ TGs and HDL
Smoking or inactivity	None (history only)	↓ (mild; 5%–10%) HDL
Pregnancy	Urine β-HCG	↑ TGs, ↓ (mild) HDL

HCG = human chorionic gonadotropin; HDL = high-density lipoproteins; LDL = low-
density lipoproteins; OCPs = oral contraceptive pills; TGs = triglycerides; TSH = thyroid-stimulating hormone.

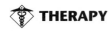 **THERAPY**

Setting Target Lipid Levels

A patient's target lipid level can be determined by the presence of known CAD or the number of CAD risk factors if the patient does not have known CAD (Table 13–6). Smoking cessation and exercise, unlike most medications, can usually raise HDL. Thus, the NCEP II chose LDL as the primary target lipoprotein.

The target level for TGs is variable. For an isolated dyslipidemia, a cutoff point of 400 mg/dl is acceptable. For a combined dyslipidemia, a target level of 150 mg/dl is preferred because combined dyslipidemias carry a high risk of future CAD. Patients should know their target levels. You should reinforce their target levels at each visit.

NOTE

TGs that contribute to a combined dyslipidemia may be more atherogenic than those that lead to an isolated dyslipidemia.

Setting Management Goals

The following questions should be considered when deciding on an initial management course for a patient with dyslipidemia:

- Has the patient been screened for dyslipidemia?
- What is the patient's future risk for CAD?
  - □ How many CAD risk factors does the patient have?
  - □ Is cardiovascular disease of any kind present (e.g., coronary, peripheral, cerebral)?
- Is the patient's lipid disorder acquired or genetic?
  - □ Screening of children and siblings must be considered when a lipid disorder is genetic.

TABLE 13–6. Target Lipoprotein Levels for Dyslipidemia*

Patient Characteristics	LDL (mg/dl)	HDL (mg/dl)	TGs (mg/dl)	TC (mg/dl)
Known CAD with any dyslipidemia	< 100†	> 35	< 150	< 170
No CAD with ≥ 2 risk factors	< 130	> 35	< 150	< 200
No CAD with < 2 risk factors	< 160	> 35	< 400	< 240

CAD = coronary artery disease; HDL = high-density lipoproteins; LDL = low-density lipoproteins; TC = total cholesterol; TGs = triglycerides.

*These levels are based on the second consensus report of the National Cholesterol Education Program.

†Patients with known CAD have a very low LDL target level to promote plaque stabilization and regression.

□ Acquired dyslipidemias need to have the conditions that lead to them identified and treated first, before implementing lipid-lowering medications.

■ What are the patient's target lipid levels? Does the patient know the levels?

■ What is the treatment plan to achieve the target lipid levels (e.g., diet, exercise, medication), and does the patient understand the plan?

□ Dyslipidemias are usually best treated in the context of the family. Even "food preparers" without dyslipidemia need to be counseled on a low-fat, low-cholesterol diet. Involvement of the whole family may lead to improved adherence.

■ If the target lipid level is not being met, why not?

□ How adherent is the patient to the treatment plan?

■ Is the diagnosis correct (e.g., unrecognized acquired disorder)?

Nonpharmacologic Therapy

Exercise, smoking cessation, and stress reduction play a role in dyslipedemia therapy (see Chapter 11, Nonpharmacologic Therapy; p 119).

Dietary recommendations are also part of therapy. For patients with mild dyslipidemia who are not on a cholesterol-lowering diet when first tested, it is reasonable to prescribe a step 1 diet for 6 to 12 months. Adherent patients can usually achieve their target lipid levels within this period. For those who cannot, the trial period may help them adjust to the fact that unless appropriate nonpharmacologic therapy can be instituted or advanced in the future, life-long drug therapy will be necessary to achieve healthier target levels.

Diets for HDL disorders

A restricted dietary fat intake can lower HDL levels. If HDL is already low, encourage the patient to keep total fat as calories at 30% and to use monounsaturated fat (e.g., olive and canola oils).

Diets for TG disorders

For TG disorders, controlling dietary fat is critical to lower the TG level. For some patients, just a few adjustments (e.g., cutting out most fast foods) may result in a significant decrease in TG levels. Other patients may require more extreme changes.

Pharmacotherapy

Drug therapy is indicated if a patient fails to achieve the chosen lipoprotein target level after an adequate trial of nonpharmacologic intervention. For patients with severe dyslipidemia at screening (i.e., needing more than a 50 mg/dl reduction in fasting LDL), it may be reasonable to initiate both diet and drug therapy at the outset. It is important that patients get a sense of how much nonpharmacologic measures alone can achieve before initiating medications.

Choosing medication

Table 13–7 lists the various drugs used in the treatment of dyslipidemia and their indications. In addition to the guidelines suggested in Table 13–7, drug choice can be initially assessed by answering the following questions:

- Which components of the lipid profile (i.e., LDL, HDL, TGs) need to be lower?
- How severe is the problem?
  - ☐ Identify how great a reduction is necessary to achieve the target levels.
  - ☐ There are differences in drug potency for LDL lowering that help guide selection (Figure 13–1).
- What are the concomitant conditions and how may therapy effect these conditions?
  - ☐ **Niacin** can worsen glucose tolerance and can increase uric acid, precipitating gout attacks.
  - ☐ **Bile acid sequestrants** indirectly increase hepatic TG synthesis and should not be used in patients with elevated TGs. Bile acid sequestrants can also cause severe constipation.
  - ☐ The **statins** can all increase hepatic transaminases and should be used cautiously or avoided in patients with chronic liver disease. As of this writing, the only statin not associated with rhabdomyolysis is pravastatin. If any of the other statins or niacin are used, patients should be educated about the symptoms related to rhabdomyolysis. Some clinicians still monitor any statin every 3 months with total creatine phosphokinase (CPK) determination.

TABLE 13–7. Drugs of Choice for High Cholesterol

Dyslipidemia	First-Line Agents	Second-Line Agents
Isolated Dyslipidemia		
↑ LDL	Statin	Niacin, bile acid resin
↓ HDL	Niacin	Statin (to lower LDL and improve TC/HDL ratio), fibric acid
↑ TGs	Fibric acid	Niacin, fish oil
Combined Dyslipidemia		
↑ LDL, ↑ TGs	Statin	Niacin, fibric acid
↑ TGs, ↓ HDL	Niacin	Fibric acid
↑ LDL and TGs, ↓ HDL	Niacin, atorvastatin	Other statin, fibric acid

HDL = high-density lipoproteins; LDL = low-density lipoproteins; TC = total cholesterol; TGs = triglycerides.

Drug	0%	10%	20%	30%	40%	50%	60%
Cholestyramine		4 ········ 6 g					
Niacin		750 ······ 1500 mg					
Cholestyramine + niacin		4/750 ···· 8/2000 mg					
Cerivastatin		0.2 ······· 0.3 mg					
Fluvastatin		20········ 40 mg					
Pravastatin			10····20···40 mg				
Lovastatin			10····20···40···80 mg				
Simvastatin		5 ····· 10···20···40······ 80 mg					
Atorvastatin					10···· 20····40 ···· 80 mg		

FIGURE 13–1. Dose-related low-density lipoprotein (LDL) lowering abilities of various drugs. Atorvastatin is the most potent single agent for LDL lowering, and is a reasonable choice for patients who require more than a 40% reduction. For a 10% to 20% reduction in LDL, many other agents can be selected.

- Are there any drug side effects or interactions that might cause problems in this patient?
- How much will this drug cost the patient or health care plan formulary?

Combination therapy

If a patient fails to achieve target lipid levels with a maximized single-drug therapy, combination therapy may be necessary.

For isolated dyslipidemia with severe LDL elevations, a statin with a bile acid sequestrant is the most potent combination.

Combined dyslipidemias are difficult to treat and often require two or more lipid-lowering medications. If an initial trial of atorvastatin fails, then adding gemfibrozil with or without pravastatin may also be an effective combination.

The combination of a **statin and fibric acid,** however, should be avoided in patients with renal disease or severe illness and in those patients older than 70 years. Patients who are likely to have problems with adherence, patients on multiple medications, and patients who do not understand the danger of myopathy also should not use a statin and fibric acid combination. Patients on simvastatin or atorvastatin or any other statin plus fibric acid should be advised to stop these medications if myalgias develop, at which time they should present for laboratory evaluation (see Urgencies and Emergencies, p 156).

Follow-up care

After starting lipid-lowering therapy, patients should be monitored with lipid profiles every 2 to 3 months. As long as there is no evidence of major abnormalities after two or three lipid profiles, the monitoring interval may be increased.

Testing for adverse metabolic effects can be relaxed after 15 to 18 months on a stable dose of medication. The specific blood tests of choice should be based on the therapy:

- **Statins**—hepatic profile, CPK, fasting lipid profile
- **Fibric acid derivatives**—CPK, prothrombin time/partial thromboplastin time/international normalized ratio, fasting lipid profile
- **Niacin**—hepatic profile, uric acid, fasting lipid profile, glucose

If a patient has not achieved the target lipid profile, upward titration of the drug dose may be indicated. If the target level is not reached with the maximal dose of the medication, consider reviewing the history to be sure that the medication has been taken appropriately and that there is not an undetected acquired cause. If these possible sources of failure are ruled out, add a second agent.

 ## URGENCIES & EMERGENCIES

The most common urgencies directly caused by dyslipidemias or their treatment are acute pancreatitis and drug-induced rhabdomyolysis. These urgencies and their serious sequelae can be prevented if patients are educated about the early warning signs.

Acute pancreatitis can occur in association with hypertriglyceridemia (i.e., TGs > 1000 mg/dl). Simplification of the diet or fasting at the first sign of acute epigastric pain may prevent a patient from developing severe acute pancreatitis. This condition should always be considered in patients with hypertriglyceridemia who present with the classic physical signs and symptoms (i.e., acute, severe epigastric or left upper quadrant pain that radiates to the back and is associated with vomiting and anorexia). In more advanced stages, signs of peripheral circulatory collapse may also be present.

Drug-induced rhabdomyolysis caused by the statins alone or in combination with gemfibrozil is rare; however, if neglected it can lead to acute renal failure. Patients should be advised to stop lipid-lowering agents and greatly increase hydration at the onset of unexplained, diffuse myalgia in the absence of fever or a mechanism of injury. Patients should get a serum CPK to assess for myositis, a urinalysis for proteinuria (myoglobinuria), and a renal profile to determine renal function and identify the presence of hypokalemia. If these abnormalities are present, the patient should be treated with vigorous hydration to maintain a good urine output, and the hypokalemia should be corrected.

 ## SPECIAL POPULATIONS

Children

Lifestyle behaviors begin in childhood, and most CAD risk factors track into adulthood. For the family physician, the primary concerns in the pediatric patient are to encourage healthy lifestyle behaviors, identify CAD risk factors, and screen for dyslipidemia if indicated.

Promote healthy lifestyle behaviors

Smoking should be discouraged and can be introduced between 6 and 10 years of age. **Regular exercise** should be promoted, particularly if the child spends a considerable amount of time watching television or playing video games. Obesity is the most common nutritional and behavioral disorder in children, and lack of physical activity is an important contributor.

Diet can also contribute to obesity. Common problems seen in children are diets high in calories because of large amounts of fat and simple sugars as well as overeating. Evaluating the fat and carbohydrate content of the child's diet may be necessary. Diets high in fat and simple sugars should be discouraged. After 2 years of age, the step 1 diet should be encouraged and skim milk should be introduced. This is also the time to address obesity with the parents if a problem develops. Attention to the weight-for-height portion of the growth chart can alert you to a developing obesity problem.

CAD risk factor identification

It is important to identify risk factors for CAD. Blood pressure evaluation should begin at approximately 3 years of age. A child has hypertension if the blood pressure is greater than the 95th percentile for the child's age and height (see Chapter 16).

Screening for dyslipidemia

Screening should be selective rather than universal. Screening is indicated if there is a family history of premature CAD or if the parents have a known dyslipidemia (e.g., familial hypercholesterolemia). The presence of other CAD risk factors in a child is associated with a higher likelihood that an elevated LDL will be found. A quantifiable definition of pediatric dyslipidemia can be found in Table 13–8.

If a child is diagnosed with dyslipidemia, secondary causes should be ruled out first by the family doctor. If a primary dyslipidemia is identified, the child should be referred to a lipid specialist for treatment. The bile acid sequestrants can be used starting at 10 years of age.

Seniors

Screening

Eighty-five percent of CAD deaths occur in individuals older than 65 years. Thus, the elderly are a targeted population for intervention. However, there are few studies that evaluate the efficacy of lipid lowering in this age-group.

TABLE 13–8. **Cutoff Points for Pediatric Dyslipidemia**

Lipid Parameter	Dyslipidemia	Borderline	Acceptable
Total cholesterol	> 200 mg/dl	170–200 mg/dl	< 170 mg/dl
LDL-C	> 130 mg/dl	110–130 mg/dl	< 110 mg/dl
HDL-C	< 35 mg/dl	≥ 35 mg/dl	≥ 35 mg/dl
TGs	> 150 mg/dl	150 mg/dl	< 150 mg/dl

HDL = high-density lipoproteins; LDL = low-density lipoproteins; TGs = triglycerides.

The data support primary and secondary prevention for individuals between the ages of 65 and 75 years. Secondary prevention is generally supported in individuals older than 75 years, but data are lacking for primary prevention in this age group.

Therapy

The target lipid levels for seniors are the same as for younger adults. Lifestyle modifications (e.g., diet, exercise) should be initiated before starting drug therapy. Because of the increased potential for malnutrition in some elderly patients, serious consideration should be given to obtaining a dietary assessment and low-fat diet recommendations from a registered dietitian.

The use of drugs in patients older than 65 years should be accompanied by a heightened concern for adverse effects. Most adverse reactions to lipid-lowering medications occur in elderly patients with reduced hepatic and renal function.

Elderly patients often respond well to lower doses of the statins because of longer drug half-life; therefore, these are the drugs of choice. Fibric acid derivatives are also safe, but aging is associated with increased intolerance. Over-the-counter psyllium or methylcellulose, both bulk-forming agents, can be used to achieve a 5% to 10% reduction in cholesterol and are appropriate in elderly patients with mild dyslipidemia.

Pregnancy

Plasma lipids are all increased with the hormonal changes associated with pregnancy. LDL drops until 8 weeks' gestation, at which time it begins to rise gradually, reaching 50% to 60% above prepregnancy levels at term. TGs can double or triple, and HDL can increase by 15% during pregnancy.

Women who wish to conceive or who conceive while taking a lipid-lowering medicine are encouraged to stop taking the drug. Bile acid resins can be used during pregnancy to treat elevated LDL.

COMPLEMENTARY/ALTERNATIVE MEDICINE

Chromium supplements may increase HDL. A common dose is 600 μg/day.

Fish oil from fish or supplements (between 10 and 18 g/day) has been found to decrease the likelihood that arteries will become blocked after coronary angioplasty. It appears that the effect is proportional to the intake of fish oil. Oily fish include salmon, sardines, mackerel, and bluefish. These fish appear to be particularly helpful in hypertriglyceridemias.

Garlic may help reduce LDL and TGs by as much as 20%, and increase HDL minimally. The effect may be achieved with as little as half of a clove per day. However, of the controlled studies done, only some have supported this conclusion. There is still much debate, even among alternative medicine practitioners, about fresh garlic versus supplements.

Niacin reduces TGs and LDL and increases HDL. It is also used in conventional western medicine. It may be hepatotoxic, especially in sustained-release preparations. Side effects include flushing, headache, lethargy, nausea, and diarrhea.

Soy products, particularly tofu, appear to help lower LDL and TGs. The effect may be associated with the fact that soy products contain large amounts of phytoestrogens.

 CONSULTS

Referral to a **lipid specialist** is appropriate if the family physician has addressed all of the necessary management goals but the target lipid level has not been achieved. Lipid specialists may assist with a genetic diagnosis of the disorder, medication adjustment, addition of a third agent, or more specialized therapy (e.g., plasmapheresis). Referral is also helpful for severe lipid disorders (i.e., LDL greater than 300 mg/dl or TGs greater than 1000 mg/dl) in adolescents and young adults and for primary care physicians who feel uncomfortable prescribing or initiating combination therapy.

For TG disorders, total dietary fat of less than 20% to 25% is necessary for some patients and often requires the assistance of a registered **dietitian.** Registered dietitians typically have food lists with brand name items that are separated into three categories: acceptable, in moderation, and avoid. These patient education materials are helpful for patients who need to significantly reduce dietary fat and cholesterol.

CHAPTER **14**

Headache

Robert Smith

OBJECTIVES

- Compare and contrast the general features of migraine, tension, and cluster headaches in terms of history and physical examination
- Identify the clinical indications for imaging and other studies
- Identify dietary and psychosocial interventions that may be indicated in preventing or reducing the intensity and frequency of headaches
- Demonstrate a working knowledge of the general classes of pharmaceuticals used in treating headaches

◆ INTRODUCTION

The term "headache" refers to any pain felt within the head or on its surface. The International Headache Society (IHS) standardized the classification of headaches in 1988, identifying them as either primary or secondary (Table 14–1). In family practice, the vast majority of headaches seen and evaluated are primary headaches. This chapter concentrates on three types of headache: migraine headache, tension-type headache, and cluster headache. Research suggests that tension-type headaches are the most common, followed by migraines. As migraine criteria continue to expand, they may eventually take the lead. Cluster headaches, though far less common, are included in this chapter because, when unrecognized, their severe pain can lead to needless, expensive, time-consuming, and fear-inducing workups.

Migraine headaches are of two major types—with aura ("classic" migraine) and without aura ("common" migraine). If left untreated, migraines can last several days. Rarely, they have been known to last 1 week.

Tension-type headaches are also called "muscle contraction" headaches. If left untreated, a tension headache can last from 20 minutes to longer than 1 week.

Cluster headaches are usually unilateral and severe. If left untreated, they can last from 15 minutes to 3 hours. The term "cluster" is used because the headaches occur regularly (e.g., once every other day, eight times a day) for a period of days, weeks, or (rarely) months, often at the same time of day, followed by long intervals of remission that usually last from

160

TABLE 14–1. **The International Headache Society Headache Classifications**

Primary Headaches
- Migraine
- Tension headache
- Cluster headache
- Other headaches without underlying pathology

Secondary Headaches
Headache associated with:
- Head trauma
- Vascular disorders
- Nonvascular intracranial disorders
- Substance abuse or withdrawal
- Noncephalic infection
- Metabolic disorders
- Disorders of the cranium or head, neck, facial, or oral structures
- Cranial neuralgias
- Nerve trunk pain or nerve deafferentation

several weeks to several months. Some patients with cluster headaches have recurring clusters in the spring or fall.

Table 14–2 compares and contrasts these three common types of primary headaches.

TABLE 14–2. **Comparison of Common Presentations of Primary Headaches**

	Migraine	Tension	Cluster	Red Flags for Secondary Headaches
Location	Unilateral (may radiate after onset)*	Bilateral, frontal, occipital, periorbital, "all over" (may radiate after onset)	Unilateral, orbital, temporal	Over temporal artery, in one eye but not periorbital
Duration	4–72 hours	30 minutes to 7 days	15–180 minutes	Longer than 1 week, minutes to days after hit on the head
Quality	Pulsating, throbbing	Pressure, ache, pulsating	Boring into one eye or temple	"Worst headache ever"

(continued)

TABLE 14–2. **Comparison of Common Presentations of Primary Headaches (*Continued*)**

	Migraine	Tension	Cluster	Red Flags for Secondary Headaches
Severity	Moderate to severe	Mild to moderate	Very severe	Unremitting and progressively increasing
Signs and symptoms	Nausea, pallor, photophobia, phonophobia, vomiting, abdominal pain[†]	Photophobia or phonophobia (both are rare), neck and shoulder pain without meningismus	Nausea, bradycardia, unilateral conjunctival injection, facial sweating, lacrimation, ptosis, miosis, nasal congestion, rhinorrhea	Diplopia, papilledema, meningismus, unexplained vital sign changes or vomiting, patient worsens during observation, pain with tapping on paranasal sinus or on temporal artery
Prodrome and aura[‡]	Adults: 50% have pro-dromes and 20%–30% have auras[§] Children: < 20% have either	Often preceded by an increase in emotional stress or tension	None	Unusually severe headache without prodrome or aura in someone who usually has prodrome or aura with their headaches
Time of occurrence	Anytime	Anytime	Nighttime more often than daytime, similar time for each attack	Unremitting, after exertion
Age of onset	10–30 years	Any age	Adulthood	Onset of first severe headache before 10 or after 50 years of age
Gender pre-dilection	Adult: female > male Children: male > female	Female > male	Male:female = 6:1	None

(*continued*)

TABLE 14–2. **Comparison of Common Presentations of Primary Headaches (Continued)**

	Migraine	Tension	Cluster	Red Flags for Secondary Headaches
Family history of head-aches	40% have family member with migraine	50%–60% have parent with migraine; 80% have a first-degree relative with migraine	None	First-degree relative with cerebral aneurysm
Behavior during attack	Passive; rests in a quiet, dark room; falls asleep	Variable	Active, pacing, head banging	Bizarre, lethargic, disoriented
Recognized precipi-tating or associated factors	Bright lights, fatigue or poor sleep, food additives, menstruation, stress, diet, alcohol, travel[†], exercise[†], start of school[†], minor head trauma[†], illness[†], nocturnal enuresis[†], poor concentration	Emotional stress, vascular dilation, fever, weather, menstruation, altitude, school changes or problems[†]	Alcohol, smoking, nitroglycerin, stress	Preceded by trauma, focal neurological lesions, history of heart disease or cancer, symptoms of otitis or URI, exposure to airborne chemicals, new medication, caffeine cessation, rapidly increasing need for analgesics (rebound headache), fever, coincident rash, history of cancer

URI = upper respiratory infection.
*The location of a migraine headache may be hard to specify in children.
[†]More common in children than in adults.
[‡]Aura can include scintillating scotomas, vertigo, transient global amnesia, mood disorders, and cardiac arrhythmias.
[§]Prodrome can include extreme fatigue, changes in food preferences, mood alterations, or vague, difficult to describe feelings. Prodrome or aura may be the only symptom of migraine in older patients.

TERMINOLOGY

Aura: a visual disturbance that occurs before a migraine headache, commonly lasting 30 to 60 minutes and ending when the headache begins; although most often visual in origin, aura can also occur as numbness or tingling of the face or upper or lower limb weakness

Diplopia: double vision

Dysmenorrhea: pain associated with the menstrual period

Dysphasia: difficulty understanding or using speech

Fortification spectrum: jagged, bright lines associated with a visual migraine aura

Hemiparesis: motor weakness of the upper and lower limbs on the same side

Meningismus: pain from irritation of the meninges around the brain and spinal cord

Migraine attack: the symptoms that occur from the prodrome through the postmigraine period

Migraineur: a person who gets migraine headaches

Papilledema: swelling or protrusion of the optic disc (i.e., choked disc)

Paresthesia: an abnormal neurologic sensation such as pricking, hyperasthesia, burning, numbness, or tingling

Phonophobia: increased sensitivity to loud noise

Photophobia: increased sensitivity to bright light

Primary headache: a headache that is not a symptom of an underlying disease

Prodrome: vague feelings of discomfort hours to days before a migraine attack begins; can include depression, food cravings, fluid retention, a vague feeling of the headache "coming on," or often hyperperception

Rebound headache: a chronic, frequent (i.e., often daily) headache associated with discontinuation of analgesics after overuse

Scintillation: a shimmering crescent of light associated with a visual migraine aura

Scotoma: a black spot in the visual field associated with a visual migraine aura

Secondary headache: a headache that is a symptom of an underlying disease

BACKGROUND

Most people have experienced a headache. Results from a recent survey of 15,000 people ranging in age from 12 to 29 years indicated that 57% of the males and 77% of the females had experienced a headache in the previous 4 weeks.

PREVENTION

Headaches can often be prevented or lessened in severity. General patient education about the need to identify and eliminate the factors that cause headache (i.e., triggers) is an important part of initial prevention. Triggers can include:

- Diet (e.g., chocolate, strong cheeses, red wine, beer, excessive caffeine, monosodium glutamate)
- Hunger, missed meals
- Environmental factors (e.g., bright lights, loud noises) ˉStrong aromas (e.g., perfume, cigarette smoke, cooking)
- Fatigue
- Emotional stress
- Too much or too little sleep (poor sleep may be a result of or an instigator for headaches)
- Physical exertion
- Hormonal effects of exogenous estrogen and menses

NOTE

> Many women have headaches associated with menses or the start of oral contraceptives.

Headache prevention, particularly for migraines, often involves pharmacotherapeutics (see PHARMACOTHERAPY, p 171).

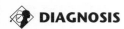 **DIAGNOSIS**

Since the diagnosis of a primary headache implies exclusion of the possibility of a secondary headache, the initial diagnostic work-up includes assessment for both. Most of the assessment focuses on excluding secondary causes.

Presentation

Patients may present with complaints similar to the following: "I can't get rid of this headache," "I think I have sinus problems," and "My eye hurts and my vision is weird."

History

When taking a history of a patient with headaches, several considerations, if kept in mind, can result in a more focused history.

Headaches may be closely associated with psychiatric disorders. For example, the lifetime prevalence of major **depression** is approximately three times higher in persons with severe headaches, and major depression is four times more likely to occur in migraineurs. Persons with migraine also have an increased prevalence of **panic and anxiety disorders**. Chronic tension headaches are highly associated with depression and chronic anxiety. Episodic tension headaches are often a physiologic response to stress, anxiety, depression, emotional conflicts, fatigue, or repressed hostility.

It is also important to consider possible triggers to focus history taking (see PREVENTION, p 164).

History of present illness

Questions to consider asking can be found in Table 14–3.

Past medical history

Ask if the patient has any of the pathologies listed in Table 14–4. If so, consider exploring for a related secondary headache.

TABLE 14–3. **Questions to Consider Asking When Taking a History of Present Illness Focused on Headache**

- How long have you had this headache?
- Is this the first time that you have experienced this kind of headache?
- How long do most of your headaches last? How frequently do they occur?
- How would you describe the headaches (e.g., stabbing, aching, pressure)?
- How severe is the pain relative to other headaches you have had?
- Where is the pain located? Is it in the eye?* Is it over the temporal artery?* Is it unilateral or bilateral, occipital, or frontal?
- Have you recently hurt your head in any way?*
- Is the headache constant and unremitting?*
- Has your sight been affected?*
- Have you had any nausea or vomiting?
- Is this your first severe headache?*
- If the patient is older than 50 years, this question is especially significant.
- Do you ever have bad headaches preceded by an aura (i.e., unusual symptoms or strange feelings)?
- Have you had any numbness, tingling, or other strange feelings in your arms, legs, or face?* Have you had any problems using your arms or legs?* Have you had any changes in your face recently?*
- What makes your headache worse? Does it become worse during exertion?*
- What makes your headache better?
- How does the headache affect your daily functioning?
- What medications, supplements, or vitamins have you taken during the last month? Did any of them begin when the headaches began?
- What do you think causes the headache?

*An affirmative answer suggests increasing one's suspicion of a secondary headache.

TABLE 14–4. **Pathologies Noted in the Past Medical History That May Suggest a Secondary Headache**

Pathology	Associated Signs and Symptoms
Arthritis of the cervical spine	Radiating pain
Cancer	Thrombus or mass
Carbon monoxide poisoning	Hypoxemia
Cerebrovascular accident (CVA)	Thrombus
Dental infection	Radiating pain
Diabetic medication	Hypoglycemia
Recurrent ear or sinus problem	Radiating pain
Head trauma	Contusion
Hemophilia or other bleeding problem	Bleeding or thrombus
Human immunodeficiency virus.	Mass or meningitis
Hypertension	Transient ischemic attack, CVA, high blood pressure readings
Hyperventilation	Hypoxemia
Pseudotumor cerebri	Increased cerebrospinal fluid pressure
Pulmonary embolism	Thrombus
Sickle cell anemia	Bleeding
Temporomandibular joint dysfunction	Radiating pain

Family history (see Table 14–2)

Most migraneurs (80%) have a first-degree relative with migraine, usually a mother, aunt, or grandmother. Many people with tension headaches grew up in a home where an adult had them as well. On the other hand, cluster headaches do not appear to be familial.

Social history

- Are you experiencing any new or worsening stress at home or work (e.g., strained family or marital relationships, new job, death in the family)?
- How much alcohol do you drink? Do you smoke or chew tobacco? Do you drink caffeine? Do you use any illicit drugs?
- What is your occupation? Can you identify any work-related triggers (e.g., exposure to drugs or toxins, visual strain and poor posture from long hours at a computer, continual wearing of a phone headpiece, exposure to cigarette smoke or noise, exposure to dust and chemical odors, constant deadlines)?

Review of Systems (Table 14–5)

Physical Examination (Table 14–6)

Laboratory Tests

Except in acute emergencies, studies to rule out secondary headache are only indicated if a secondary headache is still suspected after a thorough history and physical examination.

> **NOTE**
>
> Costly tests should not replace careful history taking and physical examination.

The **erythrocyte sedimentation rate** (ESR) is markedly elevated in temporal arteritis (i.e., giant cell arteritis). If a temporal headache is associated with tenderness in a temporal artery, consider obtaining the ESR.

Lumbar puncture may be needed to detect a small or old (i.e., 3–5 days) subarachnoid hemorrhage not seen with computed tomography (CT), to quantify increased cerebrospinal fluid pressure with pseudotumor cerebri, or to get cerebrospinal fluid for a suspected meningitis. Most clinicians wait for CT results before attempting a lumbar puncture, even if no physical signs of increased intracranial pressure (ICP) are present.

TABLE 14–5. Review of Systems in the Diagnosis of Headaches

System	Common Patient Complaints
Constitutional	Malaise, fatigue, fever*, chills*, changes in weight*,†
Dermatologic	Rash*
HEENT	Jaw pain*; sight disturbances*; sinus pain*; red, itchy eyes*; nasal congestion that is white or yellow-green*; ear pain or pressure*
Cardiovascular	Arrhythmias*, intermittent claudication*
Gastrointestinal	Nausea, vomiting
Genitourinary	Premenstrual syndrome, nocturia*
Musculoskeletal	Neck and upper back pain or tension, stiff neck*, additional acute* or chronic† pain sites
Neurologic	Irritability, photophobia, phonophobia, vertigo, paresthesia*, dystonia*
Psychiatric	Mood changes or increased emotional stress (even when headache is not present), recent insomnia

*This finding suggests increasing one's suspicion of a secondary headache.
†This finding is often associated with a somatization syndrome (see Chapter 19).

TABLE 14–6. Physical Examination Findings in Patients with Headaches*

System	Findings
General appearance	Pallor, distraction, psychomotor retardation, grimacing
Vital signs	Acute and severe high blood pressure, fever, tachypnea
HEENT†	*Head:* Tenderness over the temporal artery
	Eyes: Tearing, red conjunctiva, papilledema
	Ear: Fluid behind tympanic membrane, red tympanic membrane, hyperemia over ossicles
	Nose: Stuffy, mucus-filled nose
	Throat: Pharyngitis
Dermatologic†	Purpura, vesicular lesions in a radicular distribution of cranial nerves IV or V
Cardiovascular	Persistent irregular pulse; systolic "honk," diastolic opening "snap," of mitral valve prolapse; carotid bruit
Respiratory	Tachypnea with circumoral or peripheral paresthesia
Musculoskeletal	Temporalis or trapezius tender points
Neurologic	Neck rigidity, positive Kernig's or Brudzinski's sign, diplopia, photophobia, new focal neurologic deficits (e.g., limb weakness, cranial nerve or vision abnormalities, facial weakness, speech problems, gait and balance difficulties)
Psychiatric	Anxious or depressed mood, agitation

*Any pertinent positives, other than "general appearance," suggest the possibility of a secondary headache.
†Always note bilateral (i.e., across midline) versus unilateral (i.e., confined to left or right of midline) findings.

Imaging Studies

CT without contrast will identify 85% to 90% of cases of acute subarachnoid hemorrhage. Magnetic resonance imaging (MRI) is a more costly and lengthy procedure. However, MRI offers better detection of small lesions, especially in the brainstem and cerebellum, and of old intracranial bleeds. In addition, the contrast material used in CT contains iodine and, therefore, produces more side effects than the contrast material used in MRI (i.e., gadolinium).

In many instances neither an MRI nor a CT scan is indicated (Table 14–7).

 DD$_X$

Mild strokes and transient ischemic attacks must be carefully distinguished from complex migraine auras.

Rebound headache is in the differential when a patient already taking headache medications presents with a worsening headache. The history

TABLE 14–7. Evaluating the Need for Imaging Studies in the Diagnosis of Headache

- Previous identical headache
- Normal vital signs
- No acute neurologic abnormalities
- Supple neck
- Alert with cognition intact
- Observed significant improvement in headache without analgesics or headache abortive medications

When all six of these criteria are present, it is not necessary to consider CT or MRI. If five or less are present, neither CT nor MRI is absolutely indicated; however, the abnormal finding must be carefully evaluated.

CT = computed tomography; MRI = magnetic resonance imaging.

tends to include headaches that began sporadically but are now daily, often resulting in a need for increased frequency of medication to resolve the headache. These headaches are worse in the morning and are commonly accompanied by nausea, abdominal symptoms, insomnia, restlessness, depression, memory problems, and difficulty with concentration.

Cervical strain (i.e., whiplash) and **subdural hematoma** resulting from trauma (e.g., motor vehicle accidents) need to be ruled out initially by history.

Glaucoma that presents with headache is usually the rare primary angle-closure glaucoma, which includes eye pain. Many other symptoms of the headache caused by angle-closure glaucoma can mimic migraine, including blurred vision, nausea and vomiting, lacrimation, and increased severity with stress. The headache may be associated with beginning a medication with anticholinergic effects.

Temporal arteritis (i.e., giant cell arteritis) produces a severe, persistent headache associated with a temporal artery that is tender on palpation. It usually occurs in older female patients.

Sinus congestion can often present as a unilateral or bilateral headache, but usually also includes other signs of upper respiratory infection or allergy.

Brain tumor can often be ruled out early with a complete history and neurologic examination.

Iatrogenic headache can be induced by a variety of prescription and over-the-counter (OTC) medications (e.g., antihypertensives, antidepressants, decongestants, bronchodilators, stimulants, estrogen).

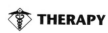 **THERAPY**

Nonpharmacologic Therapy

Patients with headaches related to psychiatric disorders may benefit from **short-term counseling** in the family physician's office, in addition to analgesics.

Headache diaries can help identify possible headache triggers (see PRE-VENTION, p 164) and are valuable in recording response to treatment.

Behavioral therapy, especially relaxation therapy and biofeedback (see COMPLEMENTARY/ALTERNATIVE MEDICINE, p 175), can be used to control migraine and tension headaches linked to stress.

Treatment of rebound headaches consists of **terminating all current analgesic medications.** Even though this may initially worsen the headache and the withdrawal symptoms, the rebound headache usually subsides once the medication is totally withdrawn.

Pharmacotherapy

A wide range of OTC medications is available for the treatment of headache. Most tension headaches and many migraines respond well to simple analgesics. If nausea is a problem, analgesics can be taken in conjunction with an antinauseant, such as promethazine, prochlorperazine, or metoclopramide. Severe primary headaches unresponsive to OTC medications may require prescription anti-inflammatories or, rarely, opioids.

NOTE

Analgesic use should be intermittent and well monitored to avoid the risk of rebound or chronic daily headaches.

Migraine

Treatment

Mild or moderate migraine headaches can often be halted with use of OTC nonsteroidal anti-inflammatory drugs (NSAIDs). If these drugs are ineffective, stronger (prescription) anti-inflammatories should be considered. Severe migraines may need migraine-specific medications (e.g., triptans, ergotamines). Moderate or severe migraines often respond best when an antinausea drug is administered simultaneously.

The triptans. The triptans are the first-line agents for the treatment of severe migraine because they act rapidly and have few major side effects. Most side effects are mild and include increased blood pressure, chest and neck pressure or tightness, facial flushing, and a "rush" sensation to the head. However, particular attention should be given to patients who may be at risk for unrecognized coronary disease or those with borderline hypertension (Table 14–8). Triptans are available in four forms: subcutaneous injection, oral tablets, tablets that dissolve in the mouth, and nasal spray.

NOTE

A positive response to triptans does not rule out tension headache or even subarachnoid headache.

TABLE 14–8. **Major Contraindications for the Use of Vasoconstrictive Migraine Medications**

- Ischemic heart disease (e.g., angina pectoris, prior myocardial infarction, documented silent ischemia, Prinzmetal's angina)
- Uncontrolled hypertension
- Previous stroke
- Epilepsy
- Pregnancy
- Raynaud's Disease

These contraindications pertain to the use of ergotamine, the triptans, and dihydroergotamine.

Ergotamine. Ergotamine, an ergot alkaloid, is a potent vasoconstrictor available in oral, sublingual, rectal, injection, and nasal spray preparations. Ergot alkaloids can simultaneously stimulate and antagonize receptors for α-adrenergics, dopamine, and serotonin, as well as inhibit reuptake of norepinephrine. It should only be used cautiously in patients with coronary artery or peripheral vascular disease. Although very effective, the use of ergotamine is often limited by extreme nausea, a symptom common with migraines. The addition of an antinausea medication may help quell the problem.

Although rare, serious peripheral arterial vasoconstriction (e.g., gangrene of the toes and feet) has been reported with ergotamine overuse. Contraindications to ergotamine are listed in Table 14–8.

Dihydroergotamine (DHE). DHE is available in injectable form (intramuscular or intravenous) and nasal spray (less potent but easy to self-administer) and can be used to treat severe migraine that does not respond to treatment with triptans or ergotamine. An antinauseant is usually given by injection before administration of DHE. DHE is safer than ergotamine because it has less severe arterial vasocontrictive action. Contraindications can be found in Table 14–8.

Prochlorperazine. Intravenous prochlorperazine has antinauseant, antiemetic, and antimigraine effects. It is favored in emergency departments for the treatment of acute migraine.

Prophylaxis

Prophylatic medications include β-blockers, tricyclic antidepressants, selective serotonin reuptake inhibitors, and calcium channel blockers. Prophylaxis should be considered for patients who have two or three disabling attacks or one prolonged attack per month. Other candidates are those in whom acute agents are contraindicated or who have poor responses to acute therapy. It may take 1 or 2 months of treatment before improvement is noted. Treatment may need to be maintained for 6 to 9 months, or even indefinitely.

Menstrual migraines can often be prevented or lessened by taking prostaglandin inhibitors, ergotamine, or estrogen supplements for a few days beginning 1 to 2 days before the usual time of headache onset.

Cluster headache

Treatment

Cluster headaches are the most difficult to treat and often require referral for specialist treatment. Multiple medications are usually needed. Oral preparations are of little value because of slowness of onset.

Oxygen inhalation by facemask often helps to relieve cluster headaches; 100% oxygen is delivered at 7 L/min for 20 minutes and repeated, if necessary.

Sublingual ergotamine may be given at the onset of a headache and repeated once, if necessary. An oral, injectable, or dissolving triptan, or DHE given by injection, can initially be effective, but attacks are often so frequent that safe dosages become inadequate.

Prophylaxis

Patients should avoid cigarette smoke, alcohol consumption, and exposure to triggers such as strong perfumes, volatile solvents, and gasoline fumes. They also should avoid highly stressful situations and high-pressure tasks. Cluster headache attacks may occur during air travel because of the high altitude and low oxygen level. Ergotamine (2 mg) taken 1 hour before takeoff may forestall these attacks. If an attack occurs during flight, it may be aborted by inhaling from the passenger's overhead oxygen supply.

Prophylactic medications include:

- verapamil, 120 to 480 mg/day
- lithium, 300 to 900 mg/day (monitoring of lithium levels is required)
- prednisone, 60 mg/day to start, then tapered over 3 weeks
- ergotamine, 2 mg, given 2 hours before bedtime to prevent nocturnal attacks
- divalproex sodium, 600 to 2000 mg/day

> **NOTE**
>
> A reduced dose of lithium is required if calcium channel blockers or NSAIDS are used concurrently.

URGENCIES & EMERGENCIES

Severe headache with stiff neck (many headache patients have sore but flexible necks that can flex and extend in an anterior–posterior direction) suggests meningismus. Thus, a lumber puncture after CT may be indicated.

Headache with neurologic deficits (e.g., loss of power in the limbs; loss of muscle tone, motor function, or both in the facial muscles; diplopia; numbness; balance problems; staggering gait; speech difficulty) suggests a cerebrovascular accident. Thus, acute anticoagulation after CT may be indicated.

A new temporal headache associated with temporal artery pain when that vessel is palpated suggests temporal arteritis. Thus, immediate treatment with steroids to prevent possible blindness may be indicated, followed by drawing of blood for an ESR and swift referral for a temporal artery biopsy.

SPECIAL POPULATIONS

Children

In children, headaches from both sinusitis and eye strain are fairly common. Before puberty, migraine prevalence is higher in boys than in girls; however, prevalence in girls increases rapidly at puberty.

Seniors

The incidence of headache in the elderly is inversely related to age. Migraine onset after age 50 is rare; however, established migraine may continue past the sixth decade. Patients with a history of migraine with prodrome or aura may note the disappearance of the headache with age, but may continue to experience the prodrome or aura in the absence of headache. These migraine equivalents, or "migraine without headache," consist of episodes of transient neurologic dysfunction or deficit.

Agents that have peripheral vasoconstrictive properties (e.g., ergotamine, DHE, the triptans) are not as well tolerated in the elderly. The combination tablet containing isometheptane (a sympathomimetic), dichloralphenazone and acetaminophen may be preferred for abortive therapy in older patients with migraine, although it should still be used with caution in patients with peripheral vascular or cardiac disease.

> **NOTE**
>
> A delay in the absorption of medications during a migraine attack has been observed in the elderly.

Pregnancy

Although pregnancy does not always transform headache presentations, it often does. Both tension and migraine headaches can begin or exacerbate during pregnancy, particularly during the first trimester, but they can also decrease in frequency or even remit.

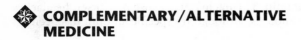 COMPLEMENTARY/ALTERNATIVE MEDICINE

Acupuncture

There is a long history in traditional Chinese medicine of acupuncture therapy for headache. Repeated visits are often required, and some patients find the treatment costly and painful. As with prophylactic medication, benefit often fades after the treatment ends.

In some people, acupressure applied to the web space between the forefinger and thumb appears to erase tension or migraine headaches within 60 seconds. It may be immediately effective even for long-term headaches accompanied by nausea. Some feel that acupressure works best in the dominant hand, with application of pressure or massage to the spot that is most tender in the "meaty" area for 1 minute. If the pain leaves, the patient is instructed to lie down and rest for 15 minutes.

Biofeedback

The biofeedback methods most often associated with migraine relief are those that lead to an increased hand temperature via inner self-control. Muscle relaxation training is also used and involves the use of an electromyogram monitor that measures muscle tension over the area of the headache (e.g., forehead, neck, shoulder).

Imagery

Treatment using imagery requires the patient to focus on warm images (e.g., sitting by a fire, sitting on a beach, holding a hot cup of tea). By focusing on these images at the first sign of headache, some patients can abort an acute attack or at least decrease the severity and duration of a headache.

Supplements and Herbs

Ginkgo is associated with increased blood flow; therefore, it is thought to help in the treatment of vascular headaches. However, studies on the benefits of ginkgo are very limited. Because ginkgo is a mild blood thinner, it should be used with caution in patients with bleeding disorders or those taking other anticoagulants (e.g., daily ginseng, high doses of garlic, aspirin, coumadin).

Feverfew (tanacetum parthenium) is said by herbalists to constrict the cephalic blood vessels and prevent cranial blood vessel spasms. This herb has been shown, in a few good trials, to help prevent migraine if one eats a few leaves each day. Unfortunately, in some individuals, this practice can also induce mouth swelling and ulcers, as well as decrease the ability to taste.

Vitamin A and **vitamin B₃ (niacin)** may cause or worsen headaches when taken in large amounts, although no specific amount has been established.

◆◆ CONSULTS

Headache specialization is a relatively new field. The number of headache clinics and education and research organizations is growing. An increasing number of neurologists are specializing in headache, as are some primary care physicians. Referral to a headache specialist should be considered in all of the following situations:

- When a patient presents with severe, sudden onset of headache without previous significant headaches
- When a secondary headache (see Table 14–1) is suspected but not yet clearly identified
- When the patient has a new chronic daily headache
- When the diagnosis is uncertain
- When the patient has not responded to treatment with usual measures
- Migraines with comorbid conditions that have confounding symptoms
- Increasing requests by the patient for narcotic analgesics

With the first four situations, referral is often initiated after a CT of the head is performed to assess if another consultant is more appropriate.

CHAPTER **15**

Human Immunodeficiency Virus Infection

Susan Louisa Montauk

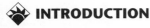 **INTRODUCTION**

OBJECTIVES

- Inject appropriate prevention efforts into routine office visits for all patients
- Describe the basics of the initial work-up of adults with the human immunodeficiency virus
- Explain the appropriate use of antiretroviral medications
- Initiate suitable referrals, discerning between routine and urgent cases

In a patient with acquired immune deficiency syndrome (AIDS) or advanced infection with the human immunodeficiency virus (HIV), it is often difficult to discern which signs, symptoms, and laboratory abnormalities are caused directly by HIV and which are caused by other infections, cancers, or medications. HIV infection notoriously disrupts many immune system functions. Its pathologic processes include the destruction of T helper (CD4) cells. Without medical intervention, infected persons often develop multiple opportunistic infections and cancers within 10 years and die within 15 years.

The major routes of transmission of HIV are penile-anal and penile-vaginal sexual intercourse and needle sticks with contaminated products. Although uncommon, oral-vaginal and oral-penile intercourse can transmit HIV as well. It can also be acquired *in utero,* during birth, and through breast-feeding. Most (i.e., 75% to 85%) HIV infections are transmitted through unprotected (i.e., no condom) vaginal or anal sex.

TERMINOLOGY

Acquired immune deficiency syndrome (AIDS): a syndrome characterized by a positive test for HIV plus either 1) a current or past CD4 cell count of less than 200 or 2) a diagnosis of an "AIDS-defining illness" as defined by the Centers for Disease Control and Prevention (CDC)

CD4 cell: the white blood cell that regulates cell-mediated immunity

CD4 cell count: a count of the number of CD4 cells in serum that is generally reported in 10^6/L; thus, a count of 425 implies 425×10^6/L of serum

Highly active antiretroviral therapy (HAART): a term used to identify the newer antiretroviral regimens, which often include three or four antiretroviral agents and at least one protease inhibitor

Opportunistic infection: an infection not usually seen in someone with a healthy immune system; once the defenses are down, it seizes the "opportunity" to flourish

 ## BACKGROUND

The exact incidence of AIDS is unknown, and quantifying HIV is even more difficult. Experts generally assume that there are approximately seven to ten times as many persons with HIV as there are persons known to have AIDS. As antiretroviral agents become more effective, the ratio of persons with pre-AIDS HIV infection to persons with AIDS will increase.

NOTE

There appears to be approximately 1 million people with HIV in North America and approximately 20 million people with HIV in Africa.

 ## PREVENTION

Primary Prevention

All sexually active individuals should be encouraged to use condoms when engaging in intercourse, unless in a long-term, committed, monogamous relationship. Those who are decidedly not sexually active may benefit from reassurance that waiting for the "right" person, or choosing celibacy, is a healthy choice. At the same time, patients can be educated about condoms by encouraging them to discuss their use with sexually active friends.

A key time for HIV-related education is when a patient decides to get an HIV test. The Centers for Disease Control and Prevention (CDC) has published criteria for pre- and posttest counseling that includes several important, relevant topics.

Based on CDC criteria, strong indicators for HIV screening include:

- A history of illicit intravenous drug use
- Multiple anonymous or minimally known sexual partners
- Rape
- Pregnancy

- A clinical presentation that suggests immunosuppression
- A diagnosis of chlamydia, gonorrhea, syphilis, lymphogranuloma inguinale, genital herpes, or genital condyloma
- A history of HIV in a sexual partner
- A patient expressing fear of having HIV

Based on CDC criteria, moderate indicators for HIV screening include:

- Adolescents who may be sexually active
- A history of sexual abuse
- Recipients of blood products in the United States between 1968 and 1985
- Sexual activity in a high-incidence area (e.g., San Francisco, New York, Miami)

NOTE

HIV testing should follow the legal parameters set by your state. If you are unfamiliar with these parameters, ask your preceptor or the legal counsel at your hospital.

Secondary Prevention

All patients should be aware that it is possible to be reinfected with HIV once infected, and that multiple exposures may lead to highly resistant HIV. Thus, safer sex techniques (e.g., condoms, abstinence from sexual acts that result in exposure to body fluids) are always indicated.

Vaccinations should include pneumococcal vaccine, influenza vaccine (seasonal), tetanus toxoid, and, if studies indicate, hepatitis B vaccine. Although it is a live virus, the measles, mumps, and rubella (MMR) vaccine has not been noted to cause problems great enough to outweigh its benefits in immunosuppressed pediatric populations. However, MMR vaccination in adults with HIV is controversial. The injectable polio vaccine (IPV) is acceptable in both children and adults, but the oral polio vaccine (OPV) should not be given because it is a live virus with a well-known negative impact on persons with immunosuppression.

Although persons with HIV can present in unusual ways with highly unusual complications, there are many commonly seen and well-categorized infections and cancers (Table 15–1). Prophylaxis for opportunistic infections is based on initial laboratory testing and medical history and includes medications for *Pneumocystis carinii*, toxoplasmosis, tuberculosis, and *Mycobacterium avium-intracellulare complex* (Table 15–2).

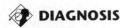 **DIAGNOSIS**

Presentation

A mononucleosis-like syndrome (e.g., malaise, fever, macular rash, lymphadenopathy) may characterize initial infection. For a short period (i.e.,

TABLE 15–1. **HIV-Related Complications and Their Association with CD4 Cell Count**

CD4 Cell Count	Infections	Other
> 500 cells	Aseptic meningitis, primary HIV infection	Idiopathic thrombocytic purpura, progressive multifocal leukoencephalopathy
< 500 cells	Candidiasis (oropharyngeal and vaginal), *Cryptosporidium parvum* (diarrhea), Epstein-Barr virus, *Haemophilus influenzae* (pneumonia), Herpes simplex virus (orogenital), *Streptococcus pneumoniae* (pneumonia), recurrent pneumonia, tuberculosis (pulmonary)*, varicella-zoster virus (shingles)	Non-Hodgkin's lymphoma*, cervical intraepithelial neoplasia, anemia, Kaposi's sarcoma
< 200 cells	*C. parvum* (pneumonia), variable bacteria (chronic diarrhea)	
< 100 cells	Candidiasis (disseminated, esophagitis), *Cryptococcal meningitis* CMV, Epstein-Barr virus, herpes simplex virus (disseminated or aggressive), microsporidia, *Mycobacterium avium-intracellulare complex* (disseminated: encephalitis, GI, dementia, myelopathy, retinitis, wasting), *Toxoplasma gondii,* tuberculosis (disseminated or extrapulmonary, varicella-zoster virus (disseminated or aggressive), variable bacteria (meningitis)	Diarrhea (wasting syndrome), HIV encephalitis, lymphoma (primary CNS)

CMV = cytomegalovirus; CNS = central nervous system; GI = gastrointestinal; HIV = human immunodeficiency virus.
*These conditions are defined by the Centers for Disease Control and Prevention as AIDS-indicator conditions, even when the CD4 cell count has never been below 200 cells/mm³.

days to weeks), an HIV test may be positive. However, the test then often reverts to negative for many months. Unrecognized chronic HIV infection generally is not associated with any specific chronic physical or emotional complaints until many years into the disease process.

A more common initial presentation is stated something like, "I just need to get checked," and is based on the patient's own knowledge of his or her sexual or drug history.

TABLE 15–2. **Guidelines for Prophylaxis of Opportunistic Infections in Persons With HIV**

	Who	What
PCP prophylaxis	HIV-seropositive persons with one or more of the following: ■ CD4 count < 200 cells/mm³ ■ A history of prior PCP ■ Constitutional symptoms suggestive of advanced immunodeficiency	One of the following: ■ TMP-SMX (drug of choice) ■ Dapsone (alternative recommendation) ■ Aerosolized pentamidine (alternative recommendation) ■ Atovaquone (alternative recommendation)
Toxoplasmosis	HIV-seropositive persons with a CD4 count < 100 cells/mm³ who are seropositive for *Toxoplasma gondii*	Choice depends on PCP prophylaxis* and includes one of the following: ■ TMP-SMX ■ Pyrimethamine and leucovorin
Tuberculosis	All HIV-seropositive persons with ■ A positive PPD skin test (5 mm of induration) ■ A history of positive skin test but no previous prophylaxis ■ Close contact with someone with active tuberculosis	One of the following: ■ Isoniazid with pyridoxine for 9 months ■ Rifampin with pyrazinamide for 2 months
MAI complex	All HIV-seropositive persons with a CD4 count < 50 cells/mm³	One of the following: ■ Clarithromycin plus azithromycin (drug of choice) ■ Rifabutin (alternative recommendation)

HIV = human immunodeficiency virus; MAI = *Mycobacterium avium-intracellulare*; PCP = *Pneumocystis carinii* pneumonia; PPD = purified protein derivative; TMP-SMX = trimethoprim-sulfamethoxazole.
*Although clarithromycin, azithromycin, and atovaquone each have in vitro activity against toxoplasmosis, efficacy is not yet substantiated.
Adapted from the 1999 USPHS/IDSA Guidelines for the Prevention of Opportunistic Infections in Persons Infected with Human Immunodeficiency Virus. *MMWR* 48(RR-10);1–59, 1999.

History

History of present illness

Untreated HIV may later be accompanied by almost any symptoms in a primary care visit, but often eventually includes one or more of the following:

■ Chronic cough or dyspnea on exertion (pneumonia)
■ Weight loss with or without diarrhea (idiopathic-, oncologic-, or infection-related wasting)

- Headache or focal neurologic signs (cryptococcal meningitis, lymphoma, toxoplasmosis)
- Dysphagia or whitish mouth lesions (candidiasis)
- Skin lesions (Kaposi's lesions, herpes zoster, or other cancers or infections)
- Sight changes (cytomegalovirus (CMV) retinitis)
- Chronic diarrhea (HIV, cryptosporidium, CMV, *Mycobacterium avium* complex (MAC))

Past medical history

HIV can affect all organ systems. However, you may want to emphasize questions that focus on the following topics:

- Obstetrics—infected child, family completed?
- Gynecology—condyloma, Pap smears, sexually transmitted diseases?
- Urology—sexually transmitted diseases?
- Dermatology—atopic dermatoses, shingles?
- Gastroenterology—diarrhea?
- Respiratory—asthma, chronic obstructive pulmonary disease, cigarettes?
- Allergy—drugs, seasonal?
- Neuropsychiatric—mood and anxiety disorders, memory problems, gait disturbances?
- Other infections—chickenpox, hepatitis, tuberculosis?
- Previous vaccinations

Family history

The family history presented in Chapter 3 is appropriate (see FAMILY HISTORY, p 17).

Social history

NOTE

Although rare, some persons with HIV were infected during their first sexual encounter.

The social history commonly includes either sexual intercourse with multiple individuals who were not well known or the use of needles to inject illicit drugs. Blood transfusions were a significant source of transmission for the 6 to 8 years before April, 1984, after which the blood supply began to be monitored for HIV. Some health care professionals have been infected by needle sticks and by HIV-positive serum coming into contact with their mucous membranes (e.g., eyes, abraded skin).

In general, the social history in Chapter 3 is appropriate (see LIFESTYLE ISSUES, p 17). Lifestyle and psychosocial topics should also include past and present sexual and drug history, chemical abuse (nicotine, alcohol, recreational drugs), diet, exercise, and support systems.

Review of Systems (Table 15–3)

All systems need to be carefully reviewed early in the disease process.

Physical Examination (Table 15–4)

Laboratory Tests

Initial laboratory screening should include the following:

- **Complete blood count** with platelets and differential to evaluate for anemia, leukopenia (immune status), and thrombocytopenia
- **Cholesterol** and **albumin** to evaluate nutritional status
- **Renal** and **liver** profiles plus **hepatitis serology** (i.e., HBsAg, HBsAb, anti-HCV, anti-HAV)
- **Toxoplasmosis immunoglobin G (IgG) titer** to determine if prophylaxis is necessary and to help with future differential diagnoses
- **Glucose-6-phosphate dehydrogenase (G6PD)** [controversial; some clinicians rarely do, some do only in African Americans and those of Mediterranean descent, and others do in all patients]

TABLE 15–3. **Review of Systems in the Diagnosis of HIV Related Infections**

System	Common Patient Complaints
Dermatologic	Pruritus (eczema, seborrhea, psoriasis), bumps (folliculitis)
HEENT	Mouth sores (aphthous ulcers, herpes simplex virus), sore gums (gingivitis), sinus pain, white lesions (hairy leukoplakia, thrush)
Cardiovascular	Chest pain, dyspnea (HIV cardiomyopathy)
Respiratory	Dyspnea, cough (pneumonia)
Gastrointestinal	Dysphagia (esophageal candidiasis), abdominal pain (CMV, MAC), rectal pain (STD, cancer)
Urogenital	Discharge (urethritis, vaginitis), pruritus (pubic lice, candidiasis), masses (cancer), irregular menses
Musculoskeletal	Myalgias, arthralgias (HIV myopathy or arthropathy)
Neurologic	Ataxia (meningitis, toxoplasmosis, lymphoma), headache (meningitis), memory loss (dementia), paresthesias (HIV, medication), visual changes (CMV retinitis)
Psychologic	Concentration or mood changes (depression, dementia), sleep changes (depression)

CMV = cytomegalovirus; HIV = human immunodeficiency virus; MAC = mycobacterium avium complex; STD = sexually transmitted disease.

TABLE 15–4. **Physical Examination Common to Untreated, Advanced HIV Infection**

System	Findings
Vital signs	Fever, weight loss, increased respiratory rate
Hematologic	Lymphadenopathy*, inguinal versus noninguinal adenopathy
Dermatologic	Seborrhea, purpura, petechiae, Kaposi's, herpes, psoriasis, molluscum, oncomycosis, folliculitis
HEENT	*Eyes:* retinopathy, visual field defects
	Oral: thrush, hairy leukoplakia, ulcers, gingivitis
	Nose: sinus pressure, pain
Gastrointestinal	Organomegaly; masses; rectal fissures, lesions, discharge, condyloma
Genitourinary	Rashes, vaginitis, cervicitis, masses, urethritis, ulcers, condyloma
Neurologic	Ataxia, dysgraphia, focal neurological signs, mental status changes, paresthesias, psychomotor retardation, weakness
Psychologic	Depression, anxiety

*Although localized lymphadenopathy should be evaluated further because it may be a sign of infection or malignancy, persistent generalized lymphadenopathy does not correlate with prognosis or disease progression.

- **Varicella-zoster virus IgG** if chickenpox history is unclear, for future consideration of vaccine or postexposure prophylaxis
- **Cytomegalovirus IgG** (rarely negative but, when it is, suggests use of cytomegalovirus-negative blood products if a transfusion is ever needed)
- **β-Human chorionic gonadotropin**
- **Tuberculosis-purified protein derivative (PPD)**
- **Venereal Disease Research Laboratory (VDRL)**
- **HIV RNA** (viral load)
- **HIV antibody** if unsure of confirmation
- **CD4 cell count** to stage HIV, assess the risk of specific HIV-associated complications (see Table 15–1), guide prophylaxis, and evaluate likely response to antiretroviral therapy

When testing for HIV antibody, the two most common tests are the **enzyme-linked immunosorbent assay (ELISA),** also called the enzyme immunoassay (EIA), and the **Western blot test.** Although the ELISA is a very sensitive test (i.e., few false negatives), it has low enough specificity (i.e., many false positives) that no one should ever be told that they have HIV based on the ELISA alone. That is why most laboratories automatically repeat a positive ELISA. If both ELISAs are positive, a confirmatory Western blot test is performed. The Western blot test is very specific. A "positive" Western blot test after two "positive" ELISAs equals a "positive" HIV test.

> **NOTE**
>
> The CDC recommends testing initially at 6 weeks, then 3 and 6 months after initial exposure. At 6 months, the test is more than 95% sensitive; however, it is only about 50% sensitive at 6 weeks.

Many factors in addition to HIV affect both CD4 and HIV RNA, including diurnal variations, seasonal variations, steroids, laboratory methods, acute illnesses, and recent vaccinations. Most medical research has used the absolute CD4 cell count to evaluate immunologic status; however, it is also possible to use CD4 cell percentages. CD4 cell counts of 200 and 500 cells/mm³ generally correspond to CD4 percentages of 14% and 29%, respectively.

> **NOTE**
>
> When the total white blood cell count is uncommonly high, CD4 percentages may be more accurate for assessing immunologic status than CD4 count.

Imaging Studies

Many clinicians still get a baseline chest x-ray, even if the patient is asymptomatic, but most do not.

THERAPY–ANTIRETROVIRAL

Nonpharmacologic Therapy

Many of the prevention measures outlined in Chapter 3 may be helpful for quality, and perhaps quantity, of life for patients with HIV.

Pharmacotherapy

> **NOTE**
>
> Adherence to HIV-related medication regimens is often difficult but extremely important to help avoid resistant strains of HIV.

Once started, the goals of antiretroviral therapy include:

- A sustained minimal viral load and maximum CD4 cell count
- Restoration or maintainence of healthy immunologic function

- Maximal quality of life
- Minimal morbidity and mortality

Classification of antiretrovirals

Most experts suggest using two or three antiretrovirals when initiating therapy. Four or five in someone who has failed a previous regimen is not uncommon. Many antiretroviral medications, identified by class, are listed in Table 15–5. Recommended antiretroviral combinations are listed in Table 15–6.

> **NOTE**
>
> Most antiretroviral regimens are complex. Even for the most committed patients, several education and follow-up sessions on how to administer these drugs appropriately will be necessary.

Protease inhibitor regimens have been well documented to maintain clinical effectiveness and positive virologic and immunologic marker responses. In addition, resistance requires multiple mutations concurrently, and the virus is targeted at two different replication steps.

Nonnucleoside reverse transcriptase inhibitor (NNRTI) regimens usually have significantly fewer major side effects and are much easier to adhere to than those that contain protease inhibitors.

Triple nucleoside reverse transcriptase inhibitor (NRTI) regimens are usually much easier to adhere to than those that contain protease inhibitors and have fewer major side effects than even the NNRTIs. Also, resistance to one NRTI does not confer cross-resistance to all NRTIs.

> **NOTE**
>
> Many antiretrovirals have potentially dangerous or problematic drug-drug interactions or side effects, so rapid access to knowledge about them is important.

Initiation of therapy

One set of decision-making criteria for initiation of therapy can be found in Table 15–7.

Arguments supporting early therapy (i.e., therapy prior to a significant drop in CD4 count or increase in viral load) include:

- Early treatment prevents the loss of immune function and allows for more effective immune reconstitution.
- Patients with low viral loads tend to respond better to antiretrovirals, as judged by immunologic markers and side effects.

TABLE 15–5. Antiretroviral Therapies by Category*

Major Category	Medication
Nucleoside reverse transcriptase inhibitors	Abacavir (ABC), didanosine (ddI), emtricitabine (FTC), lamivudine (3TC), stavudine (d4T), zalcitabine (ddC), zidovudine (ZDV, AZT), zidovudine/lamivudine (3TC)
Nonnucleoside reverse Transcriptase inhibitors	Delavirdine (DLV), efavirenz (EFV), nevirapine (NVP)
Protease inhibitors	Amprenavir (APV), indinavir (IDV), nelfinavir (NFV), ritonavir (RTV), saquinavir (SQV)
Other	Hydroxyurea

*These agents were available in 2000.

Arguments against early therapy

- Some people (possibly 5% to 10%) infected with HIV never show signs of progression.
- Side effects are common with antiretrovirals and can cause a fair amount of morbidity.
- Some denial can be beneficial with a new, asymptomatic illness. Antiretroviral schedules can result in multiple painful reminders of the HIV diagnosis.
- Because resistance is a major concern, pharmaceutical options may deplete before they are most needed.

TABLE 15–6. Recommended Antiretroviral Combinations in 2000

	Column A	Column B
Strongly recommended	Efavirenz	Stavudine + lamivudine
	Indinavir	Stavudine + didanosine
	Nelfinavir	Zidovudine + lamivudine
	Ritonavir + saquinavir	Zidovudine + didanosine
Recommended as alternates	Abacavir	Didanosine + lamivudine
	Amprenavir	Zidovudine + zalcitabine
	Delavirdine	
	Nelfinavir + saquinavir	
	Nevirapine	
	Ritonavir	
	Saquinavir	

From each column, choose one drug not connected with a +, or two drugs with a + between them.

TABLE 15–7. **Indications for Antiretroviral Therapy**

Consider antiretrovirals for all HIV-infected persons with one or more of the following*:
- Symptomatic disease
- < 6 months of acute infection
- CD4 counts < 500 cells/mm³
- HIV RNA > 10,000 copies/ml by the DNA assay
- HIV RNA > 20,000 copies/ml by the PCR assay

DNA = deoxyribonucleic acid; HIV = human immunodeficiency virus; PCR = polymerase chain reaction.

*Many experts suggest antiretrovirals for all HIV-seropositive individuals.

NOTE

Strive for full patient appreciation of the importance of adherence to medication regimens. When relevant, clarify the arguments for and against early therapy before beginning antiretroviral therapy.

 ## URGENCIES & EMERGENCIES

In general, emergencies are detectable using the same criteria used in persons without HIV (e.g., angina-like chest pain, severe shortness of breath). For the exceptions, the chief complaint or a thorough history can help you to recognize urgent situations that may differ for persons with HIV (Table 15–8).

If a patient's CD4 count has ever been less than 300, urgent concerns that need careful, close follow up include symptoms of meningitis, pneumonia, brain masses, and gastrointestinal problems that can lead to dehydration and malnutrition.

 ## SPECIAL POPULATIONS

Children

Most family physicians caring for young children with HIV closely collaborate with a pediatric HIV specialist. In many cases, management is turned over to the specialist.

Seniors

The percentage of persons with HIV who are seniors is increasing every year. In 1997, close to 4000 persons living with AIDS in the United States were over 65 years of age.

HIV appears to advance much more rapidly in seniors. There is evidence

TABLE 15–8. **Signs and Symptoms of Possible Urgent Concerns**

Urgent Concerns	Signs and Symptoms
Cryptococcal meningitis or toxoplasmosis	Persistent headache, balance problems, sight problems, or any sudden inability to use a part of the body
PCP	Shortness of breath with exertion or a chronic cough
CMV retinitis	Floaters or vision changes
Parasitic infection, mycobacterium, or HIV enteropathy	New and persistent diarrhea
Peripheral neuropathy	Numbness, tingling, and/or pain in the feet or hands
Various side effects	Correlation between initiation of medication or supplement (herb, vitamin) and symptom onset

CMV = cytomegalovirus; HIV = human immunodeficiency virus; PCP = *Pneumocystis carinii* pneumonia.

that the time from infection to full-blown AIDS may be half of that for younger counterparts; in fact, many untreated seniors may present with a severe opportunistic infection within 5 years of initial infection. Do not allow the common misconception that seniors are not sexually active, and rarely promiscuous, deter you from asking about sexual activity when it is appropriate to the medical or prevention history.

Pregnancy

All women should be encouraged to get a test for HIV during pregnancy. Children born to HIV-seropositive women have approximately a 12% chance of being positive if their mother was taking antiretroviral medication during pregnancy. The side effects on the child, both short and long term, appear minimal.

NOTE

Administration of antiretrovirals to an HIV-infected pregnant woman greatly decreases (i.e., by threefold) the chance that her child will be born HIV positive.

❖ COMPLEMENTARY/ALTERNATIVE MEDICINE

One small, noncontrolled study has suggested that **garlic** concentrate may help with the treatment of **cryptosporidiosis,** a problematic, diarrhea-producing opportunistic infection. Note that toxicity can occur from very large amounts of raw garlic (not quantified, but likely to be at least several full bulbs daily), possibly because of its high sulfur content.

Acupuncture has been used in many HIV-related health programs, particularly for pain and fever, both of which have well-documented response to acupuncture in general populations. Because acupuncture needles should always be sterilized between patients, there is no risk of transmission from the needles when handled by skilled and knowledgeable practitioners.

◆◆ CONSULTS

- As with all patients, urge consideration of a **living will** and a **durable power of attorney** for health care. Most family physicians handle this without consult, but in some cases a legal referral is desirable.
- An **AIDS clinical trials unit** or **AIDS specialist** will need to be considered by many practitioners, depending on their level of comfort with HIV-related care.
- Patients who need initial HIV testing should be informed about **anonymous test sites.**
- A **case manager** or **social worker** familiar with HIV resources in your locale can be invaluable.
- **Dental care** will be most effective if done at regular intervals with a practitioner familiar with the patient's HIV status.
- **Home health care** or **hospice care** needs to be considered in appropriate patients.
- Careful ophthalmologic follow up can prevent major morbidity, so a referral to an **ophthalmologist** or **optometrist** for regular dilated slit-lamp examinations is important, particularly for persons with CD4 cell counts less than 300 or with a history of cytomegalovirus retinitis.
- Both **psychologic counseling** and **support groups** can be very helpful for many patients.

CHAPTER 16

Hypertension

Rick E. Ricer

OBJECTIVES

- Describe the differences between essential hypertension, hypertension associated with syndrome X, and secondary hypertension
- Explain the relationship between hypertension and atherosclerotic disease
- Differentiate between the effects of acutely elevated blood pressure and the long-term risks, complications, and treatment of hypertension
- Devise a plan to control hypertension over the lifetime of the patient, including lifestyle modifications and medications specific for each patient

 INTRODUCTION

Hypertension is a term that refers to high blood pressure. Although hypertension is often thought of as a "disease," it is not; it is a risk factor for atherosclerosis. Hypertension is often quantitatively defined as a systolic blood pressure greater than or equal to 140 mm Hg and/or a diastolic blood pressure greater than or equal to 90 mm Hg on three separate occasions.

Although a quantifiable definition of hypertension is often helpful, there is no clear cutoff value for "normal" blood pressure. The Framingham Heart Study showed that although some persons with a blood pressure of 120/80 mm Hg will experience strokes, kidney failure, and heart attacks, a substantially larger percentage of persons with a blood pressure higher than 140/90 mm Hg will have these complications. Plotting deaths caused by the complications of high blood pressure against blood pressure readings produced a logarithmic curve. The quantitative definition of hypertension was defined by where the curve began to precipitously steepen.

NOTE

Recently, a new descriptive term (i.e., "high normal blood pressure") has suggested for adults with a systolic blood pressure of 130 to 139 mm Hg or a diastolic blood pressure of 85 to 89 mm Hg.

Hypertension can be classified as essential (idiopathic) or secondary (has a known cause). Currently, an important new concept in essential hypertension is emerging. Approximately half of the cases that were once considered essential hypertension are not. They are part of syndrome X. Persons with syndrome X produce extra insulin to compensate for their peripheral insulin resistance, often in association with specific dyslipidemias (e.g., low high-density lipoprotein, slightly elevated triglycerides). It is theorized that the hyperinsulinemia is responsible for the hypertension and lipid abnormalities. Obesity further increases insulin resistance in persons with syndrome X. See Chapter 12 for more information on syndrome X.

In practice, patients who present early in the course of syndrome X often have only one or two of its manifestations; a patient can present with hypertension without overt diabetes, and vice versa. It is important to be aware of syndrome X when diagnosing hypertension, and differentiating between essential hypertension and hypertension associated with syndrome X can be extremely important in treatment.

TERMINOLOGY

Angioedema: an allergic reaction causing swelling of the lips, mouth, or tongue
Atherosclerosis: the progressive narrowing and hardening of the arteries over time due to fibrosis, calcium deposition, or cholesterol plaques
End-organ damage: in hypertension, the major "end organs" are the brain, heart, and kidneys
Hypertension, essential: hypertension that has no identifiable cause
Hypertension, secondary: hypertension that has an identifiable cause, such as medications, pheochromocytoma, renovascular disease (e.g., renal artery stenosis), polycystic kidney disease, coarctation of the aorta, Cushing's disease, primary aldosteronism, or syndrome X
Isolated systolic hypertension (ISH): quantitatively defined as a systolic blood pressure greater than 140 mm Hg and a diastolic blood pressure less than 90 mm Hg

 ## BACKGROUND

At least 50 million adults in the United States have the diagnosis of hypertension. Hypertension is the number one reason for adult outpatient office visits. The incidence increases with age. African Americans are at much higher risk than Caucasians.

 ## PREVENTION

Primary Prevention

Children whose parents have syndrome X are at risk for developing the syndrome. Primary prevention for these children includes a lifetime of proper diet and exercise to ensure that they remain near ideal body weight.

Secondary Prevention

Secondary prevention involves keeping the blood pressure in the normal range to help avoid end-organ damage.

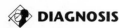 **DIAGNOSIS**

Presentation

Hypertension, the "silent killer," is almost always asymptomatic. Patients feel well and have no complaints, but their blood pressure is noted to be high on routine checks.

History

History of present illness

Questions to consider asking include:

- When was the last time you had your blood pressure checked?
- What does your blood pressure usually run?
- Do you feel you can tell when your blood pressure is up?
  - □ Use this as an opportunity to explain why hypertension is called the "silent killer."
- Have you ever been told your blood pressure was high?
- Have you gained or lost a lot of weight, become more or less active, or changed your diet since you were told your blood pressure was high?
- Are you taking any blood pressure medications? If yes, are there any side effects, and how often do you remember to take it?
- Do you take any anti-inflammatory or pain medications (e.g., ibuprofen)
  - □ Many nonsteroidal anti-inflammatory drugs (NSAIDs) can increase blood pressure in some individuals as well as interfere with angiotensin-converting enzyme (ACE) inhibitors.
- Are you taking any estrogen medications (e.g., oral contraceptives, hormone replacement therapy)?
- Do you have migraines? If yes, what medications do you use?
  - □ Ergot alkaloids and triptans can greatly increase blood pressure in some individuals.
- What other medications do you take (e.g., prescription medications, over-the-counter (OTC) medications, supplements)?
  - □ Respiratory decongestants and many OTC diet supplements or medications can markedly increase blood pressure in some people.

Also consider including questions pertaining to coronary artery disease (see Chapter 11, HISTORY OF PRESENT ILLNESS; p 112).

Past medical history

Question the patient about those pathologies often associated with hypertension, including:

- End-organ damage
  - ☐ Cerebral vascular disease
  - ☐ Coronary artery disease
  - ☐ Heart failure
  - ☐ Peripheral vascular disease
  - ☐ Retinopathy
- Components of syndrome X
  - ☐ Diabetes
  - ☐ Dyslipidemia
  - ☐ Gout

Family history

Ask about family members with blood pressure problems or with any potentially associated pathologies (see PAST MEDICAL HISTORY; p 194).

Social history

Questions to consider asking include:

- Do you engage in regular exercise? If so, what kind?
- What does your diet consist of on a usual day?
- Do you usually salt foods at the table?
- How many times each week do you eat fast food?
- How much alcohol do you drink? Have you or anyone close to you ever felt that you overuse alcohol or other drugs?
- Do you currently smoke? Did you ever smoke in the past?
- What are the major sources of stress in your life? How do you deal with stress?
- What is your occupation? Do you work outside of the home? What is a normal workday like for you?
- How do you pay for your medical care, including medications?

Review of Systems

All systems should be carefully reviewed to establish a baseline, but an initial focused review to assess for atherosclerotic disease is particularly prudent (Table 16–1).

Physical Examination

An overview of the physical examination can be found in Table 16–2.

TABLE 16–1. Systems to Review After Hypertension is Diagnosed

System	Common Patient Complaints
Constitutional	Recent weight gain or loss (diabetes, thyroid disease), polyuria or polydipsia (diabetes)
HEENT	Transient vision loss (TIA)
Cardiovascular	Chest, jaw, or left arm pain; palpitations; orthopnea; PND; dyspnea on exertion; dizziness; claudication (peripheral vascular disease, CAD, CHF)
Respiratory	Shortness of breath, cough (CHF, asthma), perioral or fingertip tingling (hyperventilation)
Gastrointestinal	Abdominal pain or heartburn (atypical angina)
Neurologic	Temporary focal neurologic deficits (TIA)
Psychologic	Anxiety or panic-type symptoms (atypical chest pain), erectile dysfunction (vascular disease, medication side effect)

CAD = coronary artery disease; CHF = congestive heart failure; PND = paroxysmal nocturnal dyspnea; TIA = transient ischemic attack.

Vital signs

Blood pressure should be measured using an appropriate sized cuff. If the blood pressure is high, repeat the measurement in at least one arm after the patient has been sitting for 15 to 30 minutes.

To rule out coarctation of the aorta, measure the blood pressure one

TABLE 16–2. Focus of the Physical Examination for Hypertension

System	Common Findings
Vital signs	Blood pressure > 140/90 mm Hg, changes in height or weight
HEENT	Pale conjunctiva (anemia), changes in the retina
Dermatologic	Abdominal purple striae
Cardiovascular	▪ Neck: carotid bruits (atherosclerosis), jugular venous distention (heart failure), thyroid enlargement or nodules (hyperthyroidism) ▪ Heart: S_3 gallop (heart failure), murmurs (valvular disease) ▪ Torso: abdominal bruits over the aorta or the renal vessels ▪ Legs: bruits in the inguinal area of the femoral arteries, edema, diminished peripheral pulses (PVD)
Respiratory	Rales (heart failure)
Gastrointestinal	Masses in the abdomen (polycystic kidneys)
Musculoskeletal	Buffalo hump in the posterior neck (Cushing's disease)

S_3 = third heart sound; PVD = peripheral vascular disease.

time in both arms. The normal variation between arms is up to 10 mm Hg. A difference of more than 10 mm Hg may signify coarctation of the aorta between the brachiocephalic artery on the right and the left subclavian artery. If the coarctation occurs after the left subclavian artery, then there will be a difference in the strength and timing of the peripheral pulses. Therefore, check an upper extremity pulse and a lower extremity pulse at the same time.

NOTE

A blood pressure cuff that is too small will give a falsely high reading, and a cuff that is too large will give a falsely low reading.

Height is needed for estimating appropriate weight and body mass index (BMI).

Weight should be periodically updated on the chart.

HEENT

Eyes

The **palpebral conjunctivae** are examined for signs of anemia (i.e., pale), which causes hypertension only rarely but can complicate its effects. If there is a question after checking the conjunctivae, examine the palms and nail beds for signs of anemia (i.e., pallor).

The **fundoscopic examination** is performed to look for both early and late hypertensive retinal changes (Table 16–3). An ophthalmoscope allows you to look directly at the blood column. The blood vessel walls are invisible.

NOTE

Advanced hypertensive changes in the eye grounds are consistent with many years of uncontrolled hypertension.

Cardiovascular system

Any process that increases blood volume in the left ventricle can increase systolic pressure.

Gastrointestinal system

Abdominal masses directly relevant to hypertension include a **midline pulsatile mass** (abdominal aneurysm) and **lateral masses** (polycystic kidneys).

Abdominal **purple striae** may suggest Cushing's disease, and a **central obesity** pattern may suggest Cushing's disease or an increased risk of atherosclerotic disease.

TABLE 16-3. Ophthalmologic Changes Seen in Hypertensive Atherosclerotic Eye Disease

Changes	Comments
Early changes	
Arteriolar narrowing	The arteries appear narrower than the veins because the arterial walls are thicker. As arteriosclerotic disease develops, the arterial walls become even thicker so that the blood column becomes narrower.
Arteriovenous nicking	When an artery traverses a vein, it compresses that vein. Because the walls of blood vessels cannot be seen, you will see the blood column of the vein come up to the arterial wall and seem to reappear on the opposite side of the artery.
Increased light reflex	When the ophthalmoscope's light rays strike the curved side of the patient's arteries, they are reflected away from your eye. When the light rays hit directly on top of the patient's arteries, they are reflected back to your eye, causing the light reflex. An increased light reflex is the result of arterial wall thickening, which increases the area that will reflect light, thus broadening the reflected ray.
Late changes	
Hemorrhages and exudates	These appear because of leaky vessels.
"Copper wires"	These appear when cholesterol is laid down in the wall of the blood vessel, causing the blood vessel (or at least the yellowish cholesterol) to become visible.
"Silver wires"	These appear as the process continues because of the whitish calcium deposits.

Neurologic system

A neurologic examination should be done if the history or physical examination suggests the need to rule out any evidence of prior cerebral vascular accident.

Laboratory Tests

Laboratory tests do not help with the initial diagnosis of hypertension; however, they should be done once the diagnosis has been made. Tests include:

- **Urinalysis** to check for proteinuria
- **Complete blood count** to check for anemia and polycythemia
- **Creatinine** as a baseline or a screen for severe renal disease
- **Glucose** to check for diabetes mellitus or, rarely, Cushing's disease
- **Electrolytes** to check for high sodium and low potassium associated with Cushing's disease and primary aldosteronism

- Triglycerides, low-density lipoprotein, and high-density lipoprotein to check for syndrome X or high risk of atherosclerotic disease

Additional Studies

Electrocardiogram is generally not useful for isolated hypertension (i.e., no cardiac complications) unless used as a baseline.

DIFFERENTIAL DIAGNOSIS

Because hypertension is considered a risk factor not a disease, it has no true differential diagnosis of its own. However, when it is associated with secondary causes, consider their differentials.

THERAPY

The atherogenic changes hypertension induces throughout the body usually take place over 20 to 40 years. Therefore, the practitioner usually has time to make the diagnosis, feel confident that the patient is on the best individualized treatment plan, and help the patient be an active participant in adequate follow up before any long-term complications develop.

> **NOTE**
>
> Early hypertension causes no mortality and leads to no, or little, morbidity other than some medication side effects or some emotional concerns with having a chronic diagnosis.

Nonpharmacologic Therapy

> **NOTE**
>
> Weight loss is key in the treatment of obese hypertensive patients.

Diet

- Decrease the intake of sodium, a cation.
  - □ Some individuals have a more marked blood pressure response to sodium than others, so a 2-week, monitored, "very low sodium" trial may help put sodium restriction into perspective.
- Increase other cations, such as calcium and potassium.

Exercise

- Encourage patients to engage in regular aerobic exercise.

Chemical dependencies

- Advise the patient who uses alcohol to do so only in moderation.
- Advise the patient to discontinue use of tobacco products.

> **NOTE**
>
> Know which patients have syndrome X. Although all obese hypertensive patients are likely to benefit from regular exercise and weight loss, those patients with syndrome X who lose weight and exercise regularly are likely to see their blood sugar, lipids, and blood pressure all revert toward normal without medication.

Pharmacotherapy

Many classes of medications have proved to be beneficial for the treatment of hypertension. Each class has its own benefits and drawbacks. The decision to use a specific class of antihypertensive medications should be based on individual patient characteristics.

Diuretics

There are several classes of diuretics. The **thiazide diuretics**, with more than 15 varieties, are the most frequently used. Of the thiazide diuretics, the most commonly used is hydrochlorothiazide.

Thiazide diuretics continue to be a first-line agent in the treatment of essential hypertension.

> **NOTE**
>
> Thiazide diuretics lose their effectiveness when the creatinine level is above 2 mg/dL.

The **loop diuretics** (e.g., furosemide) are much stronger than the thiazide diuretics, but must usually be taken multiple times each day. They are rarely used as first-line agents in the treatment of hypertension.

> **NOTE**
>
> Loop diuretics are useful in patients with congestive heart failure.

The **potassium-sparing diuretics** are very weak antihypertensive medications that can be combined with hydrochlorothiazide to help decrease the potassium loss associated with that medication. The potassium-sparing diuretics are rarely used as solo agents.

Diuretics are often effective in the treatment of true essential hypertension. However, they can actually worsen syndrome X because of their many negative side effects, including increased cholesterol, increased glucose intolerance, decreased potassium, increased uric acid, fatigue, and impotence.

Calcium channel blockers

The metabolic side effects of calcium channel blockers are much less common than those seen with diuretics. However, there are a few potentially significant side effects to keep in mind (Table 16–4).

Calcium channel blockers have been widely used in the treatment of hypertension. Recent data suggest that the use of short-acting calcium channel blockers may actually increase mortality in some populations.

β-Blockers

At least 15 β-blockers (e.g., atenolol) are on the market. They decrease blood pressure, but have multiple possible side effects (Table 16–5). The cardioselective β-blockers (i.e., β_2-blockers) are most often used in the treatment of hypertension. However, required doses are often so high that there is a tendency to overcome the cardioselectivity.

Angiotensin converting enzyme (ACE) inhibitors and angiotensin receptor blockers (ARBs)

ACE inhibitors have become a popular class of medications for treating hypertension. They have few metabolic side effects and multiple brands are on the market. The ACE inhibitors protect the kidneys from the damage of type 2 diabetes mellitus and are beneficial in the treatment of heart failure. The most common side effect is a cough that is unresponsive to most cough remedies.

NOTE

The cough associated with ACE inhibitors can begin more than 1 month after beginning the medication. A cough with one ACE inhibitor suggests a cough with any ACE inhibitor.

TABLE 16–4. Significant Side Effects of Calcium Channel Blockers

- Worsened conduction defects
- Worsened heart failure
- Headaches
- Constipation
- Peripheral edema unresponsive to diuretics

TABLE 16–5. **Common Side Effects of β-Blockers**

- Bronchospasm (worsens chronic obstructive pulmonary disease and asthma)
- Bradycardia
- Heart failure
- Aggravation of peripheral vascular disease
- Fatigue
- Depression
- Impotence
- Masking of the symptoms of hypoglycemia*
- Decreased exercise tolerance†

*Because β-blockers mask the symptoms of hypoglycemia, do not use them, or use them cautiously, in patients taking insulin or sulfonylureas.

†β-Blockers are not usually the best choice for younger individuals or for individuals who have been prescribed an exercise regimen.

The ARBs are the newest class of antihypertensive medications. They appear to be very similar to the ACE inhibitors, but without producing the cough. Although uncommon, both the ACE inhibitors and the ARBs can produce hyperkalemia and angioedema.

NOTE

Many consider ACE inhibitors and ARBs to be the treatment of choice for hypertension associated with syndrome X. However, both are contraindicated in patients with renal artery stenosis.

α-Blockers

The **peripheral α-blockers** have the often helpful side effect of reducing benign prostatic hypertrophy; therefore, they may be indicated in older men with symptoms of that condition. These drugs can also lead to postural hypotension and fatigue. Currently, terazosin and doxazosin are the peripheral α-blockers used.

The **central α-agonists** are an older class of antihypertensive medications that have multiple negative side effects, including sedation, dry mouth, fatigue, and impotence. Methyldopa is considered a safe drug to use in the treatment of hypertension during pregnancy. Clonidine is the only antihypertensive medication available as a skin patch, which can be changed once a week. The major drawback of clonidine is severe rebound hypertension if the drug is abruptly discontinued. Patients on this medication should be carefully educated about the risks of rebound hypertension.

Labetalol is a combined α- and β-blocker. This drug can be useful in the treatment of hypertension that is difficult to control. However, labetalol has the side effects associated with both the α- and β-blockers.

Vasodilators

The vasodilators are very powerful antihypertensive medications with numerous, bothersome side effects. They are often used intravenously to treat hypertensive emergencies.

Adherence

Adherence to medication regimens can be a major problem in the treatment of hypertension. The patient rarely is symptomatic, but is placed on a medication that requires daily dosing. Good patient education, once-a-day dosing, minimal cost, and medications with few or no side effects are all important to help patients adhere to therapy.

 ## URGENCIES & EMERGENCIES

The term "hypertensive emergency" is used to describe the condition of a patient whose blood pressure is much higher than normal and who also has symptoms of hypertensive encephalopathy, intracranial bleed, unstable angina, heart attack, heart failure, or dissecting aneurysm. This disorder requires admission to the hospital.

If a patient is seen in the office with high blood pressure but no symptoms of the conditions previously mentioned, the patient can usually be given oral doses of antihypertensive agents and evaluated over the next 1 or 2 days as an out-patient.

 ## SPECIAL POPULATIONS

Children

Hypertension diagnosed in children or adolescents should be worked-up for secondary causes. Normal blood pressure values are based on the child being at or below the 95th percentile for age and height.

Seniors

The elderly seem to have a higher incidence of purely systolic hypertension. Treatment of hypertension in the elderly decreases morbidity and mortality. Most drugs used for younger patients are appropriate for the elderly, but may need to be given in smaller doses.

Pregnancy

Hypertension in pregnancy creates problems for both mother and fetus. Chronic hypertension in a pregnant patient can be treated with methyldopa, β-blockers, or diuretics. ACE inhibitors and ARBs are contraindicated during pregnancy because they cause fetal renal abnormalities. Hydralazine is commonly the intravenous drug of choice in hypertensive emergencies during pregnancy.

African Americans

African Americans have a higher incidence of hypertension and are generally more responsive to diuretics and calcium channel blockers than to β-blockers and ACE inhibitors. Therefore, African-American patients taking ACE inhibitors may require a higher dose than that used for Caucasians. However, each patient's therapy must still be individualized.

 ## COMPLEMENTARY/ALTERNATIVE MEDICINE

NOTE

Both licorice (i.e., real black licorice that contains anise) and ginseng, when used regularly, can induce or exacerbate hypertension. Licorice may also decrease potassium levels.

Studies have shown a correlation between lowered blood pressure and **meditation, yoga, massage,** and **biofeedback.** Most of the studies suggest that the effects are short-term. A recent study found a significant decrease in carotid artery wall thickness (relative to controls) in 30 African Americans practicing regular transcendental meditation. Soothing music (as defined by the patient) and owning pets may also have an effect on lowering blood pressure.

 ## CONSULTS

If a patient's blood pressure cannot be controlled on maximum doses of three or four different classes of medications, referral to a cardiologist, nephrologist, or hypertension center may be helpful.

CHAPTER **17**

Knee Injuries

Todd S. Carran

OBJECTIVES

- Describe the anatomy and function of the knee
- Recognize the signs and symptoms of specific types of knee injuries
- Be familiar with the physical examination techniques necessary to efficiently and accurately locate damaged structures in the knee
- Know the general treatment guidelines for the more common knee injuries seen in primary care offices

 INTRODUCTION

Similar to most problems encountered in the physician's office, the diagnosis of musculoskeletal injuries and diseases is based on a thorough history and a directed physical examination. Although this chapter focuses on knee injuries, many of the principles discussed can be applied to other joint injuries.

Many specialized physical examination techniques have evolved in the field of sports medicine that aid in precisely determining the location of damage to ligaments, cartilage, and tendons within a given joint. In the past, the use of these specialized techniques was concentrated in the subspecialty fields (e.g., orthopaedics, rehabilitation medicine). However, these techniques are beginning to be used in every family physician's office.

Because even specialized physical examination techniques depend on a solid grasp of anatomy and function, this chapter includes a brief review of the anatomy and function of the knee joint that will serve as a foundation upon which to develop your physical examination skills.

Knee Anatomy and Function

The gross anatomy of the knee is shown in Figure 17–1. The knee normally has significant motion in only one plane—flexion and extension. Its susceptibility to injury comes from the tremendous amount of stress it endures, particularly during athletic activities. In addition, any relative weakness in the supporting muscles of the knee results in the ligaments, tendons, and cartilage being subjected to increased stressors. This is often the case in "weekend warrior" injuries.

The cruciate ligament

The function of the anterior and posterior cruciate ligaments (see Figure 17–1) is to hold the tibia in proper alignment with the femoral condyles while still allowing for flexion and extension of the knee joint.

The meniscus

The meniscus in the knee is a poorly vascularized, cartilaginous structure, which serves mainly as a **shock absorber and cushion** between the bony articulation of the femoral condyles and the tibial grooves in which they rest. Although it is a single structure, it is often referred to in terms of the medial and lateral portions to specify the particular area of damage.

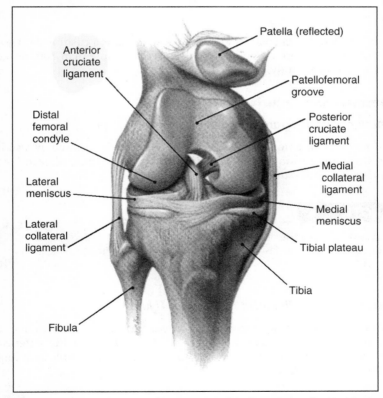

FIGURE 17–1. An anterior view of the anatomy of the knee. (Reproduced with permission from Johnson MW, Maj MC: Acute knee effusions: a systemic approach to diagnosis. *Am Fam Physician* 61:2391–2400, 2000.)

The patella

The patella provides a mechanical connection between the quadriceps femoris muscle and the tibial plateau by means of the patellar tendon, thereby allowing extension of the knee joint.

The muscles of the knee

The muscles of major movement, as in all joints, originate proximally to the joint they control. These muscles include the **quadriceps femoris** and **hamstring** muscles as well as the **adductor** and **abductor** groups, each of which can be broken down into multiple specific muscles.

The major artery and nerve

The **popliteal artery** and **common femoral nerve** should not be overlooked in the assessment for damage, particularly with severe traumatic injuries.

The bursae

A bursa is best described as a fluid-filled sac that acts as a **cushion** at major friction points within the musculoskeletal system. More than 100 bursae are in the human body.

Common Knee Injuries

Anterior cruciate ligament injuries *(see Figure 17–1)*

Injuries of the anterior cruciate ligament are most often caused by a **sudden stop** with the foot planted firmly or a **blow to the tibial plateau** (i.e., the most proximal surface of the tibia).

> **NOTE**
>
> When injury to the anterior cruciate ligament is severe (e.g., a flexed knee hitting a car dashboard), a posterior cruciate ligament tear can result.

Posterior cruciate ligament injuries *(see Figure 17–1)*

The posterior cruciate ligament is torn infrequently, relative to its anterior counterpart. The most common mechanism is a **blow to the anterior proximal tibia.** This injury can result from something as simple as falling on a flexed knee while running.

Meniscal injuries

Patients with a **meniscal tear** often have a painful **"popping," "clicking,"** or **"locking"** with activity (e.g., going up and down stairs).

Patellar injuries

The patella is susceptible to both traumatic fractures and dislocation or subluxation. Excessive tightness in the plica (i.e., the lateral connective tissues) often causes dislocation and subluxation. The patellar tendon, the connection of the patella to the tibial plateau, is susceptible to tendonitis secondary to overuse.

TERMINOLOGY

Bursitis: inflammation of a bursa from any cause
Plica: the lateral connective tissue of the knee joint
Sprain: injury to a tendon or ligament
Strain: injury to a muscle
Subluxation: short-term (i.e., seconds) dislocation of a joint
Tendonitis: inflammation in a tendon from any cause
Tibial plateau: the most superior-anterior portion of the tibia where the patellar tendon attaches

BACKGROUND

In general, musculoskeletal problems are responsible for approximately 25% of all primary care visits. Approximately 40 million Americans make 325 million visits to their primary care providers each year for musculoskeletal complaints.

PREVENTION

Primary Prevention

Body posture and form

Using the proper body posture and form for a particular sport is often very important for prevention. For instance, bending the knees more than 90° while doing "squats" can lead to patellar tendonitis. A coach or trainer can be a valuable resource for evaluating proper form and posture during a particular motion.

Strengthening and stretching

Strengthening muscles near joints is important because when a workload exceeds the limits of a muscle's strength, undue stress transfers to associated tendons, ligaments and cartilage.

Stretching is thought to have a long-term protective effect against tendon injuries. In addition, stretching appears to have a short-term protective effect against muscle injuries as a result of the heat generated within the muscle during stretching.

Proper equipment

Proper equipment is also an important part of primary prevention. For example, shin pads should be worn when playing soccer.

Secondary Prevention

Secondary prevention includes braces for weak or reconstructed joints, such as knee-stabilizing braces for patients with torn or reconstructed anterior cruciate ligaments. In addition, techniques that help with primary prevention are often helpful for secondary prevention as well.

> **NOTE**
>
> Effective prevention includes strengthening the major muscle groups around the joint over time, stretching the appropriate muscle groups before planned use, and using proper equipment.

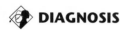 **DIAGNOSIS**

History

History of present illness

Questions to consider asking include:

- What were you doing when this happened?
- Did sudden pain follow a specific traumatic event?
- Were you moving when this happened? If so, how were you moving (e.g., straight forward versus making a sharp turn or twisting)?
- Was there repetitive use before the onset of pain?
- What are the location, timing, character, and aggravating or alleviating factors of the pain?
- Are you experiencing any numbness or tingling near the area of pain?
- Did swelling occur immediately after an acute injury or later?
- What have you been taking or doing for the injury or pain?
- Have you ever had pain or trauma to this area before? If so, did you have surgery, radiographs, or other imaging studies? What helped?

In addition to the previous questions, keep the following "pearls" in mind while you take the history:

- **Delayed pain** after use suggests the development of inflammation from tendonitis or muscle damage.
- **Acute trauma** suggests damage to ligaments, cartilage, and, occasionally, bones.
- **A lateral blow to the knee** suggests a torn medial collateral ligament. If severe, a torn anterior cruciate ligament and medial meniscal tear may also be seen. This is referred to as "the terrible triad."

- **Twisting** suggests meniscal damage.
- **Radicular pain or paresthesia** suggests nerve damage or entrapment.
- **Immediate swelling** suggests hematoma.
- **Delayed swelling** suggests inflammation.

Past medical history

Questions to consider asking include:

- Have you had other significant injuries in the past? If so, what was the nature of the injury? When did it occur and what was done about it?
- Do you have any ongoing medical problems?
- Do you regularly take any medications or supplements?
- Did you ever have an ulcer or other stomach or indigestion problem that caused pain or bleeding?
- Have you had any past problems with anti-inflammatories (e.g., ibuprofen)?

> **NOTE**
>
> Many anti-inflammatory medicines can cause or exacerbate gastro-esophageal problems.

Family history

Consider asking about a family history of any type of bleeding disorder or joint disease.

Social history

Consider asking the following questions:

- Did this injury occur at work?
- Has this injury had a significant effect on your job, exercise routine, schoolwork, or family life? If so, how?
- How active are you? What kinds of activities do you normally engage in throughout the day (e.g., on the job, at home)?
- How well are you sleeping?
- Do you exercise regularly? If so, what do you do?
- Had you been drinking alcohol or using drugs when you were injured?

Review of Systems (Table 17–1)

Physical Examination

Physical Examination

- Inspect for gross deformity, muscular atrophy, asymmetry, and any obvious swelling or erythema. Compare the injured knee with the normal knee.

NOTE

Joint effusion can be distinguished from bursal swelling by its diffuse appearance throughout the joint. Pushing on one side of the joint often creates a bulge of the synovial capsule in another area, indicating a true joint effusion.

- Palpate the underside of the medial and lateral patellar edges to elicit tenderness, a sign of possible subpatellar chondromalacia.
- Palpate the length of the patellar tendon for tenderness or defect, a sign that tendonitis or a tear may be present.
- Palpate the mobility of the patella to determine if it is dislocated.
- Palpate the medial and lateral joint lines. Tenderness is a sign of possible meniscal damage.

NOTE

Palpation that elicits pain in the corresponding areas suggests patellar tendonitis, suprapatellar bursitis, and pes anserine bursitis.

Assessing patellar pain

When comparing knees, if the knee eliciting pain appears swollen, it may be the result of a prepatellar or an intra-articular effusion (Figure 17–2).

Have your patient move the knee through a full range of motion. When the knee is near full extension, push the patella laterally to see if you elicit any notable pain and apprehension, common signs of patellofemoral syndrome.

Place one hand gently on the anterior surface of the knee to feel for crepitus, a sign of possible inflammation.

Testing for ligament tears

Test for **anterior cruciate ligament** tears using the anterior drawer test and Lachman's test (the more sensitive of the two) [Figure 17–3]. Evaluate the

---

TABLE 17–1. **Review of Systems for Large Joint Pain**

System	Symptoms
Constitutional	Fever, chills (infection)
Genitourinary	Urethritis, vaginitis (Reiter's syndrome, gonorrhea)
Musculoskeletal	Arthralgias, myalgias (infection or rheumatologic disease)
Dermatologic	Rash (infection or rheumatologic disease)
Neurologic	Weakness, numbness, tingling (neuropathy)

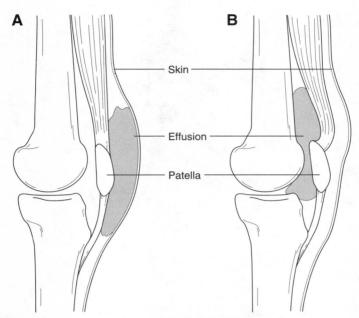

FIGURE 17–2. Patellar effusions. (*A*) Involved region with septic prepatellar bursitis. (*B*) Involved region with septic intra-articular knee effusion.

posterior cruciate ligament with the posterior drawer test, reversing the direction of forces placed on the femur and tibia. Tests for anterior cruciate ligament integrity may be particularly difficult to assess when acute injury results in much pain and swelling. In this case, your patient may be placed in a knee immobilizer to prevent further internal derangement. The patient should return for a repeat examination in 7 to 10 days.

To test for **collateral ligament** tears, place a varus (lateral) or a valgus (medial) stress on the knee (Figure 17–4). Excessive opening of the joint space, usually accompanied by pain, is a sign that one or more of the collateral ligaments are stretched or torn. This test should be performed with the knee in full extension and flexed to approximately 30°.

NOTE

Meniscal injuries often accompany medial collateral ligament tears.

Testing for meniscal damage

Perform McMurray's test by placing a valgus stress on the knee, then moving it from full flexion to full extension (Figure 17–5). Perform the maneuver at least twice, first with the tibia externally rotated and then with the tibia internally rotated to test the medial and lateral meniscus, respec-

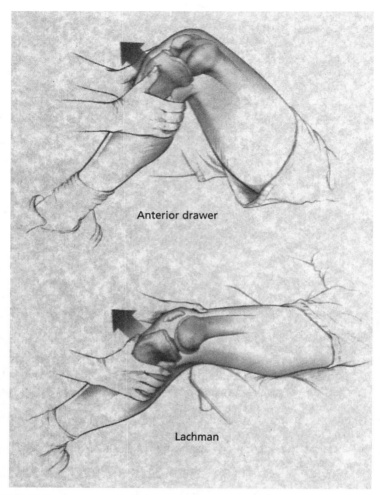

FIGURE 17–3. Assessment of anterior cruciate ligament instability. (*A*) The anterior drawer test is performed with the knee flexed to 90°. Similar to Lachman's test (*B*), in which the knee is flexed to 20°, the tibia is drawn anteriorly. Asymmetric translation is an indicator of anterior cruciate ligament injury. (Reproduced with permission from Johnson MW, May MC: Acute knee effusions: a systemic approach to diagnosis. *Am Fam Physician* 61:2391–2400, 2000.)

tively. Any pain, particularly if associated with a click, catch, or pop, is a sign of a meniscal tear and requires further investigation.

Imaging Studies

Magnetic resonance imaging (MRI) allows visualization of intra-articular soft tissue structures. Therefore, use of MRI results in more accurate diagnosis of damage to cartilage, ligaments, and tendons.

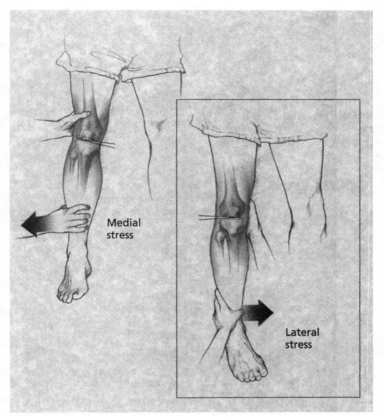

FIGURE 17–4. Assessment of collateral ligament stability. The knee should be stressed in full extension and at 30° of flexion. The amount of opening compared with the opposite knee indicates the severity of injury. (Reproduced with permission from Johnson MW, Maj MC: Acute knee effusions: a systemic approach to diagnosis. *Am Fam Physician* 61:2391–2400, 2000.)

A **computed tomography** scan is not very helpful when evaluating soft tissues, so it is not commonly used for joint evaluation.

Radiographs help identify fractures, dislocations, and changes associated with arthritis and osteopenia.

Additional Studies

Subacromial injections of lidocaine with anti-inflammatory steroids are often used to diagnose subacromial bursitis and supraspinatus tendonitis. These injections also have therapeutic effects by decreasing the inflammatory reaction and decreasing pain.

Electromyograms can distinguish muscle weakness caused by compression neuropathies from the typical muscle atrophy seen in chronic tendonitis.

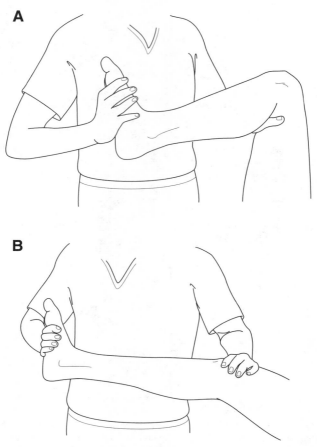

FIGURE 17–5. Assessment for meniscal tears using McMurray's test. (*A*) Flex the knee and rotate the tibia on the femur (i.e., external rotation for medial meniscus and vice versa). (*B*) Extend the knee and repeat. A clicking sound and complaint from the patient detects the flap from a meniscal tear.

Arthroscopy may be the only way of determining the exact extent of damage in some cases. For example, an MRI done to look for meniscal damage in a knee will likely provide only nonspecific information about the size and severity of the meniscal tear.

Arthrograms may help to distinguish partial from complete ligament and cartilage tears, particularly when MRI results are ambiguous.

NOTE

A careful history and physical examination remain the basis for diagnosing most joint problems.

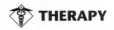 **THERAPY**

Nonpharmacologic Therapy

Caring for sprains (Table 17–2)

Physical therapy

Treatment for many knee injuries includes physical therapy. Modalities such as iontophoresis, ultrasound, and ice can often help to initially control the swelling and pain of inflammation. Exercises to restrengthen damaged or atrophied muscles are frequently important to the recovery phase. Exercises to strengthen the quadraceps femoris muscle are found in Figure 17–6.

Pharmacotherapy

The mainstay of pharmacotherapy for joint injuries is **nonsteroidal anti-inflammatory drugs (NSAIDs).** Occasionally, narcotics are used as adjuncts in pain relief for short periods (usually less than 2 weeks).

Because of their anti-inflammatory action, **steroids** (injectable and oral preparations) are also used when inflammation is the primary concern. **Acetaminophen,** although useful for pain, lacks the anti-inflammatory action necessary to reduce the swelling often associated with joint injuries.

TABLE 17–2. **How to Care for a Sprain**

Grade	Physical findings	Injury	Management*
1	Tenderness with mild swelling and no ecchymosis or laxity	Pulled ligaments or tendons without tears	Respond to conservative treatment (i.e., rest, ice, compression, elevation, and anti-inflammatories)
2	Moderate to severe swelling with ecchymosis and minor laxity	Partial tears of ligaments or tendons	Require a period of fixed immobilization (2–6 weeks) in a splint† to allow the ligament or tendon to heal at the correct length
3	Severe swelling and ecchymosis with marked laxity	Complete tears of ligaments or tendons	Tendon tears usually require surgical reapproximation; ligament tears usually require surgery but may heal with extended immobilization alone

*Return to activity is guided by assessing residual pain, strength of supporting muscles, and stability of the ligaments and tendons involved.

†Immobilization with a splint prevents laxity, which could lead to a joint that is more susceptible to recurrent sprains.

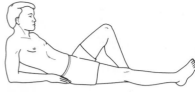

Excercise 1
Quadriceps strengthening: isometrics
Position yourself as shown. Hold your right leg straight for 10 to 20
seconds and then relax. Do the exercise 5 to 10 times.

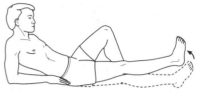

Excercise 2
Quadriceps strengthening: straight leg lift
Position yourself as shown. Raise your right leg several inches and
hold it up for 5 to 10 seconds. Then lower your leg to the floor slowly
over a few seconds. Do the exercise 5 to 10 times.

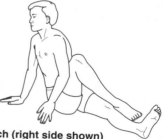

Excercise 3
Iliotibial band and buttock stretch (right side shown)
Position yourself as shown. Twist your trunk to the right and use your
left arm to "push" your right leg. You should feel the stretch in your
right buttock and the outer part of your right thigh. Hold the stretch for
10 to 20 seconds. Do the exercise 5 to 10 times.

FIGURE 17–6. Exercises to strengthen the quadriceps. (Adapted with permission from
the American Family Physicians. Copyright © 1999.)

 URGENCIES & EMERGENCIES

A **hot, swollen knee in a febrile patient** indicates septic arthritis until
proved otherwise, and usually requires immediate tapping of the effusion
for analysis and culture. These patients need intravenous antibiotics to
prevent rapid joint destruction.

Traumatic sports injuries can result in the **compromise of an artery or**

nerve. This will be evident on physical examination and requires emergent surgery to restore flow and decompress or reattach transected nerves.

Compound and open fractures are at particular risk of serious complications and require urgent consultation and treatment.

 ## SPECIAL POPULATIONS

Children

Special care should be taken to rule out growth plate (epiphyseal) injuries; radiographic evaluation is often necessary. "Comparison" films of the contralateral joint are helpful in evaluating the integrity of the growth plate in question.

Seniors

Fractures are more common in older adults as a result of bone mineral loss (i.e., osteopenia or osteoporosis). Older adults are also more likely to have degenerative changes with advancing age.

Pregnancy

Pregnant women are more susceptible to tendon and ligament injuries, perhaps because of "softening" of the tendons and ligaments that results from high levels of progesterone. NSAIDs are contraindicated during pregnancy.

 ## COMPLEMENTARY/ALTERNATIVE MEDICINE

Electrical stimulation techniques have been incorporated into many physical therapy programs; however, some clinicians still consider them to be "alternative."

 ## CONSULTS

Tears, particularly complete tears, of the tendons and cartilage of the knee joint require referral to a specialist.

Fractures that are displaced or involve joints often require referral.

Patients with **nerve and major artery injuries** should always be promptly sent to a specialist. These injuries can be identified by testing for sensation and pulses distal to the area of injury.

Recurrent patellar subluxation may require referral for arthroscopic surgery to "release" the plica, particularly if physical therapy to strengthen the medial rectus muscle proves unsuccessful in alleviating the conditions.

Growth plate injuries are extremely important to follow closely. Always refer if there is any suspicion that the growth plate has been damaged.

CHAPTER **18**

Low Back Pain

Susan Louisa Montauk

 INTRODUCTION

This chapter focuses on low back pain that is acute. Most of the information is from the Clinical Practice Guidelines series of the Agency for Health Care Policy and Research (AHCPR) [see Appendix III]. This chapter also includes information on visceral referred pain as well as some of the myofascial pain syndromes that are frequently seen in primary care, at times presenting with low back pain that is pseudoradiculopathic. Such syndromes often con-

> **OBJECTIVES**
>
> ■ Recognize the risk factors for acute low back pain
> ■ Describe the basics of the initial work-up of adults with acute low back pain, including the recommendations in the clinical guidelines of the Agency for Health Care Policy and Research
> ■ Explain the major findings in the common myofascial pain syndromes that can cause low back pain
> ■ Appropriately recommend therapy and reconditioning efforts for acute low back pain
> ■ Suggest the initiation of suitable referrals and consultations for low back pain, discerning between routine and emergent cases

found the diagnosis of true radiculopathy, leading to prolonged pain and suffering, and unnecessary work-ups.

TERMINOLOGY

Acute low back pain: low back pain that has been present for less than 3 months

Anesthesia: when sensations are not perceived

Antalgic gait: the gait that results from pain that worsens when weight is applied to one or both lower limbs; the stance is usually shorter on the affected side

Cauda equina syndrome: the constellation of signs and symptoms (e.g., bilateral motor weakness, urinary sphincter dysfunction, saddle anesthesia) seen when the nerve roots of the lower spinal cord get compressed, usually resulting from pressure from a large, central disc herniation

Contracture: in physiology (as opposed to clinical medicine), a sustained intrinsic (i.e., no motor unit action potential) activation of the contractile mechanism of muscle fibers; muscle "shortening"

Disc herniation: when the nucleus pulposus, a gelatinous substance in the center of the intervertebral discs, pushes through its fibrous outer layer (annulus fibrosis)

Ergonomics: the science of designing equipment and work or play spaces that maximize the appropriate use of body mechanics, thereby reducing user fatigue and discomfort

Low back: the spinal and peripheral low thoracic (T10 to T12) and lumbosacral regions

Neurogenic claudication: leg pain or weakness noted with standing or walking (usually with a limp) that is induced by the neurologic dysfunction associated with nerve compression

Paresthesia: when sensations are perceived as abnormal and inconsistent with external stimuli (e.g., pricking, burning, numbness, tingling)

Pseudoradiculopathic: pain or other sensations presenting in a dermatomal pattern, but not originating from pathology of a spinal nerve root

Radiculopathic pain: a neural abnormality of sensation caused by spinal nerve root compression

Radiculopathy: see *radiculopathic pain*

Range of motion: extent to which a joint can move in all six planes; **passive** implies that only the hands-on examiner executes the work necessary to test or move the joints; **active** implies that the patient alone (i.e., unassisted) executes the work necessary to test or move the joints

Saddle anesthesia: the anesthesia distribution noted over the skin when sacral nerve roots are compromised

Sciatica: pain characterized by radiation from the low back to the buttock to the posterolateral aspect of the leg that is consistent with, but not synonymous with, lumbosacral nerve root compromise

Shortening: the term used to describe the results of a contracture at a myofascial trigger point

Spinal stenosis: a stricture of the spinal canal

Spondylolisthesis: forward movement of a vertebral body relative to the vertebra below

Trigger point: a neuropathic focus of hyperirritability in tissue (e.g., myofascial, cutaneous, ligamentous, periosteal) that is locally tender when compressed

◆ BACKGROUND

Acute low back pain is usually a benign condition; 60% of patients recover or improve significantly within 1 week and 80% to 90% within 6 weeks. Yet, studies suggest that it is the most common reason for office visits to neurosurgeons and occupational medicine physicians, and one of the more common symptoms initiating office visits to primary care physicians.

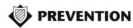 **PREVENTION**

Risk Factors

Risk factors for acute low back pain include:

- A previous history of low back pain
- Current or anticipated daily effort conducive to low back pain (e.g., lifting, turning heavy objects, driving long distances, nonergonomic sitting, repetitive bending)
- Age over 50 years
- Obesity

Occupational Precautions

Many prevention efforts need to take place on the job as well as during activities of daily living. Proper ergonomic lifting, pulling, pushing, bending, and sitting are important for many professions. Patients with a history of back problems may benefit from a lumbar corset or back belt, although the most useful preventive function of a lumbar belt may be to remind its wearer about approaching activities (e.g., lifting) with caution. In addition, good abdominal muscle tone can help to alleviate potentially harmful stress on the lower paraspinal muscles and the iliopsoas muscle by decreasing the force placed on the back during activities such as lifting and sitting up.

Aquatic Therapy

Muscles under water are not isolated; all muscles moved get a workout. Shoulder-depth water reduces body weight by 90%. The reduction in body weight combined with the fact that water resistance is more than tenfold that of air leads to a decrease in gravitational torque forces. Patients at particular risk of myofascial pain syndromes (e.g., patients with rheumatologic disorders) are likely to benefit from ongoing aquatic therapy for prevention of low back pain and other myalgias and arthralgias.

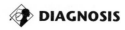 **DIAGNOSIS**

Presentation

Patients' reports of pain symptoms and treatment outcomes are strongly influenced by their unique profile and health belief model. Commonly heard complaints associated with low back pain include:

- "My back hurts."
- "My leg hurts."

- "I bent over and, as I stood up, my back went out."
- "I can hardly make it up the stairs."
- "I fell down the stairs and got a sharp pain in my back."

History

Although less than 1% of all acute low back pain presentations represent secondary processes [e.g., infection, nephrolithiasis, referred gastrointestinal (GI) or gynecologic pain, arthritis, cancer, or upper motor neuron diseases], the recognition of these causes is important. The history questions that relate to these conditions are accompanied by a **RED FLAG** designation. In addition, "radicular pearls" to consider when recording the history can be found in Table 18–1.

History of present illness

Onset

- How, when, and where did your back problem begin?
- Was any trauma involved? (**RED FLAG: Fracture**)

Pain description

- Where do or did you have pain, weakness, numbness, or tingling? (**RED FLAG: Weakness, pain, or paresthesia below the knee suggests nerve root compromise.**)

TABLE 18–1. "Radicular Pearls" to Keep in Mind for an Evaluation of Acute Low Back Pain

- Symptoms of sciatica or neurogenic claudication suggest possible neurologic involvement, as does persistent numbness or weakness in one or both legs.
- The absence of sciatica makes a clinically important lumbar disc herniation unlikely.
- Leg pain usually overshadows back pain when a clinically significant radiculopathy is present.
- Pain radiating below the knee is more likely to indicate a true radiculopathy than pain radiating only to the thigh.
- Herniations of L2–L3 and L3–L4 are difficult to diagnose with physical findings alone.
- Herniations of L2–L3 and L3–L4 make up less than 10% of disc herniation radiculopathies.
- Myofascial pain syndromes can produce low back pain with pseudoradiculopathy. A careful physical examination and observation can usually assess the likelihood of true radicular pain.

- What positions are most or least comfortable?
- How do sitting, standing still, laying down, bending, squatting, and walking affect your back pain?
- Are your symptoms constant or intermittent?
- Does your back pain improve with rest? (**RED FLAG: Cancer pain is usually unremitting.**)
- Have you ever had pain in this area before?
- What else makes the pain better or worse?

Related history

- How old are you? (**RED FLAG: Patients older than 70 years of age have an increased risk of fracture.**)
- Have you had any recent infections, fevers, or other illnesses? [**RED FLAG: Infection (e.g., pyelonephritis, prostatitis, pelvic inflammatory disease)**]
- Do you have other muscle aches or joint pain?
- Have you noticed any urinary changes? (**RED FLAG: Sign and symptoms of urinary infection may suggest pyelonephritis. New urinary retention and overflow incontinence suggest nerve root compromise.**)
- Have you noticed any abnormal vaginal/penile discharge?
- Do you have any problem holding your bowel movements? (**RED FLAG: Loss of anal sphincter tone suggests nerve root compromise.**)
- Have you had any weakness in your legs? (**RED FLAG: Progressive motor weakness suggests nerve root compromise.**)

Self-care

- What medications have you taken, and what activities have you changed to try to help your pain? How effective were these measures?
- What else have you done to try to help your pain?
- Do you sleep in a different position because of the pain?

Past medical history

When you come across a patient with low back pain that is not straightforward, look through the chart for the presence or absence of chronic pain syndromes, neuromuscular complaints, reasons for immunosuppression, mood disorders, old injuries, previous radiographic tests, abuse, or multiple physician visits for relatively minor complaints. Also consider asking the following questions:

- Have you had any previous back-related problems, studies, or therapies?
- Do you have a history of cancer? (**RED FLAG: Cancer**)
- Has your weight changed much in the past year? (**RED FLAG: Unplanned weight loss may indicate cancer.**)
- Have you had any major medical problems during the past 2 years? (**RED FLAG: Cancer, immunosuppression or fibromyalgia may suggest metastasis, uncommon infections, or fibromyalgia exacerbation.**)

- Have you been taking any medications? (**RED FLAG: Steroid use may heighten the risk of fracture.**)
- Do you have a history of pelvic inflammatory disease, urethritis, prostatitis, epididymitis, or urinary infections? (**RED FLAG: These may indicate infection.**)
- Do you have a history of other muscle or joint pains? Do you have a history of fibroids, hernias, or ovarian cysts? (**RED FLAG: Referred Pain**)

Family history

A family history of prostate cancer or rheumatic disease might suggest earlier work-up for these problems, particularly the cancer if a male patient is older than 50 years of age.

Social history

Find out what the patient does on a typical day at work or home, and what he had planned for the next 2 weeks. Then modify your suggested therapy or follow-up plans accordingly.

Review of Systems (Table 18–2)
Physical Examination
Vital signs

Blood pressure may be raised mildly because of the pain.

General appearance

Throughout the examination, observe the patient for apparent comfort level, changes in general appearance, pain-related facial expressions (e.g.,

TABLE 18–2. **Review of Systems for Acute Low Back Pain**

System	Notable Patient Complaints
Constitutional	Fever
Urogenital	Urinary incontinence; dysuria; urinary frequency, urgency, or hesitancy; vaginal, vulvar, penile, or testicular anesthesia, pain, or discharge*
Musculoskeletal	Pain in the lower back, hip, buttocks, thigh, or lower leg
Neurologic	Ataxia, cognitive change, paresthesia, anesthesia, leg weakness
Psychologic	Depression

*Be sure to ask questions to rule out pregnancy in a premenopausal woman (e.g., "When was your last normal menstrual period?").

grimacing, wincing), and flat affect. For a presentation that suggests radicular pain on a limp, perform a careful neurologic examination.

The neuromuscular examination should ideally be performed with the patient in a supine, upright, seated, and prone position. Table 18–3 describes the physical examination guidelines for the latter three.

The following procedure for the straight leg raise in a supine position has been adapted from the Agency for Healthcare Research and Quality:

1. Ask the patient to lie straight on a table in the supine position.
2. With one hand placed above the knee of the leg being examined, exert enough firm pressure to keep the knee fully extended. Ask the patient to relax the leg.
3. With the other hand cupped under the heel, slowly raise the straight limb (Figure 18–1A). Tell the patient, "If this bothers you, let me know and I will stop."
4. Monitor for any movement of the pelvis before complaints are elicited.

NOTE

True sciatic nerve root compression should elicit complaints before the hamstrings are stretched enough to move the pelvis.

5. Estimate the degree of leg elevation that elicits complaint from the patient. Then determine the most distal discomfort area (e.g., back, hip, thigh, knee, below the knee).
6. While holding the leg at the limit of straight leg raising, dorsiflex the ankle (Figure 18–1B). Note whether this aggravates the pain. Internal rotation of the limb can also increase the tension on the sciatic nerve roots.
7. A positive result occurs when the affected leg is at 70° (i.e., just before the pelvis would begin to lift) and radicular pain below the knee worsens with ankle dorsiflexion and is relieved by foot plantar flexion or external rotation.

Crossover pain occurs when lifting the "healthy" leg produces radicular pain below the knee in the opposite leg. However, the specific test for crossover pain can still be negative with neurogenic root compromise.

NOTE

Vertebral tenderness and limited spinal range of motion suggest the possibility of spinal infection, but these are also common findings in patients who have acute low back pain without infection.

If it clarifies your findings, do not hesitate to draw a picture of the location of the pain or neurologic abnormalities as part of your charted physical examination. Figure 18–2 Is a dermatome chart showing patterns

TABLE 18–3. Neuromuscular Examination Guidelines for Acute Low Back Pain When the History Does Not Suggest Red Flags

Patient in an upright position:
1. Note the patient's comfort level.
2. Examine for abrasions, ecchymoses, unbalanced lateral skin folds, swelling, contracted muscles, and atrophy.
3. Palpate for gluteal or hip trigger points.
4. Palpate for pain or masses on the spine.
5. Examine for pelvic tilt, scoliosis, kyphosis, and lordosis.
6. Observe ambulation for pace, toe walking, heel walking, and an antalgic gait.

Patient in a seated position:
1. Note the patient's comfort level.
2. Check the patient's posture.
3. Check if the knee can extend fully.
4. Check patellar and Achilles deep tendon reflexes.
5. Perform light touch and pressure testing on the medial, dorsal, and lateral aspects of the foot and on the anterior, posterior, lateral, and medial aspects of the upper and lower leg.
6. Test ankle and large toe dorsiflexion strength.

Patient in a prone position:
1. Note the patient's comfort level.
2. Note foot position and if either foot is more externally rotated.
3. Palpate for gluteal and hip trigger points.
4. Palpate spinal and paraspinal muscles.
5. Check if the hips can extend a full 20°.
6. Perform straight leg raise (Figure 18–1).

of lumbosacral radicular pain and numbness that can be referred to when illustrating the location of pain.

Laboratory Tests

An erythrocyte sedimentation rate (ESR), complete blood count (CBC), and urinalysis (U/A) should not be routine, but may be helpful in the evaluation for suspected infection, inflammation, malignancy, or other systemic illness. Older or debilitated patients who are likely to be considered for long-term nonsteroidal anti-inflammatory drug (NSAID) therapy may need a blood urea nitrogen/creatinine to identify renal contraindications.

Imaging Studies

Anatomic abnormalities of the lumbar spine increase in frequency with age, are often noted on imaging tests in subjects with no symptoms of low back problems, and can be misleading. Abnormalities on imaging must be

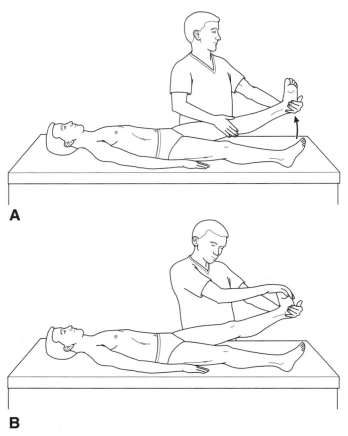

FIGURE 18–1. Positions of the straight leg procedure that stretch the L5 and S1 nerve roots and can, therefore, duplicate or exacerbate radicular disc herniation.

interpreted in conjunction with physical examination findings and physiologic testing.

NOTE

When ordering imaging studies, provide all relevant history and physical examination information, including the spinal levels involved, to help the radiologist focus on your concerns.

Plain x-rays

Plain x-rays are not effective for diagnosing lumbar nerve root impingement from a herniated disc or spinal stenosis. However, the standard an-

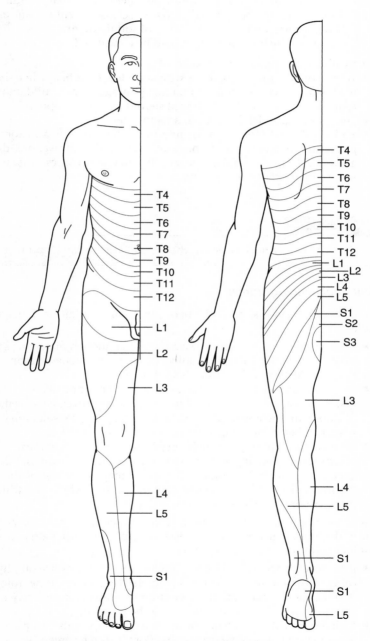

FIGURE 18–2. Approximate dermatome distribution for T4 through S4.

teroposterior and lateral views permit assessment of lumbar alignment, comparison of vertebral body and disc space size, assessment of bone density and architecture, and gross evaluation of soft tissue structures.

Plain x-rays of the lumbar spine should be considered:

- In all patients older than 70 years of age
- To rule out fractures in patients with acute low back pain when there is a history of recent significant trauma (any age), recent mild trauma (patient older than 50), prolonged steroid use, or osteoporosis
- To rule out spondylolisthesis in an adolescent
- To help evaluate for tumor or infection when there is a history of prior cancer, recent infection, fever over 100°F, intravenous drug abuse, prolonged steroid use, low back pain that becomes worse with rest, or unexplained weight loss

NOTE

Plain x-rays can be negative even when a tumor or infection is present.

Additional imaging studies

At the time of diagnosis, it may be necessary to order additional imaging studies.

- If infection or tumors are still suspected even though plain x-rays are negative, a computed tomography (CT) scan or magnetic resonance imaging (MRI) may be clinically indicated.
- If cauda equina syndrome or progressive major motor weakness is suggested, the early use of MRI is often warranted. However, because these diagnoses may require prompt surgical intervention, consultation with a surgeon before ordering tests is generally recommended.
- When clinical findings strongly suggest tumor, infection, fracture, or other space-occupying lesions of the spine, either a CT scan or MRI is generally in order. For some, a bone scan may be the test of choice. A consultation with a specialist may help clarify which test will be more useful for the particular case.

If none of the previously mentioned diagnoses were concerns at the time of diagnosis but 1 month has passed and the low back pain persists, a different approach may be necessary.

- Patients without clear evidence of nerve root compromise on physical examination may benefit from an electromyogram if neurologic dysfunction is equivocal. If the electromyogram confirms nerve root compromise, a CT scan or MRI should be pursued.
- Patients with clear evidence of nerve root compromise on physical examination may benefit from an MRI or CT scan if surgery would be considered for treatment of a herniated disc.

- Patients with low back pain who have had prior back surgery may need an MRI with contrast to help distinguish between disc herniation and old scar tissue.

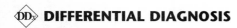

DIFFERENTIAL DIAGNOSIS

Referred Visceral Pain

The central nervous system can misread sensory input from viscera as being peripheral pain along the same dermatome level.

Pain can be perceived to be in the low back from the:

- Colon (T11-L2)
- Urinary bladder (T11-L2)
- Epididymis, ductus deferens, and seminal vesicles (T11-T12)
- Prostate and prostatic urethra (T11-L1)
- Uterus and uterine tubes (T12-L1)

Myofascial Syndromes

Myofascial pain is typified by localized pain (i.e., **trigger points**), **radiating pain** in characteristic peripheral nerve distributions, and **decreased range of motion** associated with the involved muscles. When associated with low back pain, myofascial pain is commonly worse the first hour after waking, sitting, or stooping (i.e., prolonged flexion).

In much of the medical literature, the worsening of back pain after stooping is attributed to a contracture of the muscle. Some of the literature, particularly that concentrating on physical therapy, describes palpating "taut bands" and "local twitch responses" where the trigger points are centered, but this is still controversial. On the other hand, the concept of painful trigger points is well accepted.

Iliopsoas syndrome (Figure 18–3 and Table 18–4) can confound diagnosis because contraction of the iliopsoas muscle limits performance of the straight leg raise and sitting knee extension. If this muscle is allowed to continue to shorten and eventually weaken, there will be an increase in the lordotic curve.

Piriformis syndrome (Figure 18–4 and see Table 18–4) may be diagnosed based on clinical presentation, but the most sensitive diagnostic procedure is a rectal examination to palpate for a contracted piriformis muscle. Pain from the piriformis muscle is often perceived to be deep in the buttock with a trigger point over the sciatic notch, posterior thigh, or posterior hip. It may also be perceived as general sciatica.

Quadratus lumborum syndrome (Figure 18–5 and see Table 18–4) is the most common of the myofascial syndromes mentioned in this chapter. Often seen in gardeners, it commonly begins when stooping with a twisted torso. Pain may be perceived deep in the midbuttock or over the greater trochanter, lower abdomen, iliac crest, groin, or sacroiliac joint.

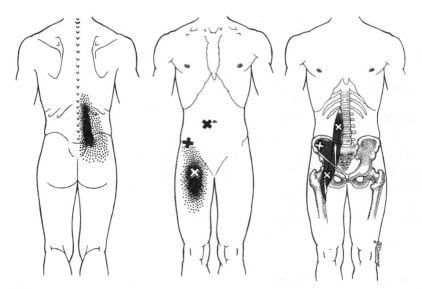

FIGURE 18–3. Pattern of pain (*light gray*) referred from palpable myofascial trigger points [*Xs*] in the right iliopsoas muscle (*darker gray*). The essential pain reference zone is *solid gray,* and the spillover pattern is *stippled.* (Adapted with permission from Travell JG, Simons DG: *Myofascial Pain and Dysfunction, The Trigger Point Manual: The Lower Extremities,* vol 2. Baltimore, Williams & Wilkins, 1983.)

TABLE 18–4. Muscles of Common Myofascial Pain Syndromes

Muscle	Major Functions	History
Iliopsoas	Hip flexion, sit-ups after the first 30°, maintain upright posture	Classic flare: prolonged car ride, truck drivers (from knees being higher than hips) Worsening pain with: upright position, getting out of a deep chair, passing hard feces, limb length discrepancy Other: limits ability to do SLR
Piriformis*	Restrains vigorous medial thigh rotation, stabilizes hips	Classic flare: after a near fall† Worsening pain with: defecation, intercourse (dyspareunia) Other: erectile dysfunction, absent Achilles reflex, pseudoradiculopathy, sciatica
Quadratus lumborum	Stabilizes lumbar spine on the pelvis, assists lateral bending	Classic flare: stooping with a twisted torso (e.g., gardening)

SLR = sitting leg raise.
*The piriformis syndrome can be initiated on the right side after a long drive with the foot on the gas pedal.
†Pain may be worse if the patient was twisting, bending, or lifting when experiencing the near fall.

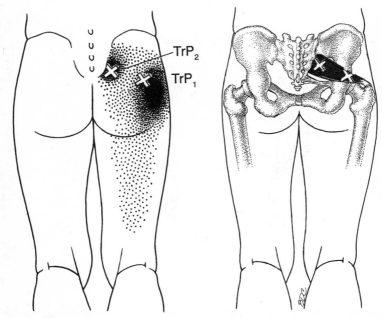

FIGURE 18–4. Composite pattern of pain (*light gray*) referred from trigger points (TrPs) [*Xs*] in the right piriformis muscle (*darker gray*). The *lateral X* (TrP$_1$) indicates the most common TrP location. The *gray stippling* locates the spillover part of the pattern that may be felt as less intense pain than that of the essential pattern (*solid gray*). Spillover pain may be absent. (Adapted with permission from Travell JG, Simons DG: *Myofascial Pain and Dysfunction, The Trigger Point Manual: The Lower Extremities,* vol 2. Baltimore, Williams & Wilkins, 1983.)

Sacroiliac Dysfunction

Sacroiliac dysfunction is a syndrome associated with unilateral pain and tenderness over the sacroiliac joint as well as a wide array of possible pseudoradiculopathic pain distribution patterns (e.g., sciatic, low lumbar, sacral, gluteal). Some clinicians have theorized that subluxation causes sacroiliac dysfunction. In clinical studies, both manipulation and surgery of the sacroiliac joint have been shown to relieve pain.

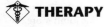 THERAPY

Nonpharmacologic Therapy

Self-care

Endurance exercises (e.g., swimming, walking, stationary biking, light running) can help avoid debilitation during healing. Exercising 10 to 20 minutes daily, beginning 2 to 3 weeks after the onset of symptoms, usually

Quadratus lumborum

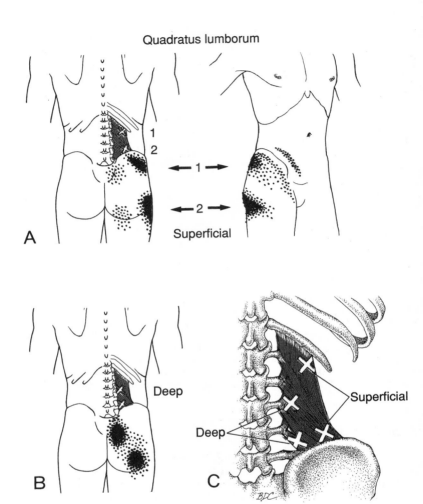

FIGURE 18–5. Referred pain patterns (*light gray*) of trigger points (TrPs) [*Xs*] in the quadratus lumborum muscle (*gray*). *Solid light gray* denotes an essential pain pattern, and *stippled gray*, a spillover pattern. (*A*) Pain patterns of superficial (lateral) TrPs that are palpable (*1*) below and close to the 12th rib, and (*2*) just above the iliac crest. (*B*) Pain patterns of deep (more medial) TrPs close to the transverse processes of the lumbar vertebrae. The more cephalad deep TrPs refer pain to the sacroiliac joint; more caudal TrPs refer pain low in the buttock. (*C*) Examples of locations of TrPs in the quadratus lumborum muscle. (Adapted with permission from Travell JG, Simons DG: *Myofascial Pain and Dysfunction, The Trigger Point Manual: The Lower Extremities,* vol 2. Baltimore, Williams & Wilkins, 1983.)

puts little stress on the back. After the first week, the patient can usually increase the time by 5 or 10 minutes each week, up to a total of 35 to 45 minutes. Other suggestions for general self-care can be found in Table 18–5.

Activity restrictions for return to work

It is often the family physician's responsibility to determine what is and is not physically appropriate for the patient. Many patients will be ready and able to return to work within 2 to 3 days, particularly if they have a note stating appropriate physical restrictions. Some patients will even return the same day. Patients in jobs with regular physical activity may be able to perform well and safely within 1 to 2 weeks, as long as they follow physical restrictions and precautions (e.g., rotate mild to moderate load-bearing work with nonload-bearing work; rest frequently; and limit twisting, bending, and reaching while lifting).

Lifting limitations

Load bearing after an episode of low back pain should be guided carefully. Even moderate lifting (approximately 15 to 20 pounds for women and 30 to 40 pounds for men) can aggravate low back pain.

Sitting limitations

Patients who have pain with prolonged sitting can be guided to increase their time intervals of continuous sitting from 10 to 20 minutes to 50 to

TABLE 18–5. **General Self-Care for Low Back Pain**

Activity	Directions
Stretching shortened muscles	Slowly initiate as soon as the patient feels up to it, often within a few days.
Aerobic exercises that mildly stress the back (e.g., walking, biking, swimming)	These can usually start within 2 weeks of the onset of acute low back problems, as long as the principle of slow-but-sure increase is heeded.
Conditioning exercises for trunk	These are not recommended during the first few weeks; later, if increase is gradual (i.e., slow-but-sure), they can be helpful, especially if symptoms persist.*
Bed rest	Resting 2–4 days may be helpful, but more than 4 days of bed rest may be debilitating.
Massage, ultrasound, ice, heat	Lack unequivocal efficacy, but are generally considered benign.†

*It is not uncommon for back exercises to produce more pain rather than less in the first 1 to 2 weeks. Exercise time and difficulty should begin slowly and then gradually increase rather than stop if pain occurs.

†Many physical therapists who practice massage, ultrasound, ice, and heat are praised by their patients.

60 minutes over 1 to 3 months. Sitting that aggravates pain may also be less problematic if the patient changes position often, slightly tilts the chair back, and uses a chair with armrests. A soft support placed near the small of the back often helps as well.

Manipulation

Manipulation is a clinician-induced loading force on the spine that uses the concept of leverage to shift pressure. It has been found to be safe and effective for patients without radiculopathy. However, if manipulation has not resulted in symptomatic and functional improvement after 4 weeks, it should be stopped and the patient should be reevaluated.

Physical therapy

A physical therapist can play an important role in the care and education of patients with low back pain. Physical therapists commonly use modalities such as massage and diathermy. Although there are no well-done studies regarding the efficacy of these modalities in the treatment of acute low back pain, many clinicians (and patients) feel that these approaches are beneficial, and there is no indication that they are harmful.

The physical therapy literature emphasizes carefully chosen techniques that stretch the muscles involved in myofascial syndromes (Figures 18–6 through 18–8).

Surgery (see SURGEONS; p 239)

Pharmacotherapy

Acetaminophen

Acetaminophen is safe and inexpensive. The maximum dose should be 4 g/day, whether as plain acetaminophen or as a combination medication (e.g., acetaminophen with codeine, hydrocodone, oxycodone), because high doses of acetaminophen can lead to liver damage.

Nonsteroidal anti-inflammatory drugs (NSAIDs)

The most frequent complication of NSAIDs is GI irritation, the degree of which appears to be dose related, but can occur with only one tablet. Fortunately, a new generation of NSAIDs, cyclooxygenase-2 (cox-2) inhibitors, appears to have few GI side effects. For patients who cannot tolerate cox-2 inhibitors, NSAIDs can be taken with misoprostol, which reduces the occurrence of gastric erosion and ulceration. However, many patients do not tolerate misoprostol's common side effect of diarrhea. All NSAIDs can interfere with platelet adhesion, renal sodium metabolism and overall renal function. They are contraindicated in patients with bleeding problems and must be used cautiously in patients with hypertension, renal disease, and edema.

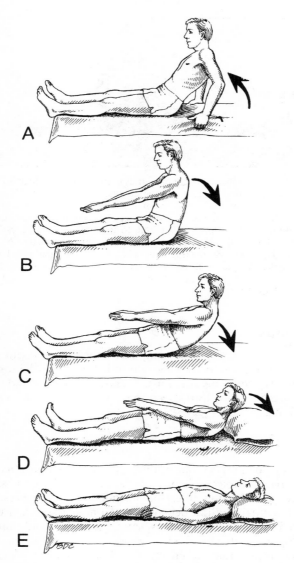

FIGURE 18–6. Slow sit-back exercise to improve strength and coordination of the abdominal and hip flexor muscles as the spine "rolls down" on the table. This exercise requires a less demanding lengthening contraction, rather than the shortening contraction of a sit-up. (*A*) Pushing the torso up (*arrow*) with the arms from the supine to the seated position. This avoids loading the flexor muscles of the trunk and hips. (*B*) Beginning of the slow sit-back, with the lumbar spine flexed. (*C*) Rolling the back down onto the table, maintaining spinal flexion so that each spinal segment reaches the table in succession. (*D*) Completion of the slow sit-back. (*E*) Period of full relaxation with abdominal (diaphragmatic) breathing. Three cycles of this slow sit-back exercise should be performed daily to provide full benefit. (Adapted with permission from Simons DG, Travell JG: Myofascial origins of low back pain. 2. Torso muscles. *Postgrad Med* 73:81–92, 1983.)

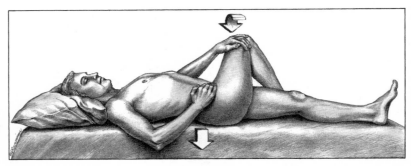

FIGURE 18–7. Self-stretch of the right piriformis muscle. The right thigh is flexed nearly 90° at the hip with the right foot on the treatment table. To adduct the thigh at the hip, pressure is exerted downward with both hands (large arrows). One hand is placed on the thigh and the other on the pelvis, pulling against each other. To perform postisometric relaxation, the individual then attempts to abduct the thigh by pressing it gently against the resisting left hand for a few seconds (isometric contraction of abductors), then relaxes and gently moves the thigh into adduction, which gradually lengthens the piriformis muscle. (Adapted with permission from Travell JG, Simons DG: *Myofascial Pain and Dysfunction, The Trigger Point Manual: The Lower Extremities,* vol 2. Baltimore, Williams & Wilkins, 1983.)

Muscle relaxants

Muscle relaxants are only infrequently useful for low back pain. Although helpful for true muscle spasms, they do little for myofascial trigger point contractures. However, because muscle relaxants are sleep inducing, they may help patients who clearly need to slow down but will likely have a problem doing so.

Opioids

The AHCPR guidelines describe opioids as being "no more effective in relieving low back symptoms than . . . acetaminophen." Opioid side effects include decreased reaction time, clouded judgment, drowsiness, constipation, and potential physical dependence. Nonetheless, when used for a time-limited course, many clinicians have found that opioids can be an appropriate option. Patients who receive opioids should be carefully educated about the potential side effects, including the danger associated with use while operating heavy equipment or driving.

Injection therapy

Although there are no large, well-done studies, several reports in both medical and physical therapy journals describe significant relief from myofascial pain syndrome with steroid injections, lidocaine injections, or ultrasound therapy directed at the trigger points. Surgeons, neurologists, physiatrists, and anesthesiologists (see CONSULTS; p 239) are skilled at

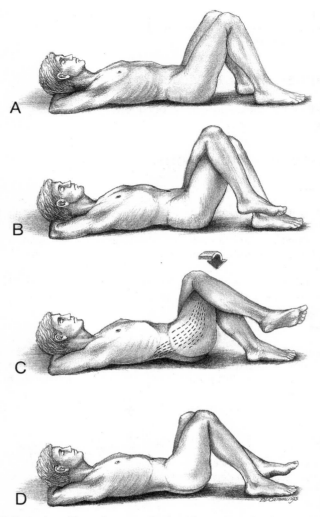

FIGURE 18–8. Supine self-stretch exercise for the right quadratus lumborum muscle. (*A*) Starting position, supine with the hips and knees bent. The hands are placed behind the head to elevate the rib cage. (*B*) Preparatory position with the controlling left leg crossed over the right thigh, the side to be stretched. After the right thigh has been adducted as far as it will go without resistance, during slow deep inhalation, the left leg is used to resist a gentle isometric abductive effort of the right thigh. (*C*) As the patient slowly exhales and relaxes the right side, the left leg gently pulls the right thigh medially and downward, which rotates and pulls the right half of the pelvis caudad; this takes up slack in the quadratus lumborum and abductor fibers of the gluteal muscles (*dashed lines*). The *large arrow* indicates the direction of applied pressure. Steps *B* and *C* may be repeated until no further increase in range of motion is achieved. (*D*) Release of stretch by slipping the controlling (left) leg off of the right knee, releasing tension and at the same time supporting the treated side. Hips and knees are then returned to the relaxed position, as in step *A*. (Adapted with permission from Travell JG, Simons DG: *Myofascial Pain and Dysfunction, The Trigger Point Manual: The Lower Extremities,* vol 2. Baltimore, Williams & Wilkins, 1983.)

epidural steroid injections, a procedure far less invasive than surgery that often has at least short-term positive results in the treatment of radicular pain.

URGENCIES & EMERGENCIES

The red flags indicated with the history questions should be considered urgent (see HISTORY; p 221).

SPECIAL POPULATIONS

Children

Significant low back pain is seldom seen in children in a family practice. In prepubertal children, low back pain usually suggests minor trauma that can be treated with acetaminophen, although it may rarely indicate infection or tumor. Postpubertal children have the same differential as adults. However, radiculopathic pain is so unusual in children or adolescents that one should have a low threshold for consulting with a specialist if it presents. A list of pediatric red flags can be found in Table 18–6.

Seniors

Seniors are much more likely to have GI complications from NSAIDs than their younger counterparts. As with many medical concerns, seniors often deserve to receive studies more swiftly than other patients do because of the higher likelihood of major pathology. Still, most presentations of acute low back pain can be watched for awhile before initiating therapy.

Pregnancy

Low back pain is often seen during pregnancy, with sciatic nerve pain being the most common dermatomal pain experienced. Because NSAIDs fall

TABLE 18–6. **Pediatric Red Flags with Low Back Pain**

- Child is younger than 4 years of age.
- Back pain causes functional disability (e.g., child asks to miss sports, gym, or recess).
- Pain has lasted more than 4 weeks.
- Child has a fever.
- The pain causes a postural shift of the trunk, with the child chronically splinting to decrease the pain.
- The pain causes limitation of motion.
- There is a neurologic abnormality.

into a variety of pregnancy categories, use them only rarely and with careful forethought.

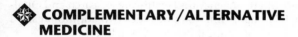 COMPLEMENTARY/ALTERNATIVE MEDICINE

Chiropractors are often useful in the treatment of low back pain (see CONSULTS; below).

Massage can be helpful, particularly for myofascial pain syndromes. Although the relaxing effects of the massaging hands of a lay person can be restful and stress reducing, many massage therapists and physical therapists have learned specific techniques that directly address the shortening of muscle fibers.

Acupuncture may lessen the need for medications and, when practiced appropriately, has virtually no side effects.

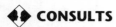 CONSULTS

Chiropractors

Manipulation appears to help patients with acute low back pain without radiculopathy when used within the first month of symptoms, although efficacy has not been proved.

Surgeons

Consultation with a surgeon should be considered for selected patients with herniated discs and nerve root dysfunction that does not respond to less invasive therapy. Emergency consultation is appropriate for patients with bowel and bladder dysfunction or progressive, severe neurologic impairment.

Neurologists

Consider a consult if a myelopathy or upper motor neuron dysfunction is suspected, and/or for a trial of epidural steroid injections.

Physiatrists

When a patient without red flags or untreated psychiatric concerns is not improving, a physiatrist may be beneficial. This referral can be particularly helpful for family physicians who cannot identify either a physical therapist with a strong interest in acute low back pain or what therapeutic modalities would be most beneficial.

Anesthesiologists

In regard to low back pain, this referral is generally for epidural steroid injection therapy.

ALGORITHMS

For those whose learning style is conducive to algorithms, we have included five algorithms from the Agency for Healthcare Research and Quality (formerly the AHCPR). Algorithm 18–2 includes two additional steps that are not found in the 1994 Clinical Practice Guidelines.

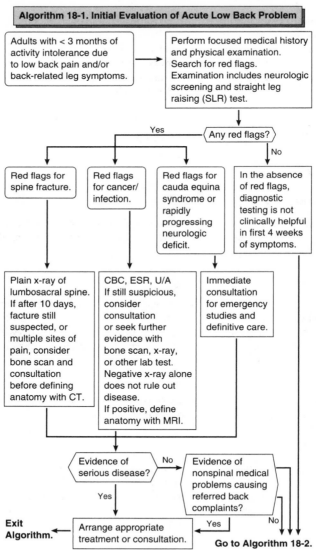

Algorithm 18-1. Initial Evaluation of Acute Low Back Problem

AHCPR: Acute low back problems in adults. Clinical Practice Guideline Number 14. Publication No. 95–0642, December 1994.

CBC = complete blood cell count; *CT* = computed tomography; *ESR* = erythrocyte sedimentation rate; *MRI* = magnetic resonance imaging; *U/A* = urinalysis.

Algorithm 18-2. Treatment of Acute Low Back Problem on Initial and Follow-up Visits

Initial visit

Adults with low back problem and no underlying serious condition (see Algorithm 18-1).

→ *Do history and physical examination suggest myofascial pain syndrome?*

No → Provide assurance; education about back problems. ← Yes → *Discuss specific myofascial pain syndromes.*

Does patient require help relieving symptoms? — Yes → Recommend/prescribe comfort options based on risk/benefits and patient preference.

No ↓

Recommend activity alterations to avoid back irritation.
Review activity limitations (if any) due to back problem; encourage to continue or return to normal activities (including work, with or without restrictions) as soon as possible.
Encourage low-stress aerobic exercise.
Encourage stretching exercises if myofascial pain is the main problem.

↓

Symptoms improving? — Yes → **Return to normal activities.**

No ↓

- -

(con't on next page)

AHCPR: Acute low back problems in adults. *Clinical Practice Guideline Number 14.* Publication No. 95–0642, December 1994.
Note: AHCPR Guideline does not include the italicized and underlined text. Those steps have been added by the author.

(con't from previous page)

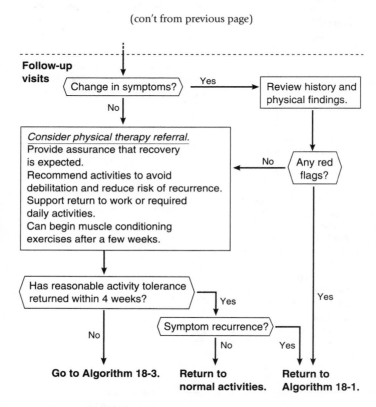

AHCPR: Acute low back problems in adults. *Clinical Practice Guideline Number 14.* Publication No. 95–0642, December 1994.

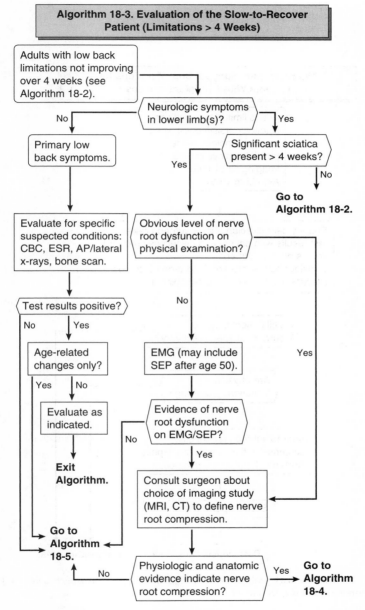

Algorithm 18-3. Evaluation of the Slow-to-Recover Patient (Limitations > 4 Weeks)

AHCPR: Acute low back problems in adults. *Clinical Practice Guideline Number 14.* Publication No. 95–0642, December 1994.

AP = anteroposterior; *CBC* = complete blood cell count; *CT* = computed tomography; *EMG* = electromyogram; *ESR* = erythrocyte sedimentation rate; *MRI* = magnetic resonance imaging; *SEP* = somatosensory evoked potential.

*These recommendations were not included in the original AHCPR *Clinical Practice Guidelines.*

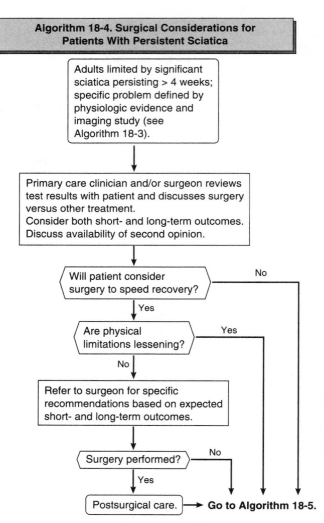

Algorithm 18-4. Surgical Considerations for Patients With Persistent Sciatica

Adults limited by significant sciatica persisting > 4 weeks; specific problem defined by physiologic evidence and imaging study (see Algorithm 18-3).

Primary care clinician and/or surgeon reviews test results with patient and discusses surgery versus other treatment.
Consider both short- and long-term outcomes.
Discuss availability of second opinion.

Will patient consider surgery to speed recovery? — No

Yes

Are physical limitations lessening? — Yes

No

Refer to surgeon for specific recommendations based on expected short- and long-term outcomes.

Surgery performed? — No

Yes

Postsurgical care. ➝ **Go to Algorithm 18-5.**

AHCPR: Acute low back problems in adults. *Clinical Practice Guideline Number 14.* Publication No. 95–0642, December 1994.

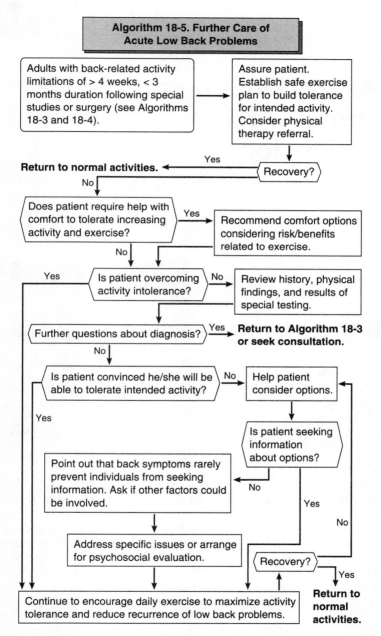

AHCPR: Acute low back problems in adults. *Clinical Practice Guideline Number 14.* Publication No. 95–0642, December 1994.

CHAPTER **19**

Mental Health and Illness—Anxiety and Depression

Timothy Freeman • Susan Louisa Montauk
• Rick E. Ricer

 INTRODUCTION

In this chapter, we compare and contrast anxiety and depression to illustrate one approach toward mental illness in a family practice setting. Based *on the 1999 report of the Office of the United States Surgeon General*, mental illness is present when a state of poor mental functioning results in the

OBJECTIVES

■ Describe the variables that affect attitudes toward mental illness

■ Be familiar with the psychologic and psychiatric terminology most often used in primary care

■ Describe the main aspects of the more common depression- and anxiety-related mental illnesses

■ Explain and contrast treatment options for the more common depression- and anxiety-related mental illnesses

inability to engage in productive activities, experience fulfilling relationships with other people, and/or adapt to change and cope with adversity successfully.

Since the inception of the specialty in 1969, many physicians chose family practice because of the discipline's emphasis on the biopsychosocial model of patient care. Long before the term "mind-body medicine" became a catch phrase, many family doctors understood, spoke of, and practiced care that strove to incorporate more than laboratory values and physical findings. Still, mental illness often goes unrecognized.

Although clinical depression is more common than hypertension, primary care physicians identify less than half of the cases of depression in their practices. Although there are many reasons for the underrecognition, we discuss three that are particularly pertinent: the stigma associated with the label "mentally ill;" the historic emphasis on the separation of mind and body; and the negative effects of somatization, especially when we misunderstand its origins.

Stigmatization

The stigma connected with mental illness appears to be the major reason why two-thirds of people with diagnosable mental disorders never seek treatment. For the majority of us, it is much easier to say "I have high blood pressure" or "My mom has cancer" than it is to say "My father became psychotic" or "I have panic attacks." Yet, statistics suggest that most families have experienced mental illness.

Separation of mind and body

In the 1600s, Descartes theorized that the mind and body were two separate entities. Despite the many scientific advances in the 1900s that disproved Descartes' perceived separation, semantics and misinformation continue to separate the two.

Somatization

Somatization may present as a single instance of a somatic complaint or a chart containing a multitude of visits for somatic symptoms. Two variables that tend to negatively influence objectivity with such patients stem from what are commonly thought of as physician (or medical student) strengths; we refer to them as "stone turning" and "stoicism."

Stone turning

Somatic complaints in unfamiliar patients often thrust physicians into the "I am afraid I am missing something so I will look for everything under the sun" mode. This type of situation can be difficult for seasoned clinicians and is often overwhelming for students.

Stoicism

Patients with a full somatization disorder may appear to suffer and complain exceedingly, and may resist any "insights" you share regarding the likelihood that their symptoms represent a specific physical disease. In contrast, physicians and medical students tend to be goal oriented and take pride in their ability to forget about a headache, an argument with a boyfriend, or bad sunburn if it interferes with work. Thus, you may have difficulty identifying and empathizing with a "whiner" or "complainer."

Fortunately, in a continuity-of-care environment, family physicians have a chance to experience how quality of life improves for patients with somatization disorder when other psychologic disorders are addressed.

TERMINOLOGY (ALSO SEE TABLE 19–1)

The descriptions of disorders in the following terminology list are brief definitions, not specific diagnostic criteria, unless otherwise specified.

Adjustment reaction: a reaction (e.g., anxiety, depression) to an identifiable experience or stressor that does not qualify for a major clinical diagnosis

Affect: the external manifestations of emotional feelings or mood

Agoraphobia: fear of being in public places without an escape

Anhedonia: the lack of pleasure from acts that would ordinarily be pleasurable

Anxiety: a sense of apprehension and fear

Biopsychosocial: the relationship of the biologic, psychologic, and social aspects of a process as opposed to strictly the biomedical aspect of a process

Cognitive-behavioral therapy: a psychotherapeutic model that combines behavioral therapy and cognitive therapy

Compulsions: repetitive, voluntary behaviors (as opposed to involuntary behaviors such as tics or twitches) performed to neutralize discomfort and anxiety

Dystonia: an abnormal tonicity in any of the body's tissues

Flight of ideas: a nearly continuous flow of speech that jumps between unrelated subjects

Functional symptom: a physical symptom without any demonstrable organic cause

Hypomania: a manic-like episode that is not of sufficient severity to produce marked impairment in function

Mind-body medicine: a clinical approach that assumes that the mind (e.g., mood, feelings, motivations, past experiences) and body (e.g., organ systems, physiologic processes) have such a strong influence on each other that they must both be considered when assessing any disorder

Mood disorder: the term used in the fourth edition of the Diagnostic and Statistical Manual of Mental Disorders to cover depressive disorders

Obsession: a condition, usually associated with anxiety and fear, in which an intrusive idea or thought repeatedly enters the mind despite one's effort to ignore or dislodge it

Panic attack: a sudden, unexpected, and unrealistic discreet period of intense fear or discomfort accompanied by symptoms of autonomic nervous system hyperstimulation

Phobia: a persistent, irrational fear of specific objects, activities, or situations

Pressured speech: abnormal verbal communication that is usually loud, rapid, and difficult to interpret

Psychosis: a mental distortion or disorganization that severely interferes with one's affect, reality recognition, and communication

Psychotherapy, behavioral: a psychotherapeutic approach to behavior that focuses on how one is acting versus how one is feeling

Psychotherapy, cognitive: a psychotherapeutic approach that centers on first examining the accuracy of one's beliefs, then shifting those beliefs that are irrational to consequently shift one's behavior

Situational anxiety: a nonpersistent (usually far less than 6 months) fear or discomfort that occurs as a reaction to a real event

Somatization: the process by which emotions are converted into physical symptoms

Suicidal ideation: having thoughts of death or suicide that may (but often do not) include suicidal intent, specific suicidal plans, or means to accomplish suicide

Tardive dyskinesia: involuntary movements of the lips or jaw that are sometimes accompanied by other dystonic gestures; can be an extrapyramidal side effect of antipsychotic medication and, although rare, can continue after the medication is discontinued

Trichotillomania: self-mutilation by pulling out one's own cephalic hair as a result of anxiety, a behavioral disorder, or psychosis

Vegetative state: a severely reduced activity level; in the extreme, only involuntary bodily functions are sustained

TABLE 19–1. **Medical Disorders: The Mind–Body Connection**

Disorder	Initiating Area	Altered Area	Clinical Example
Somatic	Body or outside of mind and body	Body	A stroke leading to limb paralysis
Psychologic	Mind	Mind	The psychologic response to limb paralysis leading to depression
Somatization	Mind	Body	Depression leading to persistent back pain
Mental	Body	Mind	A stroke leading to dementia

Note: These terms have highly variable definitions throughout medical literature. These are the definitions used in this chapter.

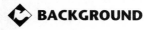 **BACKGROUND**

In the United States, mental illness accounts for more than 15% of the overall burden of disease (i.e., disability-adjusted life years, as assessed by

the United States Department of Health) from all causes. Mental illness ranks second only to cardiovascular disease, and exceeds even cancers. More than 20 million (i.e., more than 10%) Americans living today will fit the diagnostic criteria for an anxiety disorder at some time during their lifetimes and the figure is even higher for depression.

> **NOTE**
>
> The category of anxiety and depression is one of the top 10 diagnoses seen in a family practice office.

 PREVENTION

The success of primary prevention techniques for psychologic concerns has not been well verified. More is known about the success of secondary prevention; however, validation of the specifics of secondary prevention (i.e., exactly when, where, and how much) is lacking.

Primary Prevention

Exercise, stress reduction, and a strong self-image appear to help decrease the incidence of clinical anxiety and depression. Proper diet, the appropriate amount of sleep, avoidance of illicit drugs (e.g., excessive alcohol, tobacco), and a supportive family and community also may help.

Secondary Prevention

Psychotherapy and medication play an important role in secondary prevention. Education for both the patient and the patient's family appears to positively affect depression and anxiety, lessening relapse frequency and severity.

 DIAGNOSIS

When considering a diagnosis of depression or anxiety, keep in mind three important points:

1. **Psychiatric illness can have variable origins** (i.e., psychologic, somatization, or mental)

One might assume that the psychiatric disorders of anxiety and depression are always psychologic disorders. In actuality, it is more complex. Consider the following:

- A well-known sign of hypothyroidism is depression. A well-recognized result of thyroid hormone administration to a patient with hypothyroidism is remission of depression.

- A well-known sign of hyperthyroidism is anxiety. A well-recognized result of thyroid ablation therapy in a patient with hyperthyroidism is remission of anxiety.
- Strokes have been shown to cause a wide variety of psychiatric problems related specifically to the loss of neuronal function in the localized area of ischemia.
- A common result of antidepressant medication and/or counseling is the disappearance of chronic headaches, pelvic pain, or back pain.

Thus, all psychiatric disorders are disorders of mental function, but some are psychologic disorders, some are mental disorders, and others are somatization disorders.

2. "Normal" is variably defined

How does one define when "normal" becomes "abnormal?" After all, anxious feelings are common reactions to any threat. Sadness, acute sleep disturbances, and some difficulty with concentration and attention are all universal responses to subacute stress or a sad situation. Most people experience "highs" and "lows" on a daily, weekly, or monthly basis.

One helpful construct is to judge the degree of "abnormality" by the degree of interference with the individual's life, capabilities, and activities. Most often, experiences such as an acute threat or subacute stress are of relatively short duration and do not have a severe impact on activities of daily living or close relationships. When the impact of the anxiety or depression is severe enough to threaten the patient's health and well-being, (because of harsh stress, genetic loading, or both), it is considered "abnormal." If not identified, addressed, and treated, major morbidity can result.

"Normal" behavior is also defined by the culture, the politics, and the times, and is often characterized differently within subcultures in the same society. For example, many adults in the United States were raised in a time when belts and paddles were a common means of discipline. Today, a teacher or parent who whips a child with a belt is considered a child abuser and is labeled "abnormal." Similarly, some societies hold people with hallucinations in high esteem, feeling they have a special connection with higher powers. In the United States, there is little tolerance for such an outlook.

3. Anxiety and depression often occur together

Anxiety and depression often occur together; their comorbidity is the rule, not the exception. Signs and symptoms frequently overlap, and both disorders are often initiated or exacerbated in response to emotional stress. In research studies in which each disorder is defined using the fourth edition of the Diagnostic and Statistical Manual of Mental Disorders (DSM-IV) criteria, one-third to one-half of the patients with generalized anxiety disorder also fit the criteria for major depressive disorder. Likewise, two-thirds of the patients that fit the criteria for major depressive disorder also fit the criteria for generalized anxiety disorder and more than 90% of patients that fit the diagnostic criteria for panic disorder are also depressed.

> **NOTE**
>
> Comorbidity between panic disorder and depression is associated with severe emotional illness, including a significantly higher suicide risk. Thus, timely and appropriate treatment is important.

Presentation

Patients rarely present to a family physician's office stating that they have a mood or anxiety disorder. Some patients present with more classic symptoms, such as insomnia, irritability, sexual dysfunction, and anorexia with weight loss. Others present atypically with vague physical symptoms or complaints involving multiple areas of the body.

Psychiatric disorders associated with depression

Major depressive disorder

Major depressive disorder is diagnosed if the patient has had recurrent episodes of depression that last at least 2 weeks each and are not accompanied by intervening mania or hypomania. The episodes of depression are most often characterized by:

- **Diminished ability to perform activities of daily living** (e.g., poor thinking, weak concentration, inattention, decreased sex drive, lack of motivation, decreased enjoyment of pleasurable activities, decreased interest in normal activities)
- **Depressed mood** (e.g., sadness; feelings of dejection, worthlessness, or hopelessness; crying episodes; guilt)
- **Vegetative signs** (e.g., changes in appetite, changes in sleep patterns, early morning awakening, decreased activity, lethargy)
- **Suicidal thoughts or attempts**

Seasonal affective disorder (SAD)

SAD is a term used to modify the diagnosis of major depressive disorder. SAD transpires and remits with changes in the seasons. Two onset patterns have been identified:

- **Depression onset in the fall or winter** that remits in late spring or early summer and often has "atypical" signs and symptoms including significant increase in sleep, irritability, appetite, food intake (carbohydrate craving), weight, and interpersonal difficulties (e.g., rejection sensitivity)
- **Depression onset in the late spring or early summer,** often with "typical" vegetative-type signs and symptoms including decreased sleep, weight loss, and poor appetite

Bipolar disorder

A diagnosis of bipolar disorder often is first suspected when an individual has one or more manic episodes or one or more major depressive episodes accompanied by at least one episode of hypomania. To make the diagnosis, one must feel reasonably sure that a substance abuse disorder, psychotic disorder, schizoaffective disorder, or other mood disorder is not responsible for the symptoms. Because of the potential complexity of assessing for these "rule outs," patients with suspected bipolar disorder are often referred to psychiatrists.

Signs and symptoms of bipolar disorder include those of depression (see MAJOR DEPRESSIVE DISORDER; p 252) and those of mania. Signs and symptoms of mania include:

- The ability to accomplish tasks in far less time than usual
- Decreased need for sleep
- Rapid speech (often seen in hypomania, but to a milder degree)
- Sexual indiscretion that the patient would usually avoid
- Spending sprees
- Unrealistic feelings that life is nonproblematic (often seen in hypomania, but to a milder degree)
- Unusually high energy level (often seen in hypomania, but to a milder degree)

Dysthymia and cyclothymia

Dysthymia is characterized by long-standing depressed and irritable mood symptoms that are similar to but far less severe than those associated with major depressive disorder (see MAJOR DEPRESSIVE DISORDER; p 252).

Cyclothymia is characterized by at least 2 years of numerous, periodic episodes of hypomania that alternate with a depressed mood and are not associated with major depressive disorder or bipolar disorder.

Psychiatric disorders associated with anxiety

Generalized anxiety disorder (GAD)

The diagnosis of GAD generally includes at least 6 months of chronic, exaggerated worry and concern that focuses on things most people would not worry about or would be concerned about to a much lesser degree.

Obsessive-compulsive disorder (OCD)

OCD is an anxiety disorder marked by recurrent obsessions and/or compulsions that negatively impact on normal functioning. It often includes highly unsettling thoughts that arise suddenly and are very difficult to extinguish. It also includes ritual-like behaviors that have to be repeated over and over although they seem silly, counterproductive, or severely disruptive.

Posttraumatic stress disorder (PTSD)

PTSD can develop after witnessing or experiencing a terrifying event (e.g., war, rape, abuse, natural disaster) for which one is unable to emotionally compensate. It often manifests as:

- Excessive anger and irritability

- Avoidance of normally low-stress behaviors that remind one of the event
- An exaggerated startle response
- Feelings of helplessness
- Detachment in relationships
- Anhedonia
- Reliving the event in thoughts or dreams
- Sleep problems

Panic disorder

Panic disorder includes recurrent, discreet episodes of sudden, unexpected (i.e., incongruous to the situation), intense fear known as panic attacks. It also includes avoidance behaviors (e.g., agoraphobia) and frequent or persistent concern about having another attack or about the potential consequences of an attack.

The signs and symptoms of panic disorder are listed in Table 19–2.

Social phobia

Social phobia (i.e., social anxiety disorder) is present when normally mildly concerning social situations (e.g., presenting in a classroom, meeting people at a party) are frightening or disabling. Although people experiencing social phobia usually know that their response is irrational, they are unable to change.

History

History of present illness

Questions that are representative of the signs and symptoms of the various disorders (see PRESENTATION; p 252) should be included in the history.

TABLE 19–2. **Signs and Symptoms of Panic Disorder**

System	Signs and Symptoms
Cardiovascular	Chest pain or discomfort, palpitations, heart pounding, tachycardia, sweating
Respiratory	Shortness of breath, feeling of smothering or choking, tingling digits and lips (hyperventilation)
Gastrointestinal	Nausea, abdominal distress
Neurologic	Dizzy, light-headed, or unsteady feeling; fainting; paresthesias; trembling and shaking; chills or hot flashes
Psychologic	Depersonalization; fear of losing control, going crazy, or dying; feelings of unreality or doom

General questions about depression and anxiety include:

- How long have these symptoms been present?
- Have you ever had episodes like this before? If so, did you have any therapy that was helpful or any that caused problems?
- How have these symptoms effected your daily activities?
- How have these symptoms effected your ability to earn a living?
- What currently brings you the most stress?
- How is your family and your marriage?
- Where or to whom do you go for support?
- What helps you relax?
- How is your sleep?
- Are you taking any prescription medications, over-the-counter medications, herbs, or supplements? When was each initiated or changed?
- Do you use substances such as alcohol, tobacco, or illicit drugs? How long, how much, and how often do you use them?
- Have you ever received psychologic counseling?

Questions to help assess the degree of anxiety include:

- Do you tend to avoid certain places or situations?
- Are your symptoms more likely in certain situations? Are they unexpected or anticipated?

NOTE

The most common daily supplement that exacerbates anxiety is caffeine.

- What do you think is causing the symptoms?
- What do you think would help prevent or relieve the symptoms?

Questions to help assess the degree of depression include:

- Do you feel down or depressed?
- What do you do that you really enjoy (anhedonia)?
- How are your memory and decision-making abilities?
- How is your appetite (hyper- or hypophagia)?
- How is your sleep (insomnia or extended sleeping hours)?
- Are you more tired than usual? Is your fatigue the same throughout the day or does it become worse as the day goes on?

NOTE

Commonly, lethargy from a mild to moderate chronic illness is felt after the person is up for many hours while fatigue caused by depression is more constant throughout the day.

If you think a patient may be depressed, always consider the risk of suicide. Patients at risk for suicide when depressed include those with:

- Few supports
- Multiple stressors
- Chronic medical conditions
- Substance abuse problems
- Advanced age (seniors)

If questioned, suicidal patients are **not** more likely to act on their suicidal ideation. In fact, when questioned about suicide, patients are often thankful that they can finally talk about their thoughts.

Questions to consider asking when suicide is a concern include:

- Have you been feeling you would rather be dead?
- Have you thought about hurting or killing yourself? If so, how?
- Do you feel like killing yourself right now?
- Have you ever attempted suicide?

NOTE

Contemplate asking questions about suicide again during follow up. Partial treatment of a depressed patient may give that patient enough energy to actually act on their suicidal thoughts.

Past medical history

When you suspect depression, ask past history questions to rule out manic episodes that would suggest bipolar disorder. Treatment for anxiety and major depressive disorder often differs greatly from that for bipolar disorder and may even precipitate a worsening of mania associated with bipolar disorder.

Explore the presence or absence of initiating events and any past or present physical, emotional, or sexual abuse. As important as the psychosocial history is, it must always be expanded to a biopsychosocial history. Record the number and types of surgeries because there may be a history of multiple surgical attempts to treat vague complaints and symptoms. Specific questions should focus on:

- Other medical conditions (especially if chronic)
- Medications that may contribute to symptoms of depression and anxiety (Table 19–3)
- Somatic disorders that may cause or exacerbate depression and anxiety (Table 19–4)

Family history

Ask about a family history of:

- Similar problems—What therapy worked best for other members of the family who have had similar problems.
- Psychiatric admissions

TABLE 19–3. Prescription Medications That Are Known to Sometimes Cause or Exacerbate Depression and Anxiety with Chronic Use

Depression	Anxiety
Alcohol	ACE inhibitors
α-Blockers	Antidepressants
Antineoplastic agents	Caffeine (in some headache medications)
Anticonvulsants	Decongestants
Barbiturates	Digoxin
Benzodiazepines	Dronabinol
β-Blockers	Insulin (if induces hypoglycemia)
Digoxin	Steroids
Disopyramide	Stimulants (e.g., dextroamphetamine, dextroamphetamine four salt combination, or methylphenidate)
Dronabinol	
Histamine blockers	
Hydralazine	
Levodopa	
Medroxyprogesterone	
Methyldopa	
Metoclopramide	
Narcotic analgesics	
Oral contraceptives	
Procainamide	
Reserpine	
Steroids	
Stimulants (e.g., amphetamines or methylphenidate)	

ACE = angiotensin-converting enzyme.

- Nervous breakdowns
- Persons on disability
- Anxiety or mood disorders

Social history

Ask questions about:

- Rest
- Relaxation techniques
- Emotional support
- Use of alcohol, illicit drugs, tobacco, and caffeine
- Financial support

TABLE 19–4. Somatic Disorders That May Cause or Exacerbate Depression and/or Anxiety*

Adrenal dysfunction
Alzheimer's disease
Anemia
Arrhythmias
Cancer
Cerebrovascular accident
Dementia
Epilepsy
Hyperthyroidism and hypothyroidism
Hyperparathyroidism
Hypoglycemia and hyperglycemia
Hyponatremia
Malignancies
Multiple sclerosis
Pancreatitis
Parkinson's disease
Seizures
Pheochromocytoma
Postconcussion syndromes
Sarcoidosis
Stroke
Syphilis
Systemic lupus erythematosus
Vitamin deficiencies (e.g., vitamins B_6 and B_{12})

*The emotional and physical stress of any chronic illness can cause or exacerbate anxiety or depression. The disorders listed in this table have been clearly associated with these psychiatric disorders.

Review of Systems (Table 19–5)

Physical Examination (Table 19–6)

Laboratory Tests

Consider the following tests:

- Thyroid-stimulating hormone (hypothyroidism)
- Thyroxine (hyperthyroidism)
- Finger stick blood glucose (diabetes)
- Erythrocyte sedimentation rate or C-reactive protein (chronic illness and inflammation)
- Hemoglobin (anemia)

NOTE

Silent hypothyroidism can present with exactly the same symptoms and physical examination findings as depression.

TABLE 19–5. Pertinent Positives for the Diagnosis of Anxiety and Depression

System	Common Patient Complaints*	Associated Disorders†
General/Constitutional	Changes in weight Changes in sleep	Depression and anxiety (rule out an endocrine disorder)
	Changes in appetite Malaise Lethargy	Depression (rule out an endocrine disorder)
	Hot flashes and chills	Anxiety (rule out an endocrine disorder)
HEENT	Dry mouth	Anxiety
	Choking sensation	
	Lump in throat	
	Circumoral numbness or tingling	Anxiety (rule out hyperventilation)
Cardiovascular	Palpitations Tachycardia Chest pain	Anxiety (rule out a cardiopulmonary or endocrine disorder)
	Heart beating strongly	
Gastrointestinal	Nausea	Anxiety
	Vomiting	
	Diarrhea	
	Constipation	
	Stomach cramps or "in knots"	
	Abdominal distention	
	Bloating	
	Increased gas or flatulence	
	Abdominal pain	Anxiety and depression
	Heartburn	
Respiratory	Shortness of breath	Anxiety (rule out a cardiopulmonary disorder)
Muskuloskeletal	Peripheral limbs cold	Anxiety
	Clammy or tremulous	
	Twitches	
	Muscle weakness	Anxiety and depression
	Tension or pain	
	Peripheral numbness or tingling	Anxiety (rule out hyperventilation)

(continued)

TABLE 19–5. **Pertinent Positives for the Diagnosis of Anxiety and Depression (*Continued*)**

System	Common Patient Complaints*	Associated Disorders†
Urogenital/sexual function	Chronic pelvic pain	Depression
	Dyspareunia	Anxiety and depression
	Erectile dysfunction	Anxiety, depression (rule out a metabolic or systemic illness)
	Decreased libido	
Neurologic	Focal deficits	Rule out a neurologic disorder
	Tics	
Psychologic	Depressed	Depression
	Feeling "down"	
	Uncommon crying	
	Angry	
	Feeling out of control	
	Feeling explosive	
	Ruminations	Anxiety
	Obsessive behaviors	
	Anxious	
	Frightened	
	Afraid to leave the house	
	Feeling "on edge"	Anxiety and depression

*The noted complaints are representative, not all-inclusive.
†The patient's symptoms may also be associated with a more specific systemic disorder.

Additional Studies

An event monitor may be helpful in ruling out arrhythmia-induced psychiatric symptoms.

 ## DIFFERENTIAL DIAGNOSIS

The differential of disorders associated with anxiety and depression includes several uncommon psychiatric problems, somatic disorders, and medications (see Tables 19–3 and 19–4).

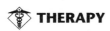 ## THERAPY

At the end of the 20th century, the rapid emergence of both available psychopharmaceuticals and managed care raised new questions related to

TABLE 19–6. Physical Examination Findings Common to Anxiety and/or Depression

System	Findings*	Anxiety	Depression
Vital signs	Tachycardia	X	
	Hypertension	X	
	Tachypnea	X	
General appearance	Poor eye contact	X	X
	Inappropriate demeanor	X	X
	Flat affect		X
	Hypervigilance	X	
	Psychomotor retardation		X
	Significant startle response or edginess	X	
Dermatologic	Skin scratches without noted causes (neurodermatitis)	X	X
	Scars (old surgical scars or from suicide attempts)		X
	Hand dermatitis or xerosis (from excessive hand washing)	X	
	Balding in unusual pattern (trichotillomania)	X	
Cardiovascular	Arrhythmia	X	
Respiratory	Difficulty catching breath	X	
Gastrointestinal	Tenderness	X	
Musculoskeletal	Muscle spasms	X	
	Tender points	X	
	Myofascial pain syndrome		X
Psychologic	Memory deficits	X	X

*The noted findings are representative, not all-inclusive. These findings may also be associated with more specific systemic disorders.

cost-effectiveness. Some studies supported the hypothesis that pharmaceuticals were more successful than counseling. Other studies disagreed. As we enter the 21st century, in addition to a continuance of research, science is beginning to address how combining the two approaches will affect the efficacy of health care.

Nonpharmacologic Therapy

Psychotherapy

As with any referral, the results of therapy will be affected by the knowledge, capability, and commitment of both the practitioner and the patient.

Whenever managed care allows, a family physician must choose the consultant thoughtfully.

Light therapy for seasonal affective disorder

Light therapy has been found to be more effective than no therapy for many people with SAD. No good studies, however, have been done to compare the efficacy of light therapy to antidepressant medications.

Pharmacotherapy

General considerations about psychopharmacology

Our ability to regulate neurotransmitters has raised important philosophical questions about psychopharmacology. For example, is it right to medicate an "overactive" sixth grader who, with the guidance of only one teacher, disrupts the work of his 27 classmates? Where is the line between "different" and "ill?" What is "normal," and should we really change who we are?

Our ability to regulate neurotransmitters has also shown us that chemical manipulation can be a two-edged sword. Pharmaceuticals have permitted millions of people to accomplish such goals as keeping their jobs, patiently nurturing their families, creating works of art, and caring for their patients. However, pharmaceuticals have also led to frightening drug discontinuation syndromes, permanent tardive dyskinesia, unexpected psychotic or manic episodes, liver failure, and hundreds of other harmful side effects.

> **NOTE**
>
> Psychopharmacology is a large component of therapy for mental illness in a family practice setting.

Many of the individual anxiolytic and antidepressant medications available to clinicians are identified in their drug circulars as being for either anxiety or depression, not both. Yet, many times, various entities in comorbid anxiety and depression improve with the same medication.

Anxiolytics (Table 19–7)

Anxiety disorders are usually treated with selective serotonin reuptake inhibitors (SSRIs), TCAs, benzodiazepines, or buspirone. OCD often responds particularly well to higher doses of SSRIs. PTSD is occasionally helped with medications used for other anxiety disorders.

Benzodiazepines have the advantage of a rapid onset. Unfortunately, they have many negative side effects. They can worsen depression, cloud the sensorium, and interact strongly with alcohol. They have a potential for addiction that can be strong in some individuals and they are associated with withdrawal symptoms after prolonged use.

TABLE 19–7. **Anxiolytic Medications**

Class	Drug	Usual Dose
AN	Diphenhydramine (Benadryl)	50–100 mg qid
AN	Hydroxyzine (Atarax, Vistaril)	50–100 mg qid
AZ	Buspirone (BuSpar)	5–15 mg bid
B	Alprazolam (Xanax)	0.5–2 mg tid-qid
B	Clonazepam (Klonopin)	0.5–2 mg bid
B	Clorazepate* (Tranxene)	3.75–15 mg tid-qid
B	Diazepam (Valium)	2–10 mg bid-qid
B	Lorazepam (Ativan)	0.5–2 mg tid-qid
B	Oxazepam (Serax)	10–30 mg tid-qid
P	Prochlorperazine* (Compazine)	5 mg tid-qid
P	Trifluoperazine (Stelazine)	1–3 mg bid

AN = antihistamine; AZ = azapirone; B = benzodiazepine; bid = twice a day; P = phenothiazine; qid = four times a day; tid = three times a day.
*These drugs are also available in a slow-release preparation.

Antihistamines that have a sedating side effect can be used acutely in place of benzodiazepines for the short-term treatment of anxiety. These include hydroxyzine and diphenhydramine.

Buspirone has no known addiction potential and can be helpful to many individuals with GAD.

Antidepressants (Table 19–8)

The pharmacologic treatment of depression includes SSRIs, TCAs, and, rarely, monoamine oxidase inhibitors (MAOIs). Patients usually do not see a positive response for several weeks on these medications, and it may take as long as 2 months to see the maximal pharmaceutical effects.

NOTE

If SSRIs are given to a person that has bipolar disorder without concomitant use of mood stabilizers, they may "unmask" a manic episode.

Although all antidepressants have the potential to be equally efficacious in the treatment of anxiety, significant differences exist in side effect profiles.

Side effects of antidepressants

The newer antidepressant agents are metabolized by the cytochrome P-450 system in the liver; therefore, they can effect the oxidative metabolism of a wide variety of other medications.

TABLE 19–8. **Antidepressant Medications***

Class	Drug	Usual Dose for Depression[†]
SSRI	Citalopram (Celexa)	20–60 mg qd
SSRI	Fluoxetine (Prozac)	10–60 mg qd
SSRI	Paroxetine (Paxil)	10–60 mg qd
SSRI	Fluvoxamine (Luvox)	50–150 mg qd
SSRI	Sertraline (Zoloft)	50–200 mg qd
AT[‡]/NSRI	Venlafaxine XR[§] (Effexor XR)	37.5–225 mg qd
TCA[//]/NSRI	Amitriptyline (Elavil)	100–300 mg qd
TCA[//]/NSRI	Imipramine (Tofranil)	100–200 mg qd
TCA[//]/NSRI	Doxepin (Sinequan)	100–300 mg qd
TCA[//]/NSRI	Trimipramine (Surmontil)	75–200 mg/day (DD)
TCA[//]/NRI	Desipramine (Norpramin)	100–300 mg qd
TC	Maprotiline (Ludiomil)	25–200 mg/day (DD)
TCA[//]/NRI	Nortriptyline (Pamelor)	75–150 mg qd
AK/NDRI	Bupropion SR[§] (Wellbutrin SR)	100–400 mg qd
AT[‡]/TC	Mirtazapine (Remeron)	15–45 mg qd
AT[‡]/PH	Nefazodone (Serzone)	50–300 mg/day (DD)
AT[‡]/TR	Trazodone (Desyrel)	100–400 mg qd
TCA[//]/NRI	Clomipramine (Anafranil)	25–250 mg qd
MAOI	Isocarboxazid (Marplan)	10–30 mg bid
MAOI	Phenelzine (Nardil)	15–30 mg tid
MAOI	Tranylcypromine (Parnate)	10–20 mg tid

AK = aminoketone; AT = atypical antidepressant; bid = twice a day; DD = divided dose; MAOI = monoamine oxidase inhibitor; NDRI = norepinephrine and dopamine reuptake inhibitor; NRI = norepinephrine reuptake inhibitor; NSRI = norepinephrine and serotonin reuptake inhibitor; PH = phenylpiperazine; qd = every day; SR = slow release; SSRI = selective serotonin reuptake inhibitor; TC = tetracyclic; TCA = tricyclic antidepressant; tid = three times a day; TR = triazolopyridine; XR = extended release.
*Most of these medications also help anxiety.
[†]These medications have therapeutic uses that may require lower or, less commonly, higher doses.
[‡]An antidepressant is labeled as "atypical" if it is the only one in a specific class.
[§]These slow-release or extended-release preparations are the most commonly prescribed forms, but there is also a regular-release tablet that is dosed tid.
[//]TCAs are associated with cardiac arrhythmias and should be used with caution in any patient with a cardiac history.

TCAs can make the symptoms of benign prostatic hypertrophy worse, and can induce or exacerbate constipation, orthostatic hypotension, tachycardia, anticholinergic effects, tremor, and weight gain.

SSRIs appear to be just as efficacious as TCAs with fewer long-term side effects. Although SSRIs can have prolonged sexual side effects (e.g., decreased libido, erectile dysfunction, anorgasmy), the body commonly develops tolerance to many of the other side effects (e.g., nausea, diarrhea, abdominal pain, headache, agitation, weight loss or gain, insomnia or sleepiness) within days or weeks.

MAOIs are rarely initiated by family physicians because they have such severe dietary restrictions and an unusually high number of significant side effects and drug-drug interactions.

Follow up

Since a positive effect is unlikely right away, it is appropriate to wait 2 to 3 weeks after an antidepressant is started or a dose is changed before another appointment. However, earlier follow up may be necessary if side effects are a strong concern, particularly if there is a significant risk of a manic episode, if suicide is a major consideration, or if there is a history of intolerance to other psychiatric medications. Further follow up can then usually be every 2 to 4 weeks until full recovery. If a full recovery has not been achieved after three months, most family physicians will then refer the patient to a psychiatrist, if they have not done so already.

Once stability is achieved, treatment for a first episode of depression usually continues for 6 to 12 months before tapering to discontinuation, or decreasing to a lower dose for chronic maintenance therapy. However, **depression is often recurrent.** Patients have a 50% chance of recurrence after the first episode, 70% after the second episode, and 90% after the third. An effective dose of medication continued for at least 6 months is associated with a decrease in the relapse rate of a first episode by 70%. **Patients experience full remission** 60% to 70% of the time after starting medication.

Mood stabilizers (Table 19–9)

Bipolar disorder and cyclothymia are often treated with mood stabilizing medications. Additional antidepressant medications may be added for severe depression with bipolar disorder, but only after stabilization with a mood stabilizer so that mania is not induced.

In addition to the medications listed in Table 19–9, anticonvulsants such as lamotrigine, topiramate, and tiagabine are sometimes used for mood stabilization. However, they are prescribed much less frequently.

 ## URGENCIES & EMERGENCIES

All patients who tell you they have recently attempted suicide or who are at high risk of doing harm to themselves or others must be treated urgently, if not emergently.

TABLE 19-9. **Mood Stabilizing Medications**

Drug	Usual Dose
Carbamazepine (Carbatrol, Tegretol)*,†	100–300 mg tid
Gabapentin (Neurontin)	300–400 mg tid
Lithium (Cibalith, Eskalith, Lithobid)*,†	900–1200 mg/day (DD)
Olanzapine (Zyprexa)§	10–20 mg qd
Valproic acid (Depakote)*,//	50–60 mg/kg/day (DD)

DD = divided dose; qd = every day; tid = three times a day. *Drug levels must be as-sessed regularly with blood draws to gauge toxicity potential.
†The complete blood count must be checked periodically for carbamazepine because it can cause bone marrow suppression.
‡Thyroid and renal function tests need to be drawn if lithium-induced iatrogenic dam-age is suspected for either organ.
§Olanzapine also has antipsychotic effects. Unlike the other medications discussed in this chapter, olanzapine has a small but important potential for tardive dyskinesia.
//Liver function tests must be periodically assessed for signs of liver failure.

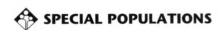

SPECIAL POPULATIONS

Children

The symptoms of mood disorders and anxiety disorders can begin in child-hood. Symptoms in children may not be typical, and may include signifi-cant mood changes, social withdrawal, worsening performance in school, aggressive behavior, multiple somatic complaints, school phobia, unac-counted school absences, runaway behavior, and weight loss. Physical or sexual abuse can present with the same symptoms and can lead to PTSD, panic disorder, GAD, or major depressive disorder.

Children usually metabolize psychoactive medications approximately twice as fast as adults do; therefore, children often need a higher dose than one might expect for their age. It is not uncommon for a 10-year-old child to be on an "adult" dose.

Seniors

It is especially important to be aware of depression in seniors because sui-cide attempts in the elderly population are usually more successful and the treatment of depression may greatly improve dementia.

Seniors have a tendency to use more medications and to experience more dementia and other chronic medical problems than younger adults do. All of these predilections can cloud the presentation of anxiety or depression.

The SSRIs are used for treatment in the elderly because of their lower side effect potential. However, they must be used in relatively lower doses because of a decrease in hepatic metabolism in this population.

Pregnancy

It is important to specifically ask all women about their mood throughout pregnancy. There is an increased risk of depression in the last trimester of pregnancy and in the postpartum period. This may be the result of fluctuating hormones during this time, or rapid changes in lifestyle.

SSRIs appear to be fairly safe for treatment during pregnancy, but any medication during pregnancy can be controversial. Mood stabilizers are not recommended when a woman is breast-feeding.

 ## COMPLEMENTARY/ALTERNATIVE MEDICINE

Saint John's Wort has been fairly well studied and has been found to be efficacious in the treatment of depression when used at 300 mg three times a day.

 ## CONSULTS

A **psychiatric consult** should be considered when bipolar disorder or psychosis is suspected, usual therapeutic protocols do not produce remission, and the patient's presentation is beyond your preceptor's expertise. A psychiatric consult should also be strongly considered for children.

A **clinical psychologist, social worker,** or **psychiatric advanced practice nurse** should be considered for all cases of anxiety or depression that are moderate or severe.

CHAPTER **20**

Obesity

Jill A. Foster

OBJECTIVES

■ Recognize the growing prevalence of obesity in the United States and the factors that led to the increase

■ Explain the genetic factors that predispose to obesity, and recognize how environmental conditions influence the ultimate outcome

■ Become familiar with the evaluation of the obese individual, and recognize when medical intervention is indicated

■ Identify diseases that obesity causes or aggravates

■ Describe the methods available for promoting weight loss, and identify their respective strengths and limitations

 INTRODUCTION

Obesity is a chronic disease. Although it is often perceived as a condition brought about by gluttony and laziness, it is actually a nutritional disorder. Abnormalities in appetite, metabolism, and energy storage all contribute to obesity. Nationally agreed upon guidelines for defining obesity have recently been established and are based on the body mass index (BMI) [Table 20–1].

TERMINOLOGY

Body mass index (BMI): weight (kg)/height squared (m^2)

Gastroplasty: a surgical procedure that reduces the size of the stomach cavity

Morbid obesity: a severe degree of obesity accompanied by obesity-related illness

Nutriceutical: compounds, many of which occur naturally in foods, that are sold as over-the-counter supplements

Obesity: a state of excess fat tissue associated with a BMI greater than 30 kg/m^2

Overweight: a body mass index of 25 to 29.9 kg/m^2

Resistance training: a nonaerobic form of exercise designed to build muscle through the use of weights or resistive devices (e.g., elastic bands)

Roux-en-Y gastric bypass: a surgical procedure that combines gastroplasty with bypass of a portion of the intestines

Visceral fat: fat surrounding the solid organs

TABLE 20–1. **Classification of Overweight and Obesity by BMI**

	Obesity Class	BMI (kg/m^2)
Underweight	—	< 18.5
Normal	—	18.5–24.9
Overweight	—	25.0–29.9
Obesity	I	30.0–34.9
Obesity	II	35.0–39.9
Extreme obesity	III	≥ 40

BMI = body mass index.
Adapted from *Obesity: Preventing and Managing the Global Epidemic.* Report of the World
    Health Organization Consultation on Obesity, 3–5 June 1997, Geneva.

BACKGROUND

Obesity is rapidly increasing in prevalence. The percentage of overweight
adults increased from 24% to 25% between 1960 and 1980 and to 33%
by 1990. Reduced activity is a major factor in the obesity epidemic. If the
present rate of obesity prevalence continues, all Americans will be obese
by the 23rd century.

Americans typically gain 9 kg (20 lb) between the ages of 25 and 55
years. Even among individuals whose weight did not increase, overall adiposity increased because of an age-related decrease in lean body mass, especially muscle. Both the increased fat mass and the loss of lean body mass
appear to be harmful.

Physical Consequences

Mild to moderate obesity has few immediate health consequences and is
often viewed as a cosmetic problem only. Unfortunately, any degree of
obesity can precipitate or exacerbate many medical conditions, including
heart disease and cancer (Table 20–2).

The pattern of fat deposition largely determines the health consequences of excess fat. Fat located in the subcutaneous areas of the hips and
buttocks has little effect on metabolism, while fat located in the upper
body and abdomen significantly effects both glucose and lipid metabolism. Most obese people with either external body composition have visceral fat. Since fat adjacent to the liver can easily influence lipid levels and
insulin sensitivity, visceral fat is a significant concern.

Psychosocial Consequences

The psychosocial ramifications of obesity are as important as the medical
consequences. Obesity carries a profoundly negative stigma. Individuals
who are obese often find themselves socially isolated and have difficulty

TABLE 20–2. **Medical Conditions Associated with Obesity**

System	Consequences Associated with Obesity
Cardiovascular	Hypertension, coronary artery disease
Respiratory	Sleep apnea, reduced lung volumes, hypoventilation syndrome
Gastrointestinal	Colon cancer, rectal cancer, pancreatic cancer, gallbladder disease, gallbladder cancer
Musculoskeletal	Osteoarthritis
Endocrine	Diabetes mellitus, hyperlipidemia
Genitourinary	Reduced fertility, breast cancer, endometrial cancer, kidney cancer
Dermatologic	Purple striae, white striae, intertrigo
Psychologic	Poor self-esteem

gaining employment compared with their nonobese peers. Lowered self-esteem and even self-loathing are common. These psychosocial undercurrents lead many normal-weight and obese individuals to become preoccupied with weight. At the extreme, this can lead to eating disorders such as binge eating, anorexia nervosa, and bulimia.

 PREVENTION

Prevention is the most effective strategy for managing obesity. Some physicians routinely screen for obesity by measuring height, weight, and waist circumference and calculating BMI. Other physicians check only the height and weight. All physicians should encourage healthy eating and physical activity.

The lifestyle practices required for weight loss and the prevention of obesity are similar. The key to both regimens is moderating caloric intake, although individuals trying to prevent weight gain do not need to restrict calories to the same degree as those who are overweight. A prudent diet is moderately low in fat, and contains a generous supply of fruits, vegetables, and whole-grain foods. The "Food Pyramid" (Figure 20–1) and the article *Nutrition and Your Health: Dietary Guidelines for Americans* (see Appendix III, p 384) are good references for individuals trying to improve their diets.

A second key to obesity prevention is regular physical activity. A structured program should include an aerobic component most days of the week and weight lifting or resistance training on alternating days. Both forms of exercise are important for maintaining weight, building lean muscle, and developing cardiovascular fitness.

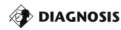 **DIAGNOSIS**

Presentation

Obesity is rarely the chief complaint in family practice. Commonly, office visits for obesity-related conditions such as hypertension, type 2 diabetes

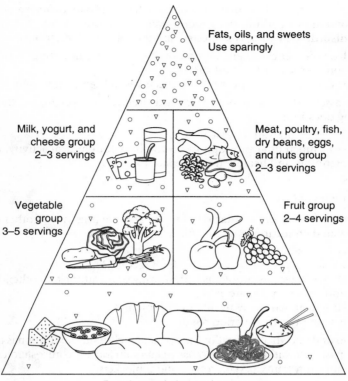

FIGURE 20–1. The "Food Pyramid." Examples of approximate serving: 1 cup milk, 2–3 oz. lean meat, one egg, ½ cup cooked beans, ½ cup cooked veg, 1 cup salad, 1 medium apple, 1 slice bread.

mellitus, back pain, and osteoarthritis present opportunities to discuss the relationship of obesity to the presenting problem.

History

History of present illness

To determine the patient's **weight history** and **dietary habits,** ask the following questions:

- When did you first develop a weight problem? How has this changed over the years?
- Have you ever seen the "Food Pyramid?"
- What are your favorite foods?
- What foods that you know are good for you do you have the most difficulty eating?
- What beverage do you usually drink and how often?
- What did you eat in the last 24 hours?

If more accurate information is desired, have the patient keep a 3- or 7-day food diary or administer a food frequency questionnaire.

If **disordered eating** is suspected, ask the following questions:

- Do you ever eat a very large amount of food at one sitting? If so, did you ever feel out of control?
- Have you ever used vomiting or laxatives to keep your weight down?

To assess whether the patient is **motivated** to lose weight, ask the following questions:

- Why do you want to lose weight?
- How much time and support do you have for physical activity, meal planning, and healthy food preparation?

Past medical history

To determine **cardiovascular risk factors** and the presence of other **obesity-related conditions,** ask the following questions:

- Do you smoke?
- What was your last cholesterol level reading?
- Do you have any problems with snoring or breathing that others have noticed when you are asleep?
- Have you had many respiratory problems?
- Is your menstrual period regular?

Also find out what medications the patient is currently taking or has taken in the past. Medications that can cause weight gain include corticosteroids, insulin, antidepressants, psychotropics, and β-blockers.

Family history

- Is anyone else in your family overweight or severely obese?
- Is there a family history of hypertension, diabetes, or heart disease?

Social history

- How often do you eat red meat, fish, chicken, vegetables, starches, and snack foods?
- How much physical activity do you do at work?
- How often do you engage in physical activity during your free time? How long does the physical activity last, and how would you rate the intensity?
- How much time do you spend watching television, working on the computer, or doing other activities that involve sitting?
- How much alcohol do you drink?
- How much of a problem will finances be in changing your diet or starting an exercise program?
- Who are your family or social supports? Will they support your weight loss?

Review of Systems (Table 20–3)

Physical Examination (Table 20–4)

The diagnosis of obesity can be made with three simple measurements: **height, weight,** (to calculate BMI) and **waist circumference** (to assess abdominal fat) [see TERMINOLOGY; p 268].

NOTE

A waist circumference greater than 102 cm (40 in) for men and 88 cm (35 in) for women is associated with an increased risk of cardiovascular disease, even if the individual is not overweight.

A more accurate assessment of an individual's degree of obesity can be obtained by taking an **anthropometric skinfold measurement.** Anthropometrics can be easily learned and performed in the office. The only instruments needed are a measuring tape and a pair of calipers. Anthropometrics may be especially useful for a muscular individual with a BMI greater than 25 kg/m^2 who may not necessarily have excess body fat.

Laboratory Tests

Routine laboratory tests are not needed when the history and physical examination do not show signs of obesity. Some clinicians check the level of

---

TABLE 20–3. Review of Systems Related to the Diagnosis of Obesity

System	Common Patient Complaints
Constitutional	Lethargy, cold intolerance (hypothyroid), daytime sleepiness (sleep apnea)
Dermatologic	Rashes under skin folds (tinea)
HEENT	Snoring (sleep apnea)
Cardiovascular	Chest pain (CAD)
Respiratory	Shortness of breath with activity or changes in position, awakening from sleep with a sense of choking (sleep apnea)
Gastrointestinal	Constipation, diarrhea, abdominal pain, chest pain consistent with gastroesophageal reflux
Musculoskeletal	Arthralgias
Urogenital/sexual function	Urinary frequency and nocturia (CHF), menstrual changes, decreased libido, erectile dysfunction (poor self-esteem, endocrine dysfunction)
Psychologic	Diminished body self-image, depressed mood

CAD = coronary artery disease; CHF = congestive heart failure.

TABLE 20–4. **Physical Examination Findings Pertinent to Obesity***

System	Findings
Vital signs	BMI $\geq$ 25 kg/m^2, waist circumference > 35 in (female) or > 40 in (male), bradycardia (hypothyroid), hypertension
General appearance	Truncal obesity (CAD risk), moon facies (Cushing's syndrome), dysmorphic features (several genetic syndromes)
HEENT	Oropharyngeal opening decrease (sleep apnea)
Dermatologic	Purple striae (rapid weight gain, Cushing's syndrome), myxedema (hypothyroid), atheromas
Cardiovascular	Bradycardia (hypothyroidism)
Respiratory	Shallow respirations, dyspnea
Gastrointestinal	Abdominal obesity, hepatomegaly (fatty liver)
Musculoskeletal	Arthralgias, back pain, antalgic gait
Extremities	Lower extremity edema, venous insufficiency
Neurologic	Delayed reflexes (hypothyroid)
Psychologic	Depressed mood, excessive drowsiness (sleep apnea)

BMI = body mass index; CAD = coronary artery disease.
*Obesity itself has few findings other than excess adiposity. Most of the examination is geared toward identifying sequelae or a rare predisposing condition.

thyrotropin to screen for hypothyroidism. Individuals older than 40 years or with a family history of type 2 diabetes should be screened with a blood glucose test.

Imaging Studies

Although useful in research, imaging studies are not currently used to assess obesity.

 DIFFERENTIAL DIAGNOSIS (Table 20–5)

 THERAPY

General Guidelines

Successful weight loss requires hard work and a long-term commitment to changing behaviors. Obesity develops gradually, and no short-term approaches to the problem are effective. A realistic initial weight-loss goal is a **10% decrease in body weight over a 6-month period.**

> **NOTE**
>
> A decrease in caloric intake and an increase in physical activity form the foundation for all successful weight-loss approaches.

TABLE 20–5. **Differential Diagnosis of Obesity**

Causes	Possible diagnoses
Endocrine	Cushing's syndrome
	Hypogonadism
	Hypopituitarism
	Hypothyroidism
	Insulinoma
Environmental	Physical inactivity
	High caloric intake
	Poor diet patterns
Genetic	Inherited predisposition
	Rare genetic syndrome
Hypothalamic disorders	Increased intracranial pressure
	Trauma
	Tumor
Iatrogenic	Antidepressants
	Antipsychotics
	Corticosteroids
	Hormone therapy
	Valproic acid
Psychologic	Anxiety
	Depression

Many individuals find that their weight hits a **plateau** after a period of successful weight loss. If a plateau lasts for 3 weeks, the patient needs to either focus on weight maintenance or make further modifications to their diet and activity patterns.

Even without weight loss, improvements in diet and activity levels can arrest further weight gain and change body composition by increasing lean muscle mass. Increased energy, enhanced muscle strength, and changes in cardiovascular risk factors may serve as tangible rewards by which to measure success. Point out these changes to help patients redirect their focus away from appearance and toward improved health.

Contraindications to weight loss

Although weight loss is generally a benign process, it is sometimes inadvisable. Individuals with uncontrolled or unstable major illnesses should not engage in a calorie-restricted weight-loss program until their condition improves. Individuals who are severely obese, have eating disorders, or have serious medical problems should only attempt weight loss with supervision.

Side effects of weight loss

Fatigue, constipation or diarrhea, hair loss, and cold intolerance can be annoying side effects of caloric restriction and the weight-loss process. Fortunately, these symptoms are usually transient and well tolerated. The risk of nutritional deficiencies can be minimized with a carefully constructed diet and the use of vitamin and mineral supplements.

Cholecystitis can be a potentially serious complication of weight loss. Individuals on severely reduced-calorie diets (i.e., less than 1000 calories each day) and other high-risk individuals (e.g., diabetics) should be monitored carefully or treated prophylactically with ursodeoxycholic acid.

> **NOTE**
>
> The risk of gallstones is markedly increased when the rate of weight loss exceeds 1.5 kg (3.3 lb) a week.

Nonpharmacologic Therapy

Diet

A diet that will support both initial weight loss and long-term maintenance must include:

- Caloric restriction
- Balance (i.e., a mix of protein, carbohydrates, and fats)
- Ample fruits, vegetables, and high fiber foods
- Sufficient appeal to promote adherence
- Opportunity to learn about healthy meal preparation and how to make healthy choices when dining out
- Guiding principles that can be readily transferred to everyday living

Calories

A low-calorie diet (LCD) is most frequently recommended for weight loss and consists of 1000 to 1500 calories each day. This should generate a 500- to 1000-calorie deficit relative to energy needs and an average of an 8.5-kg (18.5-lb) weight loss over 20 weeks. Many commercial weight-loss programs teach how to prepare balanced reduced-calorie meals. Other programs actually sell the foods needed to implement an LCD. The latter method, while easier in the short term, is expensive and does not generally promote self-sufficiency.

Very-low-calorie diets (VLCDs) consist of 600 to 800 calories each day. The classic VLCD consists of a liquid beverage consumed for several weeks followed by a gradual reintroduction of solid foods. The typical weight loss attained with VLCDs is 10 to 20 kg (22 to 44 lb) over 12 to 16 weeks. Because VLCDs are so restrictive, a physician must prescribe and supervise patients to ensure adequate nutrition and to monitor for potential complications (e.g., dehydration, electrolyte imbalances). VLCDs are difficult to adhere to and usually require the use of appetite suppressants. Although individuals on VLCDs lose weight faster than individuals on LCDs, **after 1 year there is minimal difference in the amount of weight loss maintained between the two groups.** VLCDs are best reserved for individuals who need to lose weight rapidly (e.g., persons with sleep apnea).

Fat, carbohydrates, and protein

The National Institutes of Health is funding a comparison of low-fat versus low-carbohydrate diets to help clarify how they compare.

During the past 20 years, most obesity experts and organizations have advocated a **low-fat, reduced-calorie diet as the best choice for weight loss.** Because a given weight of fat contains more calories (9 cal/g) than an equal portion of carbohydrate or protein (4 cal/g), low-fat diets usually allow consumption of a larger volume of food and result in more visually appealing and filling meals. This is especially true when fat is replaced with complex carbohydrates (e.g., whole grains, sweet potatoes, brown rice) that are high in fiber. A reduction in hydrogenated saturated fats also seems to help lower low-density lipoprotein.

In some individuals, triglycerides will increase and high-density lipoprotein will decrease on a low-fat, high-carbohydrate diet. Such patients may benefit from replacement of some carbohydrates with monounsaturated fats (e.g., olive oil, canola oil).

Many popular books (e.g., Sugar Busters, Dr. Atkins' Diet Revolution) espouse a **very-low-carbohydrate diet.** The diuresis induced by low carbohydrate reserves results in rapid weight loss initially (i.e., during the first week). When carbohydrate levels are very restricted, the body develops a state of ketosis that the authors believe suppresses appetite. Although well tolerated by many individuals, ketosis can result in fatigue, impaired thinking, or hypotension.

Adequate protein is essential during weight loss to prevent excessive nitrogen imbalance and lean muscle loss. A prudent weight-loss diet should provide a minimum of 60 g of protein each day.

Individuals consuming less than 1200 calories each day will have difficulty meeting their micronutrient requirements solely through diet and should probably take a **vitamin and mineral supplement.**

Fad diets

Many diets featured in popular magazines (e.g., the grapefruit diet) produce short-term weight loss. However, fad diets often restrict the types of foods that can be eaten and can quickly become monotonous. In addition, diets that advocate the complete elimination of certain types of foods usually fail to provide the minimum amounts of nutrients that the body needs.

Exercise

Exercise is a critical part of a sensible weight-loss regimen. Individuals trying to lose weight should exercise a minimum of 30 to 45 minutes five times a week. High-intensity exercise regimens appear to be more effective than mildly to moderately intense activities for both weight loss and reduction of cardiovascular risk factors. An ideal exercise program should include both an aerobic component and a muscle-building program.

The aerobic component enhances energy expenditure and promotes cardiovascular fitness. Warm ups, cool downs, and stretching should be incorporated into moderately high-intensity activities.

> ## NOTE
>
> Brisk walking is a good exercise for weight loss and is an excellent method for preventing osteoporosis.

Increasing muscle can help negate the decrease in basal metabolic rate that occurs during caloric restriction. Weight lifting and muscle-building activities are essential for maintaining muscle mass during weight loss. This type of exercise can be done with fancy equipment at the gym or with household items or resistance bands at home.

An exercise regimen can and should be fun. Individuals who enjoy their exercise sessions are more likely to keep them in their busy schedules. Organized sports (e.g., tennis, basketball) provide opportunities for social interaction as well as for enhancement of physical health. Activities performed around the house (e.g., mowing the lawn) can constitute important forms of exercise and provide lifestyle enhancements. In addition, "step-losing" activities (e.g., taking the stairs, parking far away and walking) can enhance the energy expenditure of daily activities.

Many organizations (e.g., American College of Sports Medicine) advocate a cardiovascular health assessment for patients older than 40 and younger patients with diabetes or hypertension before starting an exercise program. An additional examination is not needed, however, if the patient has already received one during maintenance checkups or office visits.

Behavior modification

Diet and exercise regimens for weight loss are usually most effective when paired with a behavior modification program. Your preceptor may teach behavior modification and reinforce it in the office, but the most popular method is through the use of a group-based weight-loss program. Many of these programs use regular meetings, weekly weigh-ins, and support groups in an effort to help patients remain compliant.

Programs that teach techniques for changing behavior have higher retention rates and increased weight loss. Behavioral strategies that have been most effective include the following:

- Promoting self-monitoring of food intake and exercise
- Teaching participants to recognize triggers leading to unhealthy eating
- Imparting stress management skills

Implementing behavioral techniques is also important during weight maintenance. People who participate in a formal weight-maintenance program after successful weight loss tend to have better outcomes.

Surgery

When traditional weight-loss methods fail, surgery may be an option. Surgery is most appropriate for severely obese individuals and those who have major obesity-related medical consequences. Surgical interventions essentially force individuals to restrict their caloric intake by limiting their tolerance to excess food consumption or decreasing the body's ability to absorb nutrients.

Individuals who undergo surgery lose substantial amounts of weight, especially during the first year after surgery. This may be lifesaving for individuals with sleep apnea or poorly controlled diabetes. Weight rebound often occurs after 1 or 2 years but is usually considerably less than that seen with diet and exercise alone.

Although effective at producing weight loss, surgery is not harmless. Serious complications occasionally occur. The forced semistarvation can be very frustrating for some patients. In addition, excessive weight loss and serious nutritional deficiencies can result and require screening. Because of these adverse effects, a portion of patients who have undergone surgery will seek a reversal.

Gastroplasty

In the past, gastroplasty (i.e., "stomach stapling") was a popular surgical treatment. Gastroplasty reduced the size of the stomach cavity, making it difficult to consume usual quantities of food. Unfortunately, many individuals learn to bypass the effect of this surgery by consuming energy-dense liquids and soft foods.

Roux-en-Y gastric bypass

A more aggressive surgical intervention is the Roux-en-Y gastric bypass that combines gastroplasty with bypass of a portion of the intestines. The resulting shortened gut cannot completely absorb the nutrients to which it is exposed, resulting in malabsorption. Patients who overeat experience unpleasant gastrointestinal side effects that further reinforce dietary compliance.

Pharmacotherapy

Over-the-counter (OTC) medications

A few OTC products are beneficial in promoting weight loss; however, most have little or no value. Because the dietary supplement industry is minimally regulated, the quality of OTC products is highly variable. Misleading claims are common.

Drugs scientifically proven to be effective for weight loss

Sympathomimetics, whether synthesized (e.g., decongestant medications) or found naturally in herbs (see Complementary/Alternative Med-

ICINE; p 281), can facilitate weight loss; however, they are potentially dangerous at high doses. Sympathomimetic agents may cause a small increase in metabolic rate, but they can also elevate blood pressure and heart rate, act as central nervous system stimulants in some people, and/or cause a hypertensive crisis. These risks are enhanced when drugs are combined with caffeine. Sympathomimetics are commonly used in nonprescription appetite suppressants. Their effect on appetite is not usually sustained with continued use.

Drugs with no proven benefit for weight loss

Chromium picolinate is marketed as a "fat burner" and is frequently found in diet pills, vitamin supplements, and beverages.

Theophylline creams, OTC products that claim to erase subcutaneous fat (i.e., cellulite) from the thighs, can be absorbed and cause systemic effects.

Syrup of ipecac and laxatives are widely used by people with eating disorders to "purge" the body of unwanted calories. These products can cause serious medical problems.

Prescription medications

Although pharmaceuticals can be useful adjuncts to weight loss, they generally yield little more than a 5- to 8-kg (11- to 17.6-lb) weight loss above what would be expected with diet and exercise alone. In addition, the gains achieved with these drugs are often lost after discontinuation.

Prescription medications should be reserved for individuals with a BMI greater than 30 kg/m² and individuals with a BMI greater than 27 kg/m² with obesity-related medical conditions. When drug therapy is used, it should be **a supplement to, not a substitute for,** a comprehensive weight-loss approach that emphasizes long-term changes in diet, activity, and behavior.

> **NOTE**
>
> Individuals who have not made significant lifestyle changes will experience a weight rebound after stopping prescription weight-loss drugs.

Appetite suppressants

Several medications are currently available that act as appetite suppressants by increasing catecholamines or serotonin neurotransmitters involved in appetite regulation.

Sibutramine, a serotonergic drug, was released in 1998. It is the only appetite suppressant with FDA approval for long-term use. Sibutramine frequently causes a dose-related increase in blood pressure and heart rate in some individuals. Therefore, blood pressure needs to be closely monitored when sibutramine is initiated. This drug is contraindicated in individuals with heart disease and uncontrolled hypertension.

Selective serotonin reuptake inhibitors (e.g., fluoxetine) have anorectic effects for some individuals, especially early in therapy, but the effect is inconsistent.

Drugs that affect food absorption

Orlistat, the first drug in a new category of weight-loss agents, received FDA approval in 1999. It acts by inhibiting pancreatic lipase and decreasing the gut's ability to digest and absorb fats. In high fat diets, it can also cause unpleasant side effects (e.g., oily diarrhea, fecal incontinence). The use of orlistat may cause impaired absorption of the fat-soluble vitamins A, D, E, and K and β-carotene, so supplements containing these nutrients are indicated if orlistat is prescribed.

 SPECIAL POPULATIONS

Children

Prevention of obesity can be greatly promoted by helping children and adolescents to acquire healthy eating habits and encouraging enjoyable forms of physical activity.

Adolescence is often a time when a preoccupation with weight and appearance results in the development of eating disorders. Youth engaged in sports in which weight is important (e.g., wrestling, dancing, gymnastics) are especially vulnerable.

Excessive caloric and nutrient restriction can adversely affect both current growth and later health (e.g. calcium for bones). Children and adolescents needing weight loss should receive guidance from a physician or dietician.

Seniors

Adults older than 65 years attempting weight loss should do so with supervision to help assure nutrition and health are maintained.

Pregnancy

Weight loss during pregnancy is contraindicated because it may be detrimental to the growing fetus. Obese women may need to be counseled to restrict their weight gain during pregnancy. Caloric restriction during lactation is feasible if the woman follows a balanced diet and milk production remains adequate.

 COMPLEMENTARY/ALTERNATIVE MEDICINE

Ephedrine is a sympathomimetic that occurs naturally in the herb ma huang (*Ephedra sinica*). It is commonly found in diet supplements marketed as "natural products," but like the synthetic compound phenylephrine, it can cause stimulation of the central nervous system, increased blood pressure and heart rate, and slightly increased metabolic rate.

◆▶ CONSULTS

- **Dieticians** can be of great value in educating patients about an appropriate weight-loss diet.
- **Wellness programs,** especially those that are employer-driven, often incorporate weight-control interventions.
- **Weight loss centers** can be helpful, but their quality and safety can be highly variable.
- **Group support programs** (e.g., Overeaters Anonymous) can be helpful for many patients.
- **Local exercise programs** (e.g., YWCA/YMCA), can be an important referral for many patients.

CHAPTER **21**

Otitis Media and Otitis Externa

Jeff Kirschman

OBJECTIVES

- Describe the common presentations of otitis media and otitis externa
- Evaluate the external ear, ear canal, and tympanic membrane
- Describe the appearance of the tympanic membrane in states of sickness and health
- Explain treatment protocols for common ear problems and prophylactic therapy to prevent recurrent otitis

 INTRODUCTION

Ear infections can be extremely painful. Otalgia is a common reason for children and adults to seek medical care and often leads to the administration of antibiotics. Accurate diagnosis of otalgia is essential to ensure proper treatment and prevent the overuse of antibiotics.

TERMINOLOGY

Acute mastoiditis: a bacterial infection in the mastoid process resulting in the coalescence of the mastoid air cells

Acute otitis media: the presence of fluid in the middle ear accompanied by signs and symptoms of a rapidly developing (within a few days), acute, painful, local or systemic illness (e.g., bulging tympanic membrane with otalgia, perforated tympanic membrane with purulent material)

Auricle: the largely cartilaginous projecting portion of the external ear; the outer ear

Bulging tympanic membrane: the term used to describe the appearance of the tympanic membrane under positive pressure

Chronic otitis media: permanent perforation of the tympanic membrane, with or without drainage

Chronic otitis media with effusion: otitis media with effusion that lasts more than 2 to 3 months

Conductive hearing loss: hearing loss resulting from abnormalities of the external or middle ear

Eustachian tube: the tube that connects the middle ear with the nasopharynx, equalizing the air pressure on both sides of the tympanic membrane

Eustachian tube dysfunction: refers to the inability of the eustachian tube to equalize pressure and drain middle ear effusion effectively

Landmarks: distinct visual markings associated with the tympanic membrane in healthy ears

Light reflex: reflection of light by a healthy tympanic membrane, generally seen in the anteroinferior aspect of the tympanic membrane

Mastoiditis: inflammation of the mastoid anthem and air cells

Middle ear effusion: fluid in the middle ear space from any cause

Myringitis: erythema of the tympanic membrane without middle ear effusion

Osteomyelitis: an infectious inflammatory disease of bone

Otalgia: pain or ache in the ear

Otitis externa: inflammation limited to the external ear and ear canal, generally caused by infection

Otitis media: inflammation of the middle ear

Otitis media with effusion: the presence of fluid in the middle ear in the absence of signs or symptoms of an acute local or systemic illness

Otorrhea: discharge from the external ear

Pinna: see *auricle*

Recurrent otitis media: quantitatively, three or more episodes of acute otitis media in 6 months or four episodes in 12 months

Sensorineural hearing loss: loss of hearing caused by damage in the inner ear or damage to the eighth cranial nerve

Serous otitis media: see *otitis media with effusion*

Swimmer's ear: otitis externa caused by water getting trapped in the ear canal and setting up an environment conducive to bacterial and fungal overgrowth

Tympanostomy tube (ventilating or pressure equalization tube): a manufactured tube that can be placed into (through) the tympanic membrane to maintain an opening between the middle ear and external ear

◆ BACKGROUND

There were an estimated 22.7 million ambulatory visits for otitis media and 4.7 million for otitis externa in 1996, the vast majority of cases occurring in children. Most children experience at least one episode of otitis media before first grade. The eustachian tube of young children is short, straight, and horizontal; it becomes longer, curved, and tilted as the child grows. This anatomic difference, along with lack of acquired antibody resistance, appears to be a major reason why otitis is most common in small children.

The placement of ventilating tubes for prophylaxis of recurrent otitis media is the second most common operation performed on children (circumcision is first).

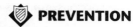 **PREVENTION**

Primary Prevention

Otitis media

In children, exposure to the following environmental risk factors may increase the chances of developing acute otitis media or otitis media with effusion:

- Bottle-feeding (especially if supine)
- Passive smoke exposure
- Group child-care facility attendance

In adults, smoking cessation, early treatment of rhinitis, and decreasing exposure to respiratory irritants aid the primary prevention of otitis media.

Otitis externa

Primary prevention of otitis externa requires that the patient avoid both swimming in areas with high bacterial counts and putting instrumentation (e.g., keys, cotton swabs) in the ears. In addition, the regular use of two to three medicated eardrops after swimming, bathing, or showering can help. Over-the-counter eardrops labeled for this purpose, homemade eardrops (i.e., 50% white vinegar and 50% rubbing alcohol), and prescription eardrops (e.g., acetic acid plus Burow's Solution) can all be used.

Secondary Prevention

Secondary problems related to otitis are rare and include epidural abscess, mastoiditis, meningitis, and temporal bone osteomyelitis. Generally, prompt appropriate treatment of otitis prevents all of these severe complications.

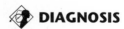 **DIAGNOSIS**

Presentation

"My ear hurts" and "I think I must have an ear infection" are common complaints when adolescent or adult patients present with otitis media or otitis externa. An infant with general fussiness and a high fever is also a presentation that may indicate otitis media or otitis externa.

History

History of present illness

- How long have you been experiencing symptoms?
  - □ Acute otitis media is characterized by recent onset of symptoms.

□ Chronic otitis media is characterized by the presence of symptoms for more than 6 weeks.
- Are you experiencing any respiratory symptoms?
  - □ A concurrent upper respiratory infection is often in the history of otitis media.
- Do you have any ear pain?
  - □ Ear pain in children with upper respiratory infections is likely caused by acute otitis media or otitis externa.
  - □ A red tympanic membrane and a history of intermittent purulence but no pain most likely indicates chronic otitis media.
- Does your child often pull at his or her ear?
  - □ Ear pulling is noted in many children with acute otitis media.
  - □ However, in several studies, less than half of all children tugging at their ears were found to have acute otitis media. Many were simply teething.
- Have you noticed any loss of hearing?
  - □ Hearing loss is associated with chronic serous otitis media.
- Does your ear itch?
  - □ Pruritus in the ear canal suggests a fungal infection, eczema, or another dermatologic disorder.
- Do you have any discharge from your ear?
  - □ Otorrhea is usually associated with otitis externa.
  - □ Clear, mucoid discharge may be associated with otitis media.
  - □ Purulent discharge may be associated with either otitis externa or otitis media.
- Have you recently been swimming, experienced trauma to your ear, or been around someone with an ear infection?
  - □ Related exposures for a history of otitis externa include water (e.g., swimmer's ear) and trauma (e.g., cotton swabs, keys, paper clips).
  - □ Related exposures for a history of otitis media include attendance at day-care or school and exposure to others with ear infections.

Past medical history

- Is there a history of many ear or upper respiratory infections?
- Do you have allergies?

Family history

- Are there any siblings with a history of ear infections or upper respiratory illnesses?

Social history

- Is your child bottle-fed while in a supine position?
- Do you smoke, or are you (or your child) exposed to second-hand smoke?

- Does your child attend day-care or school?
- Do you work in a humid or wet environment?

Review of Systems

Table 21–1 outlines the common findings and diagnoses when reviewing the systems in a patient who presents with the chief complaint of ear pain.

In addition to the possible diagnoses mentioned in Table 21–1, when performing the review of systems also focus on **malignant otitis externa.** Malignant otitis externa is a serious infection that is most common in older patients with diabetes and persons with AIDS. It is caused by *Pseudomonas aeruginosa* and is characterized by a persistent, severe earache with a foul-smelling, purulent otorrhea. Malignant otitis externa can lead to conductive hearing loss and facial nerve paralysis from osteomyelitis.

TABLE 21–1. **Review of Systems in the Diagnosis of Otitis Media and Otitis Externa: Pertinent Positives with Ear Pain**

System	Common Patient Complaints	Associated Diagnosis
Constitutional	General malaise	URI
	Fever	AOM
Dermatologic	Rash	OM or AOM with viral or streptococcal infection
HEENT	Headache	URI, meningitis
	Conjunctivitis	URI, allergies
	Hearing loss	Chronic OME
	Pain on outside of ear	OE
	"Popping" ears	OME
	Ear drainage	OE, perforation of tympanic membrane, or OM*
	Nasal congestion and drainage	URI, allergies
	Pain in the lower jaw or toothache	Dental abscess
Respiratory	Cough and congestion	URI
Gastrointestinal	Diarrhea	Viral illness
Musculoskeletal	General myalgias	Viral illness
Neurologic	Stiff neck	Meningitis (rare), viral myalgia

AOM = acute otitis media; OE = otitis externa; OM = otitis media; OME = otitis media with effusion; URI = upper respiratory infection.
*The characteristics of the discharge help determine the diagnosis. Otitis externa is associated with a thick, white discharge; a perforated tympanic membrane is associated with a clear, mucoid discharge; and otitis media is associated with discharge that is clear, thin, and barely visible.

Physical Examination

Examination of the external ear (Figure 21–1)

Visually assess the meatus for otorrhea, erythema, and surrounding skin changes.

Gently palpate the auricle and the lobe. Movement of the auricle or lobe resulting in pain without another visible source of pain (e.g., a cyst) is usually otitis externa.

Examination of the ear canal (see Figure 21–1)

Assess for the presence of otorrhea, cerumen, erythema, flaky eczematous lesions, mechanically induced scratches (e.g., from cotton swabs), edema, maceration, granulation tissue (malignant otitis), and debris (e.g., foreign bodies, sloughed keratin).

The odor and color of the otorrhea can aid in diagnosis.

- **Foul odor** often indicates otitis externa and may rarely indicate bone destruction.
- **Yellow otorrhea** almost always indicates infection.
- **White otorrhea** suggests a fungal or dermatologic condition, although otorrhea from a fungal condition can be yellow.
- A **clear, mucoid discharge** can be seen with otitis media.
- A **clear, thin discharge** can be seen with otitis media (usually quite scant) and, extremely rarely, with a leak of cerebrospinal fluid.
- **Bloody otorrhea** is generally associated with tympanic membrane perforation, trauma, or chronic infection with granulation.

Examination of the tympanic membrane

Clearing the view

If otorrhea or debris is present and obscuring the tympanic membrane, removal may be necessary for appropriate evaluation. If this is difficult because of pain from otitis externa, it may be possible to anesthetize the canal for several minutes with three to four drops of *ophthalmic* tetracaine. Cerumen often can be removed with the use of a cerumen loop or hook. However, **do not attempt this without specific permission from your preceptor.** Some clinicians do not use a cerumen loop or strong water irrigation until they have appreciated a full view of the tympanic membrane because of the possibility of tympanic membrane perforation.

Assessing the tympanic membrane

Once there is a clear view of the canal, note the position of landmarks, color, retraction, translucency, and mobility of the tympanic membrane. Keep in mind that crying (as seen with small children) can make the tympanic membrane bright red without the presence of a disease process.

A healthy tympanic membrane is translucent, without color or effusion, has visible landmarks with a bright light reflex (Figure 21–2), and is mo-

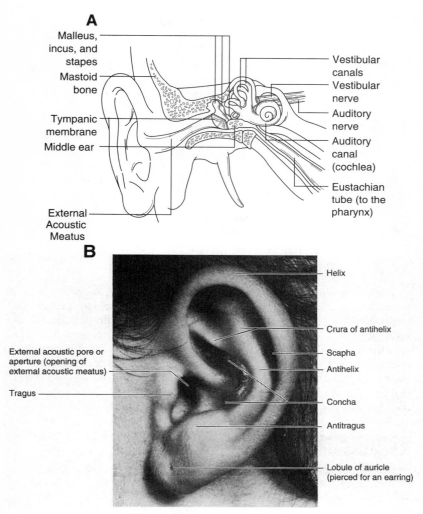

FIGURE 21–1. Anatomy of the ear.

bile. Mobility of the tympanic membrane is assessed using pneumatic otoscopy. When using a pneumatic otoscope, an airtight seal is necessary, and pressure should be supplied gently through a flexible tube attached to a rubber bulb. The examiner's mouth may supply the necessary force; however, one must be careful not to apply excess air pressure.

In otitis media with effusion, the tympanic membrane may be hyperemic over just the landmarks, and you may see the shadows of small air bubbles behind the membrane. In otitis media, the tympanic membrane is often hyperemic on the entire tympanic membrane. Other findings in otitis media can include bulging of the tympanic membrane, indistinct landmarks, diminished light reflex, and limited mobility on pneumatic otoscope insufflation.

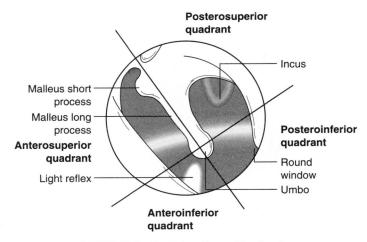

FIGURE 21-2. The light reflex and landmarks.

Further testing may include tympanometry. This procedure uses a sound source and microphone placed within the ear canal to measure the impedence (or pressure) within the middle ear. Depending on the disease state, the pressure will be increased or decreased. In patients with middle ear effusions, a flat pressure tympanogram will be generated because the pressure within the middle ear is relatively negative in comparison with the pressure within the ear canal. Tympanometry may be used to screen children for middle ear effusions when suspected, but it is not recommended as a general preventive screen.

NOTE

An erythematous tympanic membrane alone does not establish a diagnosis of otitis.

Hearing assessment

A simple office hearing evaluation with an audioscope is commonly performed if otitis media with effusion has been present for more than 2 months or if the patient or caretaker complains of decreased hearing and the canal is not completely obscured with debris.

NOTE

The tympanic membrane must be completely obscured to affect hearing clinically. Even a 0.5 mm passageway will allow the transmittal of sound waves.

If a hearing deficit is found in a small child, refer the child to an audiologist for a hearing evaluation. However, if a hearing deficit is found in an adult, perform a tuning fork examination in the office.

Rinne's test compares air conduction to bone conduction. Place a vibrating 512 Hz tuning fork on the mastoid bone until the patient no longer perceives the sound. Then place the vibrating fork next to the same ear, a few centimeters from the meatus. If bone conduction (i.e., on the mastoid bone) is better than air conduction (i.e., next to the ear), there is probably a conductive hearing loss.

Weber's test helps discern between sensorineural and conductive hearing loss when an asymmetrical hearing deficit is verified. Place a vibrating 256 Hz tuning fork on the midline of the head. If the tone is louder in the affected ear, there is a conductive hearing loss. If the tone is louder in the unaffected ear, there is most likely a sensorineural hearing loss.

Laboratory Tests

Consider checking a slide smear for fungi, and obtaining fungal and bacterial cultures of the otorrhea in cases of otitis externa that are refractory to initial trails of therapy.

Imaging Studies

A **computed tomography scan of the temporal bone** should be done if malignant otitis externa is suspected. However, because a patient with malignant otitis externa should be referred as soon as possible to a specialist, it may be best to speak with the consultant first.

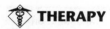 THERAPY

Nonpharmacologic Therapy

Resting on a **heating pad or hot water bottle** can give temporary pain relief for many cases of otitis media, but the heating pad should be used in only a monitored fashion.

Many clinicians instruct the patient to hold his nose so that air cannot leave the nostrils, then attempt to blow out through his nose. This maneuver increases pressure in the middle ear, which may help reposition a retracted tympanic membrane or displace some fluid in otitis media with effusion. However, because acute otitis media is associated with reflux, aspiration, and insufflation of nasopharyngeal bacteria through the eustachian tube into the middle ear, some clinicians feel this maneuver is contraindicated.

Pharmacotherapy

Otitis externa

The canal must be clear for medication to be fully effective. If removal of debris is not possible because of pain or swelling of the external canal, a wick will help facilitate removal of debris and medication placement where it is needed (i.e., the lining of the canal).

1. Place an ear wick in the canal.
2. Instill four or five drops of polymyxin B and neomycin otic suspension or a drying, acidic agent (for nonfungal infections) by moistening the wick every 4 hours.
3. Schedule the patient for a follow-up visit in 3 to 5 days for clearing of the external canal.

Ototopical medications (Table 21–2) include suspensions and alcohol-based solutions. Suspensions tend to stay in the ear longer because of their increased viscosity and are much less likely to be a problem if the tympanic membrane is perforated because they contain no alcohol. Solutions are appropriate for narrowed canals and ear wicks.

Ototopical antibiotics are most commonly "otic" preparations, but "ophthalmic" solutions are sometimes used as well. Both preparations generally include steroids to decrease the edema and inflammation of the canal. Suggested first-line therapy is outlined in Table 21–3.

If fungus is clearly identified and the infection has responded poorly to otic-specific solutions, some clinicians use antifungals such as clotrimazole 1% solution or gentian violet (2% in 95% alcohol).

Initially treat pain with acetaminophen or ibuprofen. If these medications do not control the pain, some physicians may prescribe a few days

TABLE 21–2. **Antimicrobial Coverage of Therapeutic Solutions for Otitis Externa**

Antibiotic	ST	PS	PR	AS and CA	EC	Inflammation
Ofloxacin	x	x				
Ciprofloxacin	x	x			x	x (when used with hydrocortisone)
Polymyxin B with neomycin sulfate and hydrocortisone	x	x	x			x
Gentamicin	x					
Tobramycin with dexamethasone	x	x	x			x
Clotrimazole and acetic acid (2%) and either aluminum acetate or propylene glycol diacetate (3%)				x	x	x (when used with hydrocortisone)

AS = *Aspergillus* species; CA = *Candida* species; EC = *Escherichia coli*; PR = *Proteus vulgaris*; PS = *Pseudomonas aeruginosa*; ST = *Staphylococcus aureus*.

TABLE 21–3. First-Line Therapy in the Treatment of Otitis Externa

Drug	Age-Group	Dose
Ciprofloxacin (2 mg) + hydrocortisone (10 mg/ml)	> 1 year	3 drops bid for 7 days
Polymyxin (10,000 units/ml), neomycin (0.35%), and hydrocortisone (1%)*	> 2 years	4 drops tid/qid for 10 days
Ofloxacin otic solution†	> 12 years	10 drops bid for 10 days
	1–12 years	5 drops bid for 10 days

bid = twice a day; qid = four times daily; tid = three times a day.
*Use suspension if the tympanic membrane is perforated.
†Although ofloxacin otic is a solution, it can be used in patients with a perforated tympanic membrane.

of using codeine or hydrocodone compounds. Patients requesting more pain medication should be evaluated for possible extension of the disease.

Otitis media with effusion

NOTE

Persistent otitis media with effusion after therapy for acute otitis media is expected and does not warrant repeated treatment.

If the otitis media with effusion persists after 3 months, a trial of antimicrobial therapy may be helpful (i.e., some indication that it may be helpful, but little good data). For adults, consider the addition of a short course of prednisone therapy for 7 days.

Acute otitis media (Figure 21–3)

NOTE

As many as 80% of cases of acute otitis media will resolve spontaneously, without antibiotics, within 2 weeks.

Short-course (5 day) antibiotic therapy for acute otitis media is acceptable if:

- Two years of age or older
- No perforation
- No chronic or recurrent acute otitis media

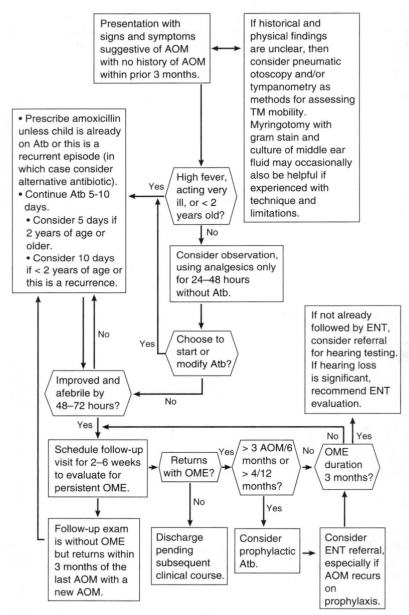

FIGURE 21–3. Management of a child 2 months to 6 years of age with signs and symptoms of a sporadic episode of acute otitis media. *AOM* = acute otitis media; *Atb* = antibiotics; *ENT* = ear, nose, and throat; *OME* = otitis media with effusion; *TM* = tympanic membrane. (Reprinted with permission from Cincinnati Children's Hospital Medical Center: *Evidence Based Clinical Practice Guideline for Medical Management of Otitis Media in Children 2 Months to 5 Years of Age.* Copyright ©1998. All rights reserved.)

- No craniofacial abnormalities
- No immunocompromised condition

Some clinicians choose to recheck the ears in 2 weeks. Recent evidence suggests that a 6-week evaluation period rather than the traditional 2 weeks decreases the necessity of retreating acute otitis media without increasing the risk.

Use **antibiotics** judiciously. The antibiotics commonly used for the initial treatment of acute otitis media are listed in Table 21–4. If the patient does not respond to initial therapy within 24 to 72 hours, consider switching to a different limited-spectrum antibiotic or to a broader-spectrum antibiotic (e.g., amoxicillin and clavulanate, azithromycin). If the patient does not respond after two to three full courses of antibiotics, consider evaluation by an otolaryngologist for myringotomy or tympanocentesis to isolate the pathogen and drain the infection.

Cases of acute otitis media that occur more than 3 months after the first infection can be treated as first-time infections. In cases that occur within 3 months of the first infection, use of a broader-spectrum antibiotic is recommended.

Prophylaxis with antibiotics is controversial and, if used, should be reserved for control of recurrent acute otitis media (three or more well documented episodes in 6 months or four episodes in 12 months). Amoxicillin or sulfisoxazole can be prescribed once a day for 3 to 6 months.

TABLE 21–4. **Antibiotics Used in the Treatment of Acute Otitis Media**

Antibiotic	Dose	Relative cost
Amoxicillin	80–90 mg/kg divided bid or tid for 5–7 days	Least expensive
Erythromycin-sulfisoxazole*	50 mg erythromycin/kg/day divided qid for 10 days[†]	Twice the cost of amoxicillin
Trimethoprim-sulfamethoxazole	4 mg/kg trimethoprim and 20 mg/kg sulfamethoxazole bid for 10 days or 8 mg/kg trimethoprim and 40 mg/kg sulfamethoxazole bid	Four times the cost of amoxicillin
Cephalosporins and macrolides (e.g., azithromycin, clarithromycin)[‡]	Variable	Seven to eight times the cost of amoxicillin

bid = twice a day; qid = four times daily; tid = three times a day.
*Erythromycin-sulfisoxazole is only indicated for microbes seen in children.
[†]The suspension is 200 mg of erythromycin/5 ml.
[‡]Cephalosporins and macrolides should be reserved for individuals who are allergic to the other antibiotics listed.

Treatment of pain is usually accomplished with acetaminophen or ibuprofen. Narcotics (e.g., codeine) may rarely be required for more advanced cases. If the tympanic membrane is intact, local anesthesia can be accomplished with the use of topical eardrops containing benzocaine, glycerine, and antipyrine.

 ## URGENCIES AND EMERGENCIES

Patients with progressive external ear infections should be evaluated in the office. If malignant otitis externa is suspected, a consult should be strongly considered.

Consider **cellulitis, perichondritis,** or **parotitis** in patients with complaints of increasing pain, drainage, and fever after 24 to 48 hours of antibiotic therapy. Such cases require urgent referral to an otolaryngologist for an evaluation.

In cases of acute **tympanic membrane perforation** from barotrauma or foreign body, have the patient evaluated that day. Patients with perforation should be started on amoxicillin (or other appropriate antibiotic) to prevent infection. Have the patient keep the ear dry. Follow up within 2 weeks and then again in 2 months. In patients without spontaneous closure, referral to an otolaryngologist is warranted.

 ## SPECIAL POPULATIONS

Children

Tympanostomy tubes are either short-term tubes (i.e., 8 to 15 months) or long-term tubes (i.e., more than 15 months). The tubes are extruded as migrating keratin from the tympanic membrane accumulates between the surface epithelium and the outer flange of the tube. Another cause of extrusion is too much pressure in the middle ear, especially if the tube's opening is clogged because of dried drainage.

Otorrhea with tympanostomy tubes

Between 10% and 30% of children with tympanostomy tubes have at least one episode of acute otorrhea. When it is associated with an upper respiratory infection, an oral antibiotic with β-lactamase coverage usually is administered. If the otorrhea is unresponsive to initial therapy within 3 to 5 days, the likelihood of infection with *P. aeruginosa* or *Staphylococcus aureus* is increased, and the patient should be started on appropriate ototopical drops. Similarly, if the otorrhea developed after exposure to water (e.g., swimming in a lake), the patient should be started on ototopical therapy. The patient may still be allowed to swim; however, while being treated, the patient should not dive.

NOTE

With tympanostomy tubes, the use of a suspension, rather than a solution, is highly recommended.

Seniors

Among this age group, impacted cerumen frequently causes hearing loss.

Pregnancy

Many antibiotics (e.g., trimethoprim-sulfamethoxazole) are contraindicated during pregnancy, although the topical agents are generally regarded as safe in pregnant women.

 COMPLEMENTARY/ALTERNATIVE MEDICINE (See Chapter 8; COMPLEMENTARY/ALTERNATIVE MEDICINE, p 92)

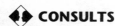 **CONSULTS**

Otolaryngologist

Otitis externa

Consider consulting with an otolaryngologist if granulation bodies or other masses are seen in the external ear canal or on the tympanic membrane, when foreign bodies cannot be removed by simple manipulation or flushing, if persistent drainage is unresponsive to medical therapy, or for continued excessive pain. Biopsy of the ear canal is often necessary to differentiate the granulation tissue typical of malignant otitis externa from a malignant neoplasm.

Acute otitis media

In cases of acute otitis media, consultation with an otolaryngologist should be considered if:

- Persistent effusion has been present for 3 months or more and is accompanied by documented hearing loss.
- Otorrhea is unresponsive to therapy within 2 weeks, including ototopical drops for *P. aeruginosa* or *S. aureus*.
- There is complete ear canal stenosis (i.e., possible malignant infection).

- There is a persistent perforation after 2 months or evidence of persistent hearing loss following a closed perforation.

Audiologist

A full audiological evaluation should be ordered if an office screen shows abnormal hearing or effusion persists for more than 4 months. The ears should be cleared of debris before testing.

Speech and Language Specialist

A speech and language specialist should be considered for evidence of speech delay or hearing loss in children or for adults dealing with hearing loss that is not correctable.

CHAPTER 22

Partner Violence

Maria M. Sandvig • Barbara Bowman Tobias • Therese Zink

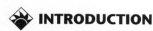 **INTRODUCTION**

Partner violence is a pattern of frightening or intimidating a sexual or intimate partner over time. Partner violence can take many forms and often includes the maintenance of power through financial control and social interactions (Figure 22–1).

OBJECTIVES

- Understand the prevalence of partner violence and its frequency in presentation in the family practice setting
- Identify appropriate and inappropriate screening questions for female victims of partner violence
- List common signs and symptoms associated with adult female victims of partner violence
- Understand the management protocol for adult female patients living in violent homes

The prevalence of violence and abuse in society is a threat to the health of all patients. Partner violence is found in 25% of all couples, including same-sex couples. Family physicians should specifically screen all patients for a history of violence and abuse, especially vulnerable groups (e.g., seniors, children, physically and mentally challenged individuals).

Although female-on-male, female-on-female, and male-on-male partner violence occurs frequently, the United States Department of Justice reports that more than 95% of the time, the victim in partner violence between a man and woman is female. Research also suggests that each year in the United States:

- Between 11% and 22% of women screened in primary care clinics are physically abused by their partners
- An estimated 1 to 4 million women are assaulted by a male partner
- More than 50% of all women murdered are killed by a current or former partner

This chapter focuses on the recognition and management of intimate partner violence against women by men; however, the information can assist your assessment and management of all cases of partner violence.

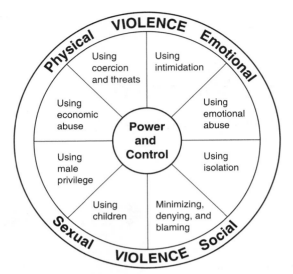

Using coercion and threats
• Making and/or carrying out threats to do something to hurt her
• Threatening to leave her, to commit suicide, to report her to welfare
• Making her drop charges
• Making her do illegal things

Using economic abuse
• Preventing her from getting or keeping a job
• Making her ask for money
• Giving her an allowance
• Taking her money
• Not letting her know about or have access to family income

Using male privilege
• Treating her like a servant
• Making all the big decisions
• Acting like the "master of the castle"
• Being the one to define men's and women's roles

Using children
• Making her feel guilty about the children
• Using the children to relay messages
• Using visitation to harass her
• Threatening to take the children away

Using intimidation
• Making her afraid by using looks, actions, gestures
• Smashing things
• Destroying her property
• Abusing pets
• Displaying weapons

Using emotional abuse
• Putting her down
• Making her feel bad about herself
• Calling her names
• Making her think she's crazy
• Playing mind games
• Humiliating her
• Making her feel guilty

Using isolation
• Controlling what she does, who she sees and talks to, what she reads, where she goes
• Limiting her outside involvement
• Using jealousy to justify actions

Minimizing, denying, and blaming
• Making light of the abuse and not taking her concerns about it seriously
• Saying the abuse didn't happen
• Shifting responsibility for abusive behavior
• Saying she caused it

FIGURE 22–1. Power and control wheel. (Reprinted with permission from the Domestic Abuse Intervention Project.)

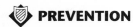 **PREVENTION**

Screening

Prevention of intimate partner violence is a societal challenge. Screening all patients for violence in the home not only raises awareness of the public health risk but can help identify families for early intervention. Usually, it is easiest to inquire about safety issues at home when taking the social history (i.e., questioning about smoking, alcohol, employment, child safety, household membership) [see HISTORY; p 304]. Just as routine questions about a patient's smoking habits identify smoking-related problems and can reinforce a patient's decision not to smoke, routine questions about violence can identify the problems of an abused woman, assess her current safety status, and reinforce her decision to confide in you.

Physicians ask questions about intimate, health-related issues all the time. Try to screen all patients, but do so when they are alone, never in front of their partners and, if acceptable to your preceptor, only cautiously in front of older children. Screening for domestic violence is simply learning to inquire during the social history about another issue that affects health and knowing what to do when you get a positive answer.

Strategies Directed Toward the Abuser

Although the victim may attempt to alter her behavior and lifestyle to please her partner, there is no way the victim can control her partner's behavior. Thus, prevention of abuse and violence must be directed at the abuser.

Conflict management skills; coping strategies; and nonviolent, nonabusive ways of expressing anger and frustration should be modeled in the home, but they can also be learned. Parenting classes and support groups; early childhood development education; and counseling and conflict management skills through schools, social agencies, and religious groups are all part of the current effort to impact violence in the home. Many communities have programs that address these issues. Find out how you and your patients can get in touch with these programs.

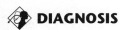 **DIAGNOSIS**

Presentation

Victims of partner violence present in various ways. Physical injuries are often the most obvious. The chronic physical (i.e., somatic) complaints and psychologic symptoms that come from living with the stress of the ongoing abuse are more difficult to identify and are often revealed with routine and universal screening. We have chosen to present several case histories to illustrate key presentations of partner violence.

Case 1: Physical Injuries

A 32-year-old woman presents with a ruptured eardrum. When asked how it happened, she reports that her fiancée boxed her ears during an argument.

Facial injuries (e.g., injuries to the teeth, jaw, eardrum) and central injuries (e.g., injuries to the chest, breasts, abdomen, pelvis, peritoneum) can suggest a screen for partner violence, as can a pattern of injury inconsistent with the patient's history (e.g., burns or bruises in unusual locations, injuries at various stages of healing, human bites, repeated visits for minor trauma, delays seeking therapy for previous assaults).

Case 2: Pregnancy Issues

A 29-year-old registered nurse, pregnant with her first child, has frequent visits for pelvic pain charted. The evaluation is always normal. When your preceptor screens her for abuse, she states that her husband has been forcing her to have intercourse.

Voicing unusually extreme worry about the health of the unborn child can indicate that a screen for partner violence is in order. Screening for partner violence is also suggested if there is a history of inadequate prenatal care, pregnancy complications, substance abuse, or inadequate maternal nutrition.

Case 3: Sexual Problems and Gynecologic Conditions

A 56-year-old woman comes to the office with vaginal complaints. She has a history of vaginitis with a negative evaluation and is on hormone replacement therapy. When screened for abuse, she reports that she has been physically and emotionally abused by her husband for many years, and now her sons are verbally abusive. Your preceptor has been her physician for 12 years, but has just started screening patients for domestic violence. Your preceptor always liked this patient's husband and never suspected an abusive relationship.

Sexually transmitted diseases, pelvic inflammatory disease, coercion in sexual relationships, sexual dysfunction, and a failure to use condoms or other contraceptives can all suggest a need for partner violence screening.

Case 4: Psychologic Problems

A 35-year-old woman comes to see you after she presented to the emergency room with chest pain, palpitations, and dyspnea. Her electrocardiogram showed sinus tachycardia. Further questioning reveals a history of panic attacks that began after her husband threatened to hunt her down if she left him.

Anxiety and panic attacks, depression, posttraumatic stress disorder, low self-esteem, suicidal ideation or attempts, eating disorders, tranquilizer or sedative use, and a history of being a "difficult" patient can all suggest that domestic violence screening is in order.

Case 5: Chronic Complaints Without Specific Diagnoses

A 41-year-old woman has just left an abusive marriage of 9 years. She needs forms completed for her insurance company. She tells you that her poorly controlled migraine headaches are better since moving out. Review of her chart shows that she denied abuse on an earlier screening.

Chronic pain (e.g., head, abdominal, pelvic, back, neck), insomnia, nightmares, fatigue, or vague complaints may point toward domestic violence.

Case 6: Behavioral Presentation

A 44-year-old teacher began crying while talking with the nurse who was checking her in. The patient disclosed that her husband had hit her teenage son to discipline him about going to bed. She reported that her husband had never hit her, but that they had talked about what type of situation would drive him to hit her.

Crying, minimizing statements, flat affect, angry or anxious body language, searching or fearful eye contact, defensiveness, and comments about emotional abuse or an abused "friend" suggest screening for partner violence.

Case 7: Change in Office Visit Patterns

The receptionist at your clinic recently attended training on domestic violence. You overhear her and your preceptor discussing two patients whose husbands continually cancel their appointments. One of these patients was previously seen for a rib fracture.

Missed or late appointments, appointments canceled by the patient's partner, a sudden change in frequency of visits, a change from office visits to the use of the emergency room, or frequent changes of health care provider can all insinuate domestic violence.

Case 8: Controlling, Coercive Behavior by a Partner or Companion

A Russian couple, both 30 years old, is waiting in your examination room. The husband explains that he came to interpret for his wife's annual examination. Later, the nurse informs your preceptor that the wife speaks English well and brings her children in all the time.

When a partner hovers (i.e., will not leave the patient unattended, attempts to minimize the time the patient is alone with the provider) or a patient is reluctant to speak in front of or to disagree with her partner, domestic violence may be the cause. If the patient's partner does not allow her to take medication or she exhibits fear of her partner, deferring to him to answer questions, domestic violence may be a health care issue.

History

History taking is the best time to screen for partner violence. When asking the patient questions, do not use words such as "abuse" and "violence" unless the patient uses them first. Because of the limitations and subjective connotations of language, specific questions about violent or controlling behavior that use words such as "hit," "hurt," and "threaten" are often more effective screening techniques.

Also remember that a person in a violent relationship may minimize or rationalize to protect the positive aspects of the relationship. Often frequency rather than severity or type of violence determines whether the patient defines her partner's violent behavior as abusive.

When taking the history, consider prefacing your screening questions with the following statements and general questions:

- "Because of the frequency of abuse and violence, I ask all patients about safety issues at home. I want them to know that there are places that can help them, their families, or their neighbors."
  - □ This introduction is especially helpful if you suspect abuse but the patient denies an abusive relationship.
- "Because relationships and living situations affect health, I have been trained to ask all patients about safety issues at home."
- "All couples fight. What happens when you and your partner fight?"
- "Has your partner ever threatened you physically or degraded you?"

To further guide the screening process, you may want to use the pneumonic **"AFRAID"** (assault, fear, rape, accused, isolation and intimidation, degraded).

- **Assault**
  - □ Have you ever been in a relationship in which you were physically hurt?
  - □ Are there weapons in your home?
  - □ Has any partner ever threatened or hurt you or your children?
- **Fear**
  - □ Have you ever been afraid that your partner was going to hurt you, your children, or your loved ones?
  - □ When you fight or disagree with your partner at home, are you ever afraid for you or your children?
  - □ Should I be concerned for your safety?
  - □ Do you feel safe returning home? If not, can you stay with family or friends, or would you consider going to a shelter?

- **Rape**
  - ☐ Has your partner ever forced you to have intercourse when you did not want to?
  - ☐ Has your partner ever touched you in ways that made you feel uncomfortable?
- **Accused**
  - ☐ Has your partner ever falsely accused you of things you did not do?
- **Isolation and intimidation**
  - ☐ Has your partner prevented you from leaving home, getting a job, having friends, or getting an education?
  - ☐ Has your partner destroyed things of importance to you?
- **Degraded**
  - ☐ Has your partner ever called you names or criticized or insulted you?
  - ☐ Has your partner dismissed your needs for care or clothing?

If during the screening process your patient confirms abuse, be ready to act appropriately by following these guidelines:

- Convey a respectful and nonjudgmental attitude.
- Tell her that you are glad she has shared this information.
- Tell her that she does not deserve to be hurt.
- Acknowledge the potential for further harm and your concerns about her safety.
- Tell her that resources and agencies can help her when she is ready.
- Discuss with your preceptor ways to assist her in putting together a safety plan (see THERAPY; below).

Documentation and reporting of abuse

If your patient confirms abuse, proper documentation and reporting is critical. Proper documentation includes the patient's own words, including name of the abuser, date, time, and place. The documentation of any examination related to confirmed or suspected abuse should give a detailed description of the injuries. Photographs of physical injuries labeled with the victim's name, date, time, and the photographer's name are useful if the patient decides to go to court in the future. If the police are involved, they will take photographs. Drawing pictures of the injuries and their locations can also be helpful.

Reporting laws vary from state to state. Some states require mandatory reporting of domestic violence to the legal authorities. Ask your preceptor the laws of the state where you practice. Special civil protection orders are now available to battered victims in every state.

✚ THERAPY

Health care professionals are often inclined to try to "fix" a situation quickly. However, partner violence is almost always a spectrum of behaviors that occurs over an extended period. Only the victim understands the complexities of her situation and the ideal timeframe for change. In fact, studies show that the female victim is often in more danger of being killed upon leaving her partner, a finding that may seem counterintuitive.

In addition to respecting the victim's autonomy, strive to empower the victim or survivor with empathy, encouragement, and community resources when she is ready to address the situation.

Safety Plans

When you encounter a patient who is ready to address her abusive situation, work with your preceptor to help her to put together safety plans to refer to when she is ready to make a change. The following safety plans can be used for assistance.

Safety during an explosive incident

- If an argument seems unavoidable, try to have it in a room or area with an exit and not in the bathroom, kitchen, or anywhere near weapons.
- Practice how to get out of your home safely. Identify which door, window, elevator, or set of stairs would be best.
- Have a packed bag ready. Keep it in a secret but accessible place so you can leave quickly.
- Identify neighbors you can tell about the violence and ask them to call the police if they hear a disturbance coming from your home.
- Devise a code word to use with your children, family, friends, and neighbors when you need the police.
- Decide and plan where you will go if you have to leave home, even if you do not think it will be necessary.
- If the situation is very dangerous, use your own instinct and judgment to keep yourself safe. Call the police as soon as it is safe to do so.

Safety when preparing to leave

- Determine who will let you stay with them or lend you some money.
- Always try to take your children with you or make arrangements to leave them with someone safe.
- Leave money, extra keys, copies of important documents, and clothes with someone you trust.
- Open a savings account in your own name to establish or increase your financial independence.
- Keep the shelter numbers close by, and keep change or a calling card with you at all times.
- Review your safety plan with a domestic violence advocate to plan the safest way to leave your batterer.

Safety once you have left

- At work, decide who you will tell about your situation, including office or building security. Provide a picture of your batterer, if possible.
- Arrange to have someone screen your telephone calls, if possible.
- Devise a safety plan for when you leave work.
  - □ Have someone escort you to your car, bus, or train.
  - □ Use various routes to go home, if possible.
  - □ Think about what you would do if something happened while going home.
- If criminal charges are filed against your batterer, let the police and court know that you want a restraining order and speak with legal counsel. You may qualify for a civil restraining order. Only this kind of order can give you temporary custody of your children. Check with your local domestic relations court.
- Inform your neighbors and landlord that your partner no longer lives with you and that they should call the police if they see your abuser near your home.
- Rehearse a safety plan with your children for when you are not with them.
- Inform school or day-care about who has permission to pick up your children. Give school authorities a copy of your restraining order.
- Change or add locks on your doors and windows as soon as possible.
- Change your telephone number.

Your safety and emotional health

- If you are thinking of returning to a potentially abusive situation, discuss an alternative plan with someone you trust.
- If you have to communicate with your partner, determine the safest way to do so.
- Have positive thoughts about yourself, and be assertive with others about your needs.
- Plan to attend a support group for at least 2 weeks to gain support from others and learn more about yourself and the relationship.
- Decide who you can call freely and openly to give you the support you need.
- Read articles, books, and poetry to help you feel stronger.

The Medical Provider as Victim

Medical students and physicians who have experienced or witnessed violence in their own homes may find that dealing with abused patients triggers complex emotions. Some may respond with rescue attempts, loss of boundaries, attempts to control the patient, or denial and doubts about the patient's story. Recognition of the personal issue and help through support and counseling can be just as essential for the medical provider as it is for the patient survivor.

URGENCIES AND EMERGENCIES

Warning signs of imminent danger for the victim and her children include:

- Escalation of the frequency and severity of the violence and abuse
- Increased use of alcohol or drugs by the victim or abuser
- The presence of a weapon in the home
- Threats of suicide or homicide on the part of the victim or the abuser
- Abuse of the children

If you find any of these signs, refer the victim to a domestic violence crisis hotline for assistance in developing a safety plan, and carefully discuss the presentation with your preceptor.

 SPECIAL POPULATIONS

Children

If partner violence is identified or suspected, it is important to evaluate for child abuse. With the guidance of your preceptor, screen the victim alone or in the company of children younger than 3 years of age. Have support staff occupy older children or take them out to the play area. Ask the victim the following questions:

- When you and your partner fight, what happens to the children?
- Does your partner ever hurt the children?
- Where are the children when you and your partner fight?
- Do you ever hurt the children?

If you suspect child abuse, involve your preceptor. It must be reported to the appropriate agency. If the person you are getting the information from is willing, she can make the report from your preceptor's office. If there is no acknowledgment of harm to the children, then talk with her about how hearing and seeing the violence affects the children. Studies suggest that children who only hear and see the violence still display various behavioral, physical, cognitive, and emotional problems and symptoms.

Seniors

Seniors represent another vulnerable population. Abuse can be physical, emotional, sexual, or financial. Neglect, such as denying the patient care, attention, or basic needs (e.g., food, water), is the most common form of abuse in this population. Throughout the United States, reporting the suspicion of any of these abuses to an agency specializing in adult protection is mandatory.

Pregnancy

All pregnant women should be screened for partner violence each trimester. Screening should be done with the woman alone, not with her partner present.

> **NOTE**
>
> Studies show that abuse during pregnancy is more common than hepatitis B, Rh incompatibility, and gestational diabetes combined.

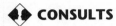 CONSULTS

Identify the major local agencies that advocate for victims and survivors of abuse. Reporting requirements vary from state to state. If you have not learned the law in your state by the time you get to your family medicine clerkship, ask!

Acknowledgment

The safety plans discussed in this chapter were developed in collaboration by the following Ohio agencies:

City of Norwood

Domestic Violence Coordinating Council

Hamilton County Department of Human Services

Norwood Domestic Crisis Committee

Norwood Police Department

Women Helping Women, Inc.

YWCA of Cincinnati

YWCA Academy of Career Women

Pruritic Skin—Common Dermatoses

Erik Powell

GENERAL INFORMATION

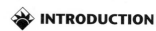 **INTRODUCTION**

Dermatologic concerns are a common reason for individuals to consult their family physicians. Pruritic rashes occur frequently. The frequent scratching, lack of sleep, and work involved in applying topical agents can be overwhelming to both patient and family. Fortunately, itchy skin is usually associated with fairly benign processes.

TERMINOLOGY

Alopecia: hair loss
Annular: ring shaped
Atopic: term used to designate a patient with a personal or family history of asthma, allergic rhinitis, or eczema
Bulla: a fluid-filled nodule
Burrow: the superficial, thread–like lesion of scabies
Dermatophyte: a group of fungi that infect the superficial layers of the skin, hair, and nails
Eczema: inflamed skin with, flaky, plaque-like, or papulovesicular lesions
Erosion: loss of the superficial layers of skin
Exanthem: a red skin eruption usually associated with infection
Fissure: a crack in the dermis

Glabrous: the smooth areas of the body where hair does not usually grow

Hive: *see wheal*

Hyperkeratosis: excessive scaling of the skin

Intertrigo: dermatitis occurring between folds of the skin

Keloid: a hypertrophied scar

Kerion: boggy inflammation of the scalp caused by tinea capitis

Lichenification: leathery thickening of the skin secondary to chronic inflammation caused by scratching

Macule: a flat lesion that is less than 0.5 cm in diameter (e.g., a freckle)

Nodule: a raised lesion that is between 0.5 and 2.0 cm in diameter

Nummular: discoid or coin shaped

Onychomycosis: a fungal infection of the nails

Papule: a raised lesion that is less than 0.5 cm in diameter

Patch: a flat lesion that is more than 0.5 cm in diameter

Petechia: a nonblanching, pinpoint macule formed from bleeding into the skin

Plaque: a raised, circumscribed, solid area

Pruritus: itching

Purpura: a lesion characterized by hemorrhage into the skin

Pustule: a pus-filled papule

Scaling: proliferation of dead epidermal cells (i.e., keratinocytes)

Secondary lesions: primary lesions that undergo transformation

Sensitization: the condition in which exposure to an allergen or irritant causes a primary immune response after the first exposure

Trichotillomania: hair pulling associated with anxiety that leads to bald spots

Tumor: a raised lesion that is more than 2 cm in diameter

Ulcer: deep erosion

Vesicle: a fluid-filled papule

Wheal: a raised area caused by dermal edema

Xerosis: dryness of the skin

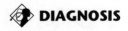 **DIAGNOSIS**

History

History of present illness

- What do you think caused the rash or the itching?
- When did you first notice the rash or itching, and how has it progressed?
- Does anything make it worse or better?
- Do you have a fever or any associated symptoms?
- Have you used any prescription or over-the-counter (OTC) medications on the rash?
- Are other family members affected?
- Are you aware of any occupational, recreational, or household exposures?

Past medical history

- Do you have a personal or family history of atopy?
- Has this condition been previously diagnosed? If so, how frequent and severe were the outbreaks, and what therapies were tried?

Social history

- How often do you bathe or shower?
- What type of soap do you use?
- How arid is your home environment?
- Are you exposed to pets?
- Is there any stress in your life?

Review of Systems

The review of systems generally includes a brief look at concurrent allergies. Associated signs and symptoms include fever, malaise, nasal congestion, sneezing, coughing, wheezing, and shortness of breath.

Physical Examination

Have the patient change into a gown to ensure adequate visualization of the rash. Describe the rash in terms of:

- Appearance (e.g., color, flat/raised, macular/papular)
- Size
- Shape (e.g., annular, nummular, linear)
- Configuration (e.g., grouped, scattered)
- Distribution

NOTE

With pruritic rashes, scratching may alter the primary lesion.

DIFFERENTIAL DIAGNOSIS

Table 23–1 is a list of common pruritic rashes not included in this chapter.

THERAPY

Nonpharmacologic Therapy

Soaps

For dry, atopic skin, use mild soaps that do not contain perfumes or dyes.

TABLE 23–1. Itchy Rashes Not Included in this Chapter

Diagnosis	Description	Severity of Itching
Cutaneous lupus	Atrophic, hyperkeratotic, erythematous plaques often seen with telangiectasia	Minimal
Dyshidrotic eczema	Papulovesicular lesions found on the palms, soles, and interdigital surfaces; risk factors are atopic, contact, and dermatophyte dermatitides	Mild–severe
Erythrasma	Reddish brown patches found in intertriginous areas that result from infection with *Corynebacterium*	Minimal
Granuloma annulare	Papular, circular or semicircular, flesh-colored lesions on the dorsal surfaces of the hands and feet and the ventral surfaces of the arms and legs	Minimal
Impetigo*	Initially appears as an erythematous, maculopapular rash that later forms vesicles; bullae; weeping, shallow, erythematous ulcers; and honey-colored crusts	Mild to severe; usually a result of primary infection
Lichen planus	Polygonal or ovoid lesions include flat-topped, shiny, violaceous papules that sometimes form linear groups and are found on flexor surfaces, male genitalia, and buccal mucosa; a white lacy pattern may be seen if oil is placed on a papule	Severe
Moniliasis (i.e., candidiasis)	A candidal dermatitis found on the perineum and marked by an erythematous, maculopapular rash with satellite lesions	Mild
Neurodermatitis†	Lichenified, skin-colored, scaly patches anywhere in reach of scratching; excoriations often present	Severe
Pityriasis rosea	Extensive, erythematous, papular rash that spares the face, hands, and feet; tends to follow the skin cleavage lines, often forming a "christmas tree pattern"; when on the trunk can last several weeks	Minimal
Psoriasis	Severe scaling on erythematous plateau usually found on knees, elbows, extensor creases and behind the ears; nail pitting is often seen	Minimal
Seborrheic dermatitis	Eczematous plaques with a yellow, greasy scale that may be found on the scalp, eyebrows, nasolabial folds, and groin	Minimal

*Impetigo may be a complication of contact dermatitis, especially in children who scratch a lot.

†Neurodermatitis can arise from primary dermatitides, including those discussed in this chapter.

Oatmeal

Nonprescription oatmeal-based bathing products added to bath water help soothe and soften itching skin.

Moisturizers

Moisturizers applied liberally several times a day, especially while the skin is still damp after bathing, help control itching. Many nonprescription moisturizers are available. Select the cheapest moisturizer that is effective.

Pharmacotherapy

Antihistamines

Sedating antihistamines (e.g., diphenhydramine, hydroxyzine) are often used to control pruritus, especially at bedtime.

Nonsedating antihistamines (e.g., cetirizine, fexofenadine, loratadine) may be less effective at controlling itching than sedating antihistamines, but they tend to be better tolerated during waking hours.

Astringents

Astringents are used for the treatment of weeping blisters, such as those associated with contact dermatitis. These lesions clear faster if helped to dry. The simplest therapy for drying is to wet the lesion with water, then leave it exposed to the evaporating effect of open air. An OTC medicated powder that consists of aluminum sulfate and calcium acetate is also a good drying agent.

Topical steroids

Topical steroids are used for the treatment of pruritus and inflammation. Part of the "art" of dermatology is learning to use the correct steroid for a given application.

> **NOTE**
>
> The potency of a steroid preparation is determined not only by the particular steroid and its concentration, but also by the vehicle used and the area of the body to which it is applied.

Classes of topical steroids

Seven classes are used to rank topical steroids in terms of potency, with class one being the most potent. It is usually clinically sufficient to know only one or two drugs in each of the following four classes: low, intermediate, high, and super high (Table 23–2).

TABLE 23–2. **Classification of Topical Steroid Preparations by Potency***

LOW POTENCY:
- Alclometasone dipropionate 0.05% (Aclovate; crm, oint)
- Fluocinolone acetonide 0.01% (Synalar; soln)
- Hydrocortisone base or acetate 0.5% (Cortisporin†; crm)
- Hydrocortisone base or acetate 1% (Cortisporin†; oint)

(Hytone; crm, lot, oint)
(Vytone†; crm)
- Hydrocortisone base or acetate 2.5% (Hytone; crm, lot, oint)
- Triamcinolone‡ acetonide 0.025% (Aristocort-A; crm) (Kenalog; crm, lot, oint)

INTERMEDIATE POTENCY:
- Betamethasone valerate 0.12% (Luxiq; foam)
- Desonide 0.05% (Desowen; crm, lot, oint) (Tridesilon; crm, oint)
- Desoximetasone 0.05% (Topicort-LP; emollient crm)
- Fluocinolone acetonide 0.1% (Derma-Smoothe/FS; oil, shampoo)
- Fluocinolone acetonide 0.025% (Synalar; crm, oint)
- Flurandrenolide 0.025% (Cordran-SP; crm) (Cordran; oint)
- Flurandrenolide 0.05% (Cordran-SP; crm) (Cordran; lot, oint)

- Fluticasone propionate 0.005% (Cutivate; oint)
- Fluticasone propionate 0.05% (Cutivate; crm)
- Hydrocortisone probutate 0.1% (Pandel; crm)
- Hydrocortisone butyrate 0.1% (Locoid; crm, oint, soln)
- Hydrocortisone valerate 0.2% (Westcort; crm, oint)
- Mometasone furoate 0.1% (Elocon; crm, lot, oint)
- Prednicarbate 0.1% (Dermatop; emollient crm)
- Triamcinolone‡ acetonide 0.01% (Aristocort A; crm, oint) (Kenalog; crm, lot)
- Triamcinolone‡ acetonide 0.2% (Kenalog; aerosol)

HIGH POTENCY:
- Amcinonide 0.1% (Cyclocort; crm, lot, oint)
- Betamethasone dipropionate, augmented 0.05% (Diprolene AF; emollient crm) (Diprolene; lot)
- Desoximetasone 0.05% (Topicort; gel)
- Desoximetasone 0.25% (Topicort; emollient crm, oint)
- Diflorasone diacetate 0.05%

(Psorcon e; emollient crm, emollient oint) (Psorcon; crm)
- Fluocinonide 0.05% (Lidex; crm, gel, oint, soln) (Lidex-E; emollient crm)
- Halcinonide 0.1% (Halog; crm, oint, soln) (Halog-E; emollient crm)
- Triamcinolone‡ acetonide 0.5% (Aristocort A; crm) (Kenalog; crm)

(continued)

TABLE 23–2. Classification of Topical Steroid Preparations by Potency* (*Continued*)

SUPER HIGH POTENCY:

- Betamethasone dipropionate, augmented 0.05% (Diprolene; oint, gel)
- Clobetasol propionate 0.05% (Temovate; crm, gel, oint, scalp application) (Temovate-E; emollient crm)

- Flurandrenolide 4 µg/sq cm (Cordran; tape)
- Diflorasone diacetate 0.05% (Psorcon; oint)
- Halobetasol propionate 0.05% (Ultravate; crm, oint)

Adapted with permission from Murphy JL (ed): *Monthly Prescribing Reference*. Prescribing Reference, Inc., New York, May 2000.

crm = cream; lot = lotion; oint = ointment; soln = solution.

*The classification is based on vasoconstrictor assays and clinical studies. Potency varies according to the steroid, its concentration, and the vehicle. In general, steroids in lotions, creams, gels, and ointments are increasingly more potent due to increased absorption from these vehicles. Absorption is increased by prolonged therapy, large areas of skin damage, and the use of occlusive dressings that may cause an increase in the incidence of side effects.

†These products have more than one active ingredient.

‡Triamcinolone is fairly inexpensive and comes in large tubes or containers, which is important if it has to be applied to extensive areas of the body.

Vehicles of suspension

The vehicle a steroid is suspended in can mean the difference between treatment success and failure. Steroid creams, gels, lotions, and ointments differ basically in their water content. A basic principle of dermatologic therapy is that if a lesion is wet, dry it; if it is dry, wet it. Prescribing the steroid in the correct vehicle allows you to do this.

Halogenation increases the strength of the steroid. Because fluorine is the halogen most often used, steroid creams are also referred to as fluorinated or nonfluorinated.

Using fluorinated steroid preparations over a long period can cause multiple local and systemic side effects (Table 23–3). These side effects are more likely when stronger steroids are used in areas prone to increased absorption (e.g., intertriginous areas, thinner areas of the skin).

NOTE

Fluorinated steroid preparations should not be used on the face, axillae, groin, or anywhere on a baby.

Color Plate

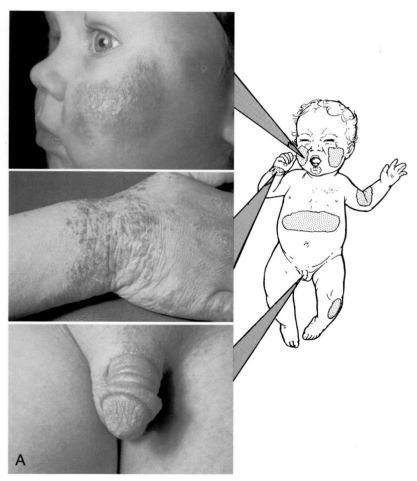

COLOR PLATE 23–1. (*A*) Atopic eczema in an infant. (Courtesy of Dome Chemicals.)

Color Plate

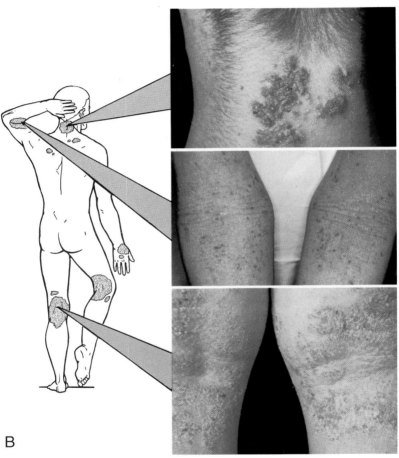

B

COLOR PLATE 23–1. (B) Atopic eczema in an adult. (Copyright 1989. Icon Learning Systems, LLC, a subsidiary of Havas MediMedia USA Inc. Reprinted with permission from Icon Learning Systems, LLC, illustrated by Frank H. Netter, MD. All rights reserved.)

Color Plate

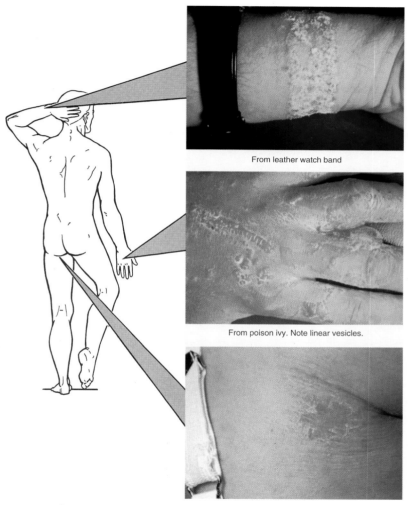

From leather watch band

From poison ivy. Note linear vesicles.

From nickel metal in garter strap

COLOR PLATE 23–2. Contact dermatitis. (Courtesy of Glaxo Smith Klein.)

Color Plate

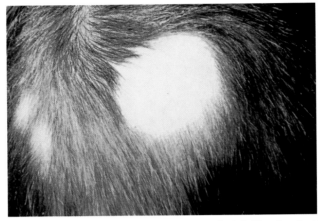

Color Plate 23–3. Tinea capitis due to *Microsporum audouinii*. (Reprinted with permission from Sauer GC, Hall JC: *Manual of Skin Diseases*, 7th ed. Philadelphia, Lippincott-Raven, 1996, p 359.)

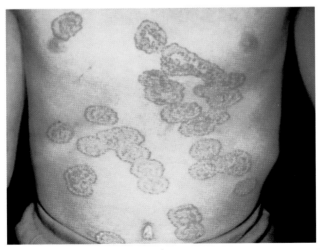

COLOR PLATE 23–4. Tinea corporis due to *Microsporum canis*. (Reprinted with permission from Sauer GC, Hall JC: *Manual of Skin Diseases*, 7th ed. Philadelphia, Lippincott-Raven, 1996, p 359.)

Color Plate

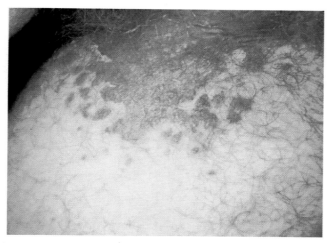

Color Plate 23–5. A close-up view of candidal intertrigo of the crural area showing satellite lesions without the sharp border seen in tinea cruris. (Courtesy of Herbert Laboratories.)

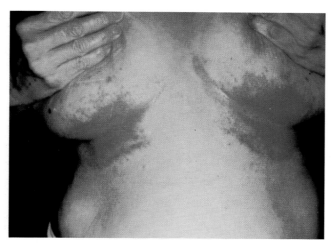

Color Plate 23–6. Candidal intertrigo under the breasts. (Courtesy of Herbert Laboratories.)

Color Plate

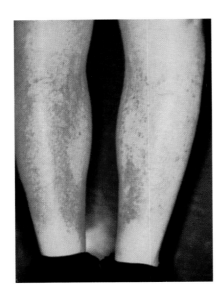

Color Plate 23–7. Redness of winter itch on the legs. (Courtesy of Johnson & Johnson.)

TABLE 23–3. **Side Effects of Chronic Fluorinated Steroid Use**

Local Side Effects	Systemic Side Effects
Telangiectasia	Hypothalamic-pituitary-adrenal axis suppression
Candidiasis	Growth retardation
Atrophy	Hypertension
Striae	Increased intracranial pressure
Delayed wound healing	Glaucoma
Discoloration of the skin	Cataracts

Creams are used most often and on most areas of the body. Being non-greasy, they have a higher patient acceptance rate. Steroid creams are halogenated or nonhalogenated.

Gels stick well without the greasiness of ointments. Unfortunately, they may irritate acutely inflamed skin.

Lotions have the highest water content and subsequently penetrate best in hairy areas. Creams and ointments stick to the top of the hair, while lotions seep down to the underlying skin. Lotions also are most effective for drying, which makes them particularly suited for application in moist, intertriginous areas.

Ointments have the least amount of water and, therefore, stick the best. When applied to damp skin, ointments are the best vehicles for preventing drying and keeping the skin moisturized. They also allow better penetration of the active ingredient. A thick, dry, scaly lesion responds best to an ointment. Some people do not like to use ointments because of the greasy feeling they leave.

Systemic steroids

When systemic steroids are needed for the treatment of pruritus or inflammation, a short burst is used. If systemic steroids are used for longer periods, they can suppress the pituitary-adrenal axis and cause adrenal insufficiency.

Antistaphylococcal antibiotics

Scratching inflamed skin that has lost its normal barrier function can deliver bacteria into the dermis. When lesions become superinfected from scratching, antistaphylococcal antibiotics are usually needed. Oral first–generation cephalosporins (e.g., cephalexin) or dicloxacillin are frequently used, often along with an OTC bactericidal ointment. Mupirocin ointment can also be used instead of oral antibiotics for less severe infections.

SPECIAL POPULATIONS

Children

Many of the pruritic rashes described in this chapter are common in children. Treatments described in this chapter are safe in children, with a few caveats.

- **Topical steroids** should not be overused.
- When treating for scabies:
  - □ **Lindane** should not be used in infants because of potential neurotoxicity
  - □ **Permethrin** is appropriate for use in infants older than 2 months
  - □ **Sulfur ointment** 6% nightly for 3 nights is preferred for infants younger than 2 months

Seniors

Scabies can be a particular problem in the institutionalized elderly. Ridding each patient of the infestation in light of the crowding and hands-on nursing care can be problematic. An organized treatment scheme needs to be adopted. All staff, family members, and frequent visitors should be treated. Laundering of all bed linens and clothes is required.

Pregnancy

None of the dermatoses discussed in this chapter have a particular predilection for pregnant women; however, treatment can differ if the patient is pregnant. Most oral antifungals are pregnancy category C; consequently, antifungals should only be used if the benefits are clearly greater than the risks. Topical therapy is preferred whenever possible. Precipitated sulfur is the treatment of choice for scabies in pregnant or lactating women. Of the nonsedating antihistamines, loratadine and cetirizine are pregnancy category B.

❖ COMPLEMENTARY/ALTERNATIVE MEDICINE

Traditional Chinese medicine, homeopathy, and other alternative modalities view rashes as manifestations of an imbalance in the body. These modalities assess the person for the imbalance and make recommendations based on the assessment.

Several herbal remedies for rashes have not been well studied but are used in countries other than the United States:

- **Primrose oil** is used for atopic dermatitis.
- **Chamomile** is used for bacterial disease of the skin and oral lesions.
- **Witch hazel** has an astringent action. Creams with witch hazel can be used for skin injuries and local inflammation of the skin.

- **Jewelweed** or **impatiens** may be rubbed onto poison ivy to neutralize the dermatitis.

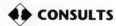 **CONSULTS**

Dermatologist

A dermatology referral is appropriate when a diagnosis is in question and a trial of a fairly benign medication is not appropriate because of time or severity. This referral is also appropriate when usual treatments fail.

Allergist

Consider an allergist for patients who need patch testing for allergic contact dermatitis and for the minority of patients with atopic dermatitis thought to be related to food.

ATOPIC DERMATITIS (Color Plate 23–1)

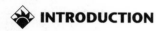 **INTRODUCTION**

Atopic dermatitis is a chronic, relapsing eczema sometimes described as "the itch that rashes." The affected skin is sensitive to a host of stimuli, including xerosis, infection, emotional stress, sweating, allergies, and local irritants (e.g., wool clothing). When exposed to irritants, the skin becomes pruritic. Scratching causes inflammation that makes the skin even more pruritic, thus perpetuating the itch-scratch-itch cycle.

BACKGROUND

Atopic dermatitis is a common condition in children, occurring in 10% of the pediatric population. The condition develops in 60% of children by 1 year of age and in 85% by 3 years of age. Asthma and allergic rhinitis are present in 50% to 80% of cases. Fortunately, a significant number of affected children outgrow the condition by puberty.

PREVENTION

Primary Prevention

Some lifestyle modifications may influence the primary prevention of eczema if they take place during the early years of life.

- A diet of only breast milk or formula for at least the first 4 months of life

- A diet containing no beef or cow's milk between 4 and 6 months of age
- Avoidance of cigarette smoke
- Avoidance of a day-care environment for the first 2 years of life

Secondary Prevention

Adherence to preventive bathing techniques and irritant avoidance will decrease exacerbations and limit the amount of topical steroid needed.

Preventive bathing

Advise patients to adhere to the following practices when bathing:

- Take short baths or showers with lukewarm water no more than every other day.
- Use only mild soap or soap substitutes, not soaps with perfumes or dyes. If possible, limit soap use to the intertriginous regions.
- Pat off water after bathing and apply moisturizer, oil, or topical steroid (if inflammation is present) while the skin is still wet.
- Reapply moisturizer at least twice a day.

Allergen and irritant avoidance

The following tips will help patients decrease exposure to common allergens and irritants:

- Consider removal of pets and stuffed toys from the home.
- Do not wear wool clothing.
- Try to replace carpeted floors with hardwood floors, which are easier to clean and retain fewer allergens.
- Use an air conditioner in the summer and a humidifier in the winter.
  - □ An inexpensive form of winter humidification can be accomplished by placing a metal pan of water over the duct or on the radiator.
- Avoid overdressing, because sweating may increase pruritus.
- Try to reduce emotional stress.
- Avoid common skin products that contain chemicals (e.g., lanolin, topical diphenhydramine) that can irritate the skin.

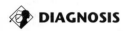 DIAGNOSIS

The diagnosis of atopic dermatitis is often straightforward. It is a clinical diagnosis; no laboratory test or diagnostic procedure confirms the condition. Itching must be present to make the diagnosis.

NOTE

If it does not itch, it is not atopic dermatitis.

Presentation

"Our child is itching and will not sleep" or "My eczema is back" are common complaints. Mild cases, particularly in children, may not be discussed until pointed out by the clinician.

History

A detailed history focusing on the age of onset (usually before 2 years of age), the nature of the disorder (e.g., chronic, recurring), and family history of atopy is a key part of the diagnosis.

Physical Examination

The physical appearance and anatomical distribution of the rash is important to the diagnosis of atopic dermatitis. The rash looks like other types of eczema. Acute lesions are erythematous, oozing, crusted plaques. Lichenification and pigment changes develop with chronic scratching.

Rash distribution varies with age. Infants usually have cheeks that appear "wind chapped." As children age, the rash localizes to include symmetrical flexural regions such as the neck, wrists, antecubital fossae, and popliteal fossae.

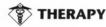 **THERAPY**

Treatment only controls the dermatitis; it is not curative. Topical steroids, antistaphylococcal antibiotics to treat bacterial superinfections, antihistamines to control itching, and good skin care are the basics of treatment (see GENERAL INFORMATION section, THERAPY; p 312).

NOTE

Do not use oral steroids for the treatment of atopic dermatitis.

CONTACT DERMATITIS (Color Plate 23–2)

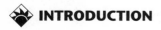 **INTRODUCTION**

Contact dermatitis is a skin reaction to a substance to which the patient is sensitive. Sensitivity may result from an irritant effect [i.e., irritant contact dermatitis (ICD)] or an immune-based effect [i.e., allergic contact dermatitis (ACD)]. ICD is more common than ACD. Causes of ICD include solvents (e.g., dishpan hands), adhesives found in dressing tape, and caustic solutions (e.g., battery acid). Causes of ACD include latex, nickel, hair dyes, and the *Rhus* family of plants (e.g., poison ivy, poison oak, poison sumac). ACD occurs only in people previously sensitized to the offending agent, whereas ICD can occur at first exposure.

BACKGROUND

The incidence of contact dermatitis varies depending on the population being studied.

PREVENTION

Primary Prevention

Avoidance of the causative agent is the prevention of choice. In the case of rhus dermatitis, this means education about the appearance of the plant and the acquisition of the rash. The rash is brought on by a reaction to the oil on the plant either through direct contact with the plant or contact with something carrying the oil (e.g., pets, gloves).

Barrier methods such as topical creams and full clothing (including gloves) may help prevent rhus dermatitis.

> **NOTE**
>
> If the stalk and leaves of a *Rhus* plant are burned, exposure to the smoke can lead to a diffuse reaction, including a reaction in the lungs.

Secondary Prevention

Exposure to irritating agents can be minimized if the area is thoroughly washed with soap and warm water soon after contact. In the case of rhus dermatitis, the fluid in the vesicles does not spread the rash.

DIAGNOSIS

Physical Examination

The location and pattern of the eczematous eruption is generally the most important feature in identifying the likely cause (Table 23–4). Chronic contact dermatitis can be differentiated from acute by the presence of lichenification, fissures, and scaling.

Laboratory Tests—Patch Testing

Patch testing may help to identify the offending agent. Potential sensitizing agents are applied to the skin and are covered with occlusive cloth

TABLE 23–4. **Rash Patterns and Causative Agents**

Causative Agent	Description of Rash
Rhus (poison ivy, poison oak)	Linear distribution consistent with where the leaf or branch touched the exposed skin
Aluminum in antiperspirants	Rash only in the axillae
Nickel in costume jewelry	Rash on ring finger, neck, wrist, or ear lobes
Hair-related chemicals (e.g., dyes, straighteners)	Rash on the scalp and upper posterior portion of the neck

patches. A true allergy will result in pruritus, vesicles, persistence of the rash beyond 24 hours, and spread of the reaction beyond the immediate site of application.

 THERAPY FOR RHUS DERMATITIS

Cool showers or baths with colloidal oatmeal may temporarily relieve itching. Topical therapies for itching include steroid creams, calamine lotion, and Burow's solution. Oral sedating antihistamines are useful at night.

Systemic steroids are recommended acutely if more than 25% of the body is affected; if there is severe itching and blistering; or if there is increased involvement of the hands, face (particularly the periocular region), or genitals. In severe poison ivy, oral steroids should start at about 60 mg/day in adults or 1–2 mg/kg/day in children, and should be tapered over at least 10 days to avoid rebound of the condition.

DERMATOPHYTE DERMATITIS

 INTRODUCTION

Dermatophytes are fungi that cause various skin infections. Transmission is by direct contact with the infected skin of persons or animals, soil, or fomites. The clinical manifestations of these infections vary among sites; consequently, the diagnosis is sometimes difficult. Although pruritus is common, it is often less severe than with contact and atopic dermatitis. The two most common fungi seen in primary care are **tinea** and *Candida.*

 BACKGROUND

Dermatophyte dermatitis is common, with an estimated 10% to 20% of the population being infected at any given time.

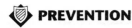 **PREVENTION**

Tinea Capitis

This fungus can exist for long periods on fomites such as hairbrushes, hair accessories (e.g., ribbons, clips), furniture, stuffed toys, and clothing. Control of the spread of tinea capitis is accomplished by examining siblings and other close contacts, eliminating the sharing of possible fomites, and cleaning and sterilizing related tools (e.g., hairbrushes, scissors).

Tinea Corporis

Tinea corporis can be prevented by decreased contact with infected individuals. If pets seem to be the cause, they will also need antifungal therapy.

Tinea Cruris

Tinea cruris can be prevented by avoiding activities that result in prolonged perspiration and by wearing lightweight, well-ventilated clothing. These measures also facilitate healing and decrease recurrence. Antifungal powders may assist in keeping the intertriginous regions dry.

Tinea Pedis

Warmth, sweat, and occlusive footwear promote fungal overgrowth. Wearing sandals in public showers, exposing feet to air while at home, and using antifungal foot powders all help prevent and treat infection.

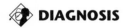 **DIAGNOSIS**

Presentation

Dermatophyte dermatitis may present in various ways. Families often have dealt with dermatophyte infections in the past; consequently, they may refer to the condition by its common name (e.g., jock itch, athlete's foot).

Physical Examination

Tinea capitis

Tinea capitis occurs most often in school–aged children. Clinically, it may appear as patches of complete alopecia, boggy inflammatory nodules (i.e., kerions), diffuse seborrheic scales, or diffuse pustules. See Color Plate 23–3 for a common presentation.

Tinea corporis

Tinea corporis (i.e., ringworm) classically appears as an annular plaque with central clearing. A raised, papular, circumscribed border is common. The lesions may be single or multiple and are usually asymmetrically distributed. Tinea corporis often presents as seen in Color Plate 23–4. Without laboratory findings, it is sometimes difficult to differentiate from other dermatitides.

Tinea cruris

Tinea cruris (i.e., jock itch) most commonly affects men, athletes, and obese people. The medial upper thighs are characteristically involved. The scrotum is not involved, which can help to differentiate it from candidal intertrigo. Tinea cruris presents as erythematous plaques with sharply demarcated borders.

Tinea pedis

Tinea pedis (i.e., athlete's foot) commonly appears as white, macerated areas in the third and fourth toe webs or as a scaly hyperkeratosis on the soles and heels (i.e., moccasin foot). Tinea pedis is the most common dermatophyte infection.

Candidal intertrigo

Candidal intertrigo of the crural area can be seen in Color Plate 23–5. Note the "indefinite" borders, which help to differentiate this from tinea cruris. Candidal intertrigo under the breasts can be seen in Color Plate 23–6.

Laboratory Tests

Microscopic evaluation is often important to the diagnosis. It is positive if hyphae or pseudohyphae are seen. Potassium hydroxide is often added to the preparation to break down cell walls, allowing the hyphae to be more easily visualized. A negative potassium hydroxide slide preparation does not rule out a fungal infection.

Potassium hydroxide yield is least likely with tinea capitis. Because the treatment for tinea capitis is systemic, culture may be warranted to confirm a diagnosis. Cultures should also be considered in recalcitrant cases, when the diagnosis is in doubt, or when required by insurance companies for treatment.

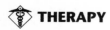 **THERAPY**

Topical Therapy for Dermatophyte Dermatitis
(Table 23–5)

Oral Therapy for Dermatophyte Dermatitis

Relative to topical agents, which are the drugs of choice for most tinea infections, oral therapies have increased cost, potential for hepatotoxicity,

TABLE 23–5. Topical Treatments and Available Formulations in the Treatment of Tinea Infections

Antifungal Agents	Rx	Crm	Soln or Spray	Lot	Pow	Gel or Oint	Apply*
Miscellaneous							
Undecylenic acid (Cruex, Desenex)		x	x		x	x	Twice daily
Tolnaftate 1% (Aftate, Tinactin)		x	x		x		Twice daily
Haloprogin 1% (Halotex)	x	x	x				Twice daily
Ciclopirox 1% (Loprox)	x	x		x			Twice daily
Imidazoles							
Clotrimazole 1% (Lotrimin, Mycelex)		x	x	x			Twice daily
Miconazole 2% (Micatin, Monistat-Derm)		x	x	x†	x		Twice daily
Econazole 1% (Spectazole)	x	x					Once daily
Ketoconazole 2% (Nizoral)	x	x	x‡				Once daily
Oxiconazole 1% (Oxistat)	x	x		x			Once daily
Sulconazole 1% (Exelderm)	x	x	x				Once or twice daily§
Allylamines							
Naftifine 1% (Naftin)	x	x				x	Once or twice daily‖
Terbinafine 1% (Lamisil)	x	x	x				Once or twice daily§
Benzylamines							
Butenafine 1% (Mentax)	x	x					Once daily

Adapted with permission from American Academy of Family Physicians. *Superficial fungal infection/cosmetic dermatology. Home study audio 201.* Kansas City, MO: American Academy of Family Physicians, 6–7, 1996.

Crm = cream; Lot = lotion; Oint = ointment; Pow = powder; Rx = prescription; Soln = solution.

*Duration of therapy varies based on the type of tinea: tinea pedis requires 4 weeks of therapy whereas tinea cruris and corporis must be treated for 2 to 3 weeks. Continue treatment for at least 2 weeks after symptom resolution.

†This lotion includes nail tincture.

‡This is available in a shampoo, which should be used twice weekly, at least 3 days apart, for a total of 4 weeks.

§Use twice daily only for treatment of tinea pedis.

‖Only the gel and ointment forms are used twice daily.

and possibility of drug interactions. Oral therapy is preferred, however, for nonlocalized tinea corporis, onychomycosis, tinea capitis, and for patients who are severely immunocompromised.

Therapy for tinea capitis

Griseofulvin is the drug of choice for tinea capitis. It is given once a day with a fatty meal (to increase absorption). A 4 to 6-week course of therapy is indicated.

Concomitant use of a sporicidal shampoo (e.g., selenium sulfide 2.5%, ketoconazole) two or three times per week may decrease fungal shedding. Kerions may require oral prednisone, 1 to 2 mg/kg/day, to curb inflammation as well as an antistaphylococcal antibiotic.

> **NOTE**
>
> Patients with tinea dermatitis may return to school or work once treatment has begun.

SCABIES

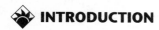 **INTRODUCTION**

Scabies is dermatitis produced by the infestation of *Sarcoptes scabiei*, a mite specific to the human host. Spread is by direct and sexual contact. Animal scabies (i.e., mange) can cause a localized reaction in humans; however, because it cannot reproduce on human skin, the rash is limited.

BACKGROUND

Scabies is found most often in poor, crowded living conditions, although it is not limited to impoverished areas. Outbreaks have also occurred in extended-care facilities.

PREVENTION

Treat all family members and contacts (including baby-sitters) simultaneously to prevent recurrence. It is also important to launder clothing and bedding in hot water and to dry them in a hot dryer. The heat of the dryer is an important scabicide.

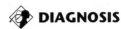 **DIAGNOSIS**

Presentation

Scabies has a myriad of presentations; all are pruritic. It has been described as "the worst itch of all."

History

- Have you previously been diagnosed with scabies?
  - □ In previously uninfected, unsensitized individuals, it may take 10 to 30 days for the hypersensitivity reaction to develop.
  - □ Individuals who have previously had the infestation (i.e., already sensitized) may develop symptoms within days of reexposure.
- Does anyone you know have scabies?
  - □ The scabies mite is usually acquired by direct contact with an infected individual.

Physical Examination

Lesions tend to be concentrated on the hands (especially the web spaces), feet, and body folds (e.g., axillae, elbows, waistband, groin). Burrows are the pathognomonic lesions of scabies; unfortunately, scratching often destroys these primary lesions. Also look for papules, nodules, and papulovesicular lesions, all of which are possible cutaneous manifestations of scabies.

Laboratory Tests

Because the clinical presentation can be so variable, seeing the mite under the microscope (Figure 23–1) is useful in providing the definitive diagnosis. With practice, the mite, eggs, and fecal pellets can be readily identified.

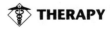 **THERAPY**

> **NOTE**
>
> Scabies therapy can be neurotoxic to children and a developing fetus.

The drug of choice for scabies is 5% permethrin lotion. Small children should apply the lotion from head to soles. Older children, adolescents, and adults should apply the lotion from the neck down, with special attention to the nails, intertriginous areas, and genital and gluteal clefts. The

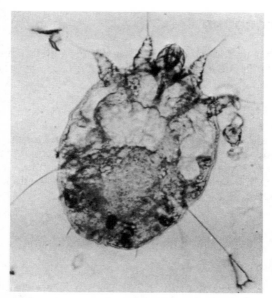

FIGURE 23–1. The female of the mite *Sarcoptes scabiei*. The small, oval, black body near the anal opening is a fecal pellet. Proximal to it is a vague, much larger, oval, pale-edged mass—an egg. (Courtesy of Dr. H. Parlette.)

lotion is then washed off after 8 to 14 hours. Some authors recommend retreatment in 1 week.

Alternative prescription therapies include 1% lindane lotion (36 times more toxic than permethrin), 10% crotamiton cream, and oral ivermectin. (Also see GENERAL INFORMATION section, THERAPY; p 312, for control of itching).

To avoid unnecessary retreatment, inform patients that even if the therapy is effective, the itching may persist for several weeks and the nodules may persist for months. To prevent recurrence and treatment failure, schedule a follow-up visit in 2 weeks, which is the lifespan of the mite.

XEROSIS (Color Plate 23–7)

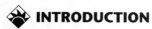 INTRODUCTION

Xerosis refers to dry, rough skin that is often pruritic. It tends to be worse in winter months because of low humidity and dry heat. Xerosis can occur on any area of the body, but is most frequently seen on the hands and lower legs. The skin typically has scaling with linear excoriations and painful fissures. The best "treatment" is prevention (i.e., keeping skin moist).

330 Common Office Problems

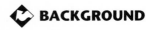 **BACKGROUND**

Incidence is greatest in the elderly (75% of those older than 64 years are affected) and individuals with Down's syndrome (up to 80% are affected).

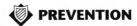 **PREVENTION**

Bathing and showering, particularly with soap, removes the natural oils from the body, exposing the skin to the drying effects of air. Preventive bathing is an essential component of patient education for any individual with a dry skin condition (see ATOPIC DERMATITIS section, PREVENTIVE BATHING; p 320).

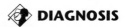 **DIAGNOSIS**

Presentation

A common presenting complaint is, "My legs itch. It happens every winter."

Physical Examination

The diagnosis is made by clinical observation. Dry, rough, scaling skin supports the diagnosis. Painful fissures may be present on the arms, hands, and lower legs.

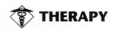 **THERAPY**

Therapy is preventive (see GENERAL INFORMATION section, THERAPY; p 312).

Sinusitis

Jeff Kirschman

OBJECTIVES

■ Differentiate between an upper respiratory infection, acute sinusitis, and chronic sinusitis
■ Describe the differences in the work-up and management of acute sinusitis versus chronic sinusitis

 INTRODUCTION

Sinusitis is inflammation of the membranes lining the paranasal sinuses. Viral infections are the most common cause of acute sinusitis. Bacterial sinusitis is much less frequent and is often preceded by a viral upper respiratory infection (URI). The most common organisms of bacterial overgrowth in the sinuses are *Streptococcus pneumoniae, Haemophilus influenzae,* and *Moraxella catarrhalis.* Chronic sinusitis can be caused by infection with these organisms as well as with *Pseudomonas aeruginosa,* group A streptococci, *Staphylococcus aureus,* anaerobes, and fungi, especially in immunocompromised patients. Sinusitis is most often classified based on the duration of symptoms (see TERMINOLOGY; below).

TERMINOLOGY

Rhinitis, allergic: an inflammatory response to an allergic stimulus in the nasal passages that often includes nasal congestion, sneezing, and a runny or itchy nose

Rhinitis, infectious: inflammation of the mucous membrane of the nose that results from an infectious process

Rhinitis medicamentosa: rhinitis induced by an overuse of nasal decongestant sprays, resulting in rebound inflammation

Rhinitis, occupational: inflammation of the mucous membrane of the nose that results from exposure to an allergen or chemical irritant at one's place of employment

Rhinitis, vasomotor: intermittent rhinitis without an identifiable allergen

Sinusitis, acute: sinusitis that lasts for less than 4 weeks (experts vary between less than 3 to less than 8 weeks)

Sinusitis, chronic: sinusitis that lasts more than 4 weeks (experts vary between more than 3 to more than 8 weeks)

Sinusitis, persistent: sinusitis that persists after 21 to 28 days of initial antibiotic therapy

Sinusitis, recurrent: sinusitis that has occurred three or more times within 1 year

Water's view: a posterior–anterior radiographic view of the face with the nose raised 2 to 3 cm off the film and the chin on the film

 ## BACKGROUND

Approximately 31 million Americans develop sinusitis each year, resulting in more than 18 million office visits to primary care physicians. Nearly 300,000 of these patients require surgery for sinusitis.

 ## PREVENTION

Primary Prevention

Control or avoidance of the predisposing factors for infectious sinusitis (Table 24–1) is often an important component of primary prevention.

Secondary Prevention

Although rare, sinusitis can lead to osteomyelitis, periorbital cellulitis, and intracranial infection. Therefore, if a patient has a probable case of infectious sinusitis, antibiotics should be prescribed to help deter such sequelae.

TABLE 24–1. **Predisposing Factors for Infectious Sinusitis**

- Increased mucus production (e.g., from smoking cigarettes or from an allergy)
- Altered mucus secretion and transport (e.g., from smoking cigarettes)
- Rhinitis (i.e., infectious, allergic, occupational, vasomotor, and rhinitis medicamentosa)
- Asthma
- Immunodeficiency
- Systemic disease (e.g., cystic fibrosis, Wegener's granulomatosis, HIV infection, Kartagener's syndrome, immotile cilia syndrome, tumors)
- Anatomic variation (e.g., deviated septum, enlarged tonsils or adenoids, previous trauma or nasal surgery, nasal polyps)

HIV = human immunodeficiency virus.

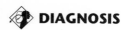 DIAGNOSIS

Understanding the natural history of the uncomplicated viral URI (Table 24–2) can aid in differentiating between simple viral infections and sinusitis.

Presentation (Tables 24–3 and 24–4)

The chief complaint generally focuses on sinus pain, with the patient complaining of pain behind or below the eyes, purulent rhinorrhea, and congestion. In addition, patients with sinusitis often describe a biphasic illness (i.e., "double sickening")—their "cold" had begun to improve when they relapsed with increased pain and congestion.

History

History of present illness

- Where on your face do you feel pain?
  - □ Table 24–5 describes the relationship of pain location, sinusitis, and URI.
- Do you have a history of asthma?

TABLE 24–2. The Natural History of Uncomplicated URI

Symptom	Duration
Sore throat	3–6 days
Sneezing	3–6 days
Fever	6–8 days
Malaise	6–8 days
Cough	14 days
Nasal discharge	14 days
Nasal congestion	14 days

URI = upper respiratory infection.

TABLE 24–3. Signs and Symptoms of Acute Sinusitis in Adults

- Purulent rhinorrhea by history or physical examination
- Failure of antihistamine or decongestant therapy
- Facial pain above or below both eyes on leaning forward, often unilateral
- Maxillary toothache
- Cough, frequently worse at night
- Hyposmia (i.e., diminished sense of smell)
- Unilateral facial pain

TABLE 24–4. **Symptoms of Chronic Sinusitis**

- Rhinorrhea
- Postnasal drainage (clear to purulent)
- Chronic congestion
- Chronic headache
- Sore throat
- Cough
- Asthma exacerbation
- Eustachian tube dysfunction (e.g., popping or ear pain without evidence of infection)
- Decreased hearing
- Tinnitus
- Vague constitutional symptoms (e.g., dizziness, fatigue, general malaise)

　□ Sinusitis is associated with asthma 40% to 75% of the time.
- Have you had these symptoms before? If so, when?
　□ Symptoms that occur only in the fall and spring suggest seasonal allergies.
- What medications or supplements have you taken for these symptoms?
- Does anyone at your home have similar symptoms?

Past medical history

- Do you have a history of allergic rhinitis, problems with your nose (e.g., deviated septum, polyps), diabetes, or blood problems (e.g., neutropenia)?

TABLE 24–5. **Physical Maturation and Adult Symptoms Specific to Involved Sinus**

Sinus	Adult Symptoms	Physical Development
Maxillary	Maxillary sinus pain, toothache, frontal headache	Pneumatization starts between birth and 12 months, adult size by 12 years of age
Frontal	Frontal sinus pain, frontal headache	Last to develop in midadolescence with greatest variation in degree of pneumatization
Ethmoid	Pain behind and between eyes, frontal headache described as "splitting"	Start to enlarge between 3 and 7 years of age, adult size by 12 to 14 years of age
Sphenoid	Frontal or occipital pain and headache	Start to enlarge between 4 and 5 years of age, adult size by 14 years of age

Family history

- Do many people in your family have allergies?

Social history

- Do you smoke or are you exposed to second-hand smoke at home or at work?
  - □ Smoking cigarettes and exposure to second-hand cigarette smoke can irritate sinuses immensely.

Review of Systems (Table 24–6)
Physical Examination (Table 24–7)
Laboratory Tests

Acute sinusitis

Blood work is not generally necessary for assessment or management of isolated acute sinusitis.

TABLE 24–6. Review of Systems for Sinusitis

System	Common Patient Complaints
Constitutional	Fever, chills, malaise
HEENT	Facial pressure or pain*, headache, ear pain or pressure, nasal congestion, nasal or postnasal drainage, tooth pain, throat pain, foul breath
Respiratory	Cough (from postnasal drip)
Gastrointestinal	Nausea (from postnasal drip)

*Facial pressure and pain often become worse when the patient bends forward.

TABLE 24–7. Physical Examination Findings in Sinusitis

System	Findings
Vital signs	Fever
HEENT	Periorbital edema, tenderness over one or more sinus cavities with percussion, mucosal edema in the nares, purulent nasal discharge*, increased posterior pharyngeal secretions, "cobblestone" pharynx, increase in facial pain when bending forward, serous otitis
Respiratory	Concurrent pulmonary problems

*The color and characteristics of a purulent nasal discharge do not help predict whether the pathogen is viral or bacterial.

Chronic or recurrent sinusitis

Nasal cytology for eosinophils may help if you are considering nasal allergies, nonallergic rhinitis with eosinophilia, nasal polyps, or aspirin sensitivity.

Immunodeficiency studies (acquired or congenital) may be helpful for patients who present with severe, recurrent sinusitis. Tests to consider include:

- Quantitative immunoglobulin (Ig) isotypes (i.e., IgG, IgM, IgE, and IgA)
- Human immunodeficiency virus (HIV) antibody
- Total complement
- Complement components

Imaging Studies

Radiographic imaging of the sinuses should be considered in cases of chronic or recurrent sinusitis or if the patient fails to respond to prolonged initial therapy. Radiographic findings that may suggest sinusitis can be found in Table 24–8. A **Waters' view** single radiograph may be substituted for a four-view sinus series when screening for isolated maxillary sinusitis.

Computed tomography (CT) is the gold standard for delineation of an obstruction of the ostiomeatal complex, because CT can demonstrate pathologic variation and anatomic defects that cannot be seen on plain radiographs. While plain radiographs are frequently ordered instead of CT in the hopes of saving money, the average four-slice, limited cut, coronal plane CT generally costs the same as the standard set of four plain radiographs.

Magnetic resonance imaging (MRI) has minimal use in imaging of the sinuses, because bone and air have similar signal intensity. In addition, it is difficult to distinguish between normal and inflamed mucosa in the nasal cavity using MRI. MRI is useful, however, in distinguishing between inflammatory disease and malignant tumors and in cases complicated by orbital or intracranial extension of disease.

Additional Studies

Transillumination may be used to evaluate the frontal and maxillary sinuses, although recent primary care studies suggest a lack of correlation between maxillary sinus transillumination and actual sinusitis.

TABLE 24–8. **Radiographic Signs Consistent with Sinusitis**

- Mucosal thickening (i.e., > 6 mm) in the maxillary sinuses
- Loss of air space volume (i.e., > 33%) in the maxillary sinuses
- Opacification or air-fluid levels in any of the paranasal sinuses

---

Endoscopic evaluation of the nasopharynx is another technique for evaluation, although its usefulness in the primary care setting has not been fully evaluated.

 ## DIFFERENTIAL DIAGNOSIS

The differential of pain in the sinus area can be found in Table 24–9.

 ## THERAPY

Nonpharmacologic Therapy

Smoking should be discouraged and assistance with smoking cessation offered (see Chapter 25, PREVENTION; p 344). In addition, symptoms may be helped with attention to hydration, which can be accomplished with:

- Water intake (e.g., 8 to 10 glasses daily)
- Steam inhalation (i.e., 20 to 30 minutes a few times each day)
- Saline irrigation
- Nose drops

Pharmacotherapy (Figure 24–1)

Antibiotics

Acute sinusitis

Because almost all cases are viral, antibiotics are generally not indicated in the treatment of acute sinusitis.

TABLE 24–9. Differential Diagnosis of Sinus Pain

Diagnosis	Distinguishing Characteristics
Dental disease	Patient most likely complains of mandibular or upper or lower jaw pain
Nasal foreign body	Seen mainly in children
Migraine or cluster headache	Generally presents with clear rhinorrhea, minimal to no posterior pharyngeal erythema, unilateral pain, and no history of fever
Temporal arteritis	Generally presents with tenderness outside the region normally associated with sinusitis and minimal rhinorrhea
Tension headache	Generally presents with minimal rhinorrhea and pharyngeal inflammation
Temporomandibular disorders	Generally present with tenderness over the temporomandibular joints, pop-and-click sound or crepitus on jaw opening, and spasms in the muscles of mastication

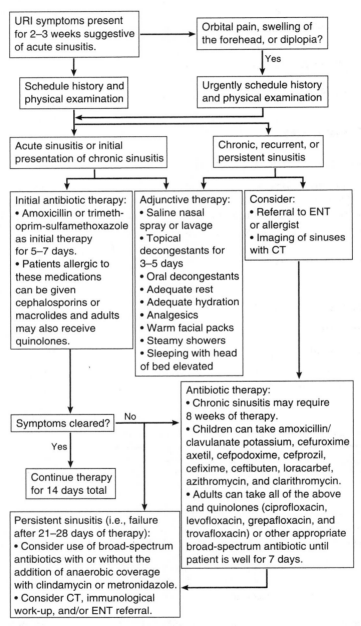

FIGURE 24–1. Algorithm for the treatment of sinusitis. *CT* = computed tomography; *ENT* = ear, nose, and throat; *URI* = upper respiratory infection.

Chronic, persistent, or recurrent sinusitis

The treatment of chronic sinusitis focuses on resolving the cause of inflammation. For patients without complicating factors (e.g., previous nasal surgery or trauma, nasal polyps, related drug allergy), an initial trial of amoxicillin or trimethoprim-sulfamethoxazole is indicated. Patients with complicating factors should be started on broad-spectrum antibiotics. Therapy should continue for a total of 10 to 14 days (see Figure 24–1).

Patients are often counseled to call back after 5 to 7 days of therapy if there has been no improvement in their condition. Because failure with first-line antibiotics is frequent, a broad-spectrum antibiotic should be given if the patient does not respond within 7 days of initial therapy.

Antihistamines and decongestants

Antihistamines can thicken mucus secretions; therefore, they are generally not appropriate for initial therapy unless the sinusitis is thought to be totally allergy-mediated. However, antihistamines may be initiated for treatment of an associated allergic rhinitis after resolving the acute sinusitis.

Oral and nasal decongestants, alone for viral sinusitis or combined with appropriate antibiotics, for suspected bacterial sinusitis, can provide relief within 3 days.

Anti-inflammatories

Treatment of sinusitis is also directed by the results of additional studies that suggest underlying disease. In the case of anatomic obstruction resulting in chronic infection or the presence of chronic allergic rhinitis, initial management with nasal or oral corticosteroid therapy along with the broad-spectrum antibiotic therapy may be necessary.

URGENCIES AND EMERGENCIES

Orbital Cellulitis and Other Invasive Infections

Complaints of diplopia, swelling, or pain around the orbits should be assessed urgently. Although rare, sequelae can include meningitis, subdural empyema, cavernous sinus thrombosis, and osteomyelitis.

High Fever

Patients with sinusitis and unrelenting (i.e., without antipyretic medication) high fever after 48 hours of antibiotic therapy should be assessed for possible extension outside the sinuses, especially patients presenting with an altered sensorium.

SPECIAL POPULATIONS

Children

On average, children have between six and eight "colds" per year. Between 5% and 10% of those URIs are complicated by sinusitis, while only 0.5% of adult URIs develop into sinusitis.

Younger children frequently do not exhibit the classic signs of acute sinusitis seen in adults (see Table 24–3), in part because sinus cavities develop at different ages. The symptoms of sinusitis that may be seen in children can be found in Table 24–10.

A sweat chloride test should be considered in children who have nasal colonization with *P. aeruginosa* and young children with nasal polyps.

Seniors

Oral decongestants containing pseudoephedrine can exacerbate urinary retention and anxiety in older patients.

Pregnancy

Nasal decongestant sprays should be used cautiously in pregnant women with borderline placental reserve. These sprays contain sympathomimetic (i.e., adrenergic) agents (e.g., oxymetazoline), which are vasoconstrictors and may cause the constriction of blood vessels in the uterine walls.

Oral decongestants (e.g., pseudoephedrine) are Class C agents and often not recommended for use during pregnancy. Women who breast-feed should generally not use antihistamines, although diphenhydramine is considered safe by most clinicians.

COMPLEMENTARY/ALTERNATIVE MEDICINE (See Chapter 8; COMPLEMENTARY/ALTERNATIVE MEDICINE, p 92)

Supplements and herbs often found in preparations that claim to be helpful for sinusitis include:

TABLE 24–10. **Symptoms of Sinusitis in Children**

	Fever	Facial Pain	Nasal Swelling	Cough	Nasal Congestion	Time Course
Acute	+	+	+	+*	++	Several days to 4–8 weeks
Chronic	++	+++	++	+	+	> 4–8 weeks

*Cough may include posttussive vomiting.

- Echinacea
- Ma Huang (ephedra)
  - □ Ma Huang is a potent vasoconstrictor in some preparations, so watch blood pressure and tachycardia.
- Vitamins A, C, and E (antioxidants)
- Zinc
  - □ Some studies suggest that zinc may help shorten the common cold, but most studies have not concurred.
  - □ Large amounts of zinc can cause problematic gastrointestinal symptoms and, used chronically, can deplete necessary copper.

◆◆ CONSULTS

Consider consulting with an **ear, nose, and throat specialist** for:
- Persistent sinusitis
- Recurrent sinusitis
- Abnormal MRI or CT scan of the sinuses (e.g., ostiomeatal obstruction)
- Clarification of immunologic or allergic contribution to sinusitis
- Sinusitis associated with unusual opportunistic infections
- A diagnostic procedure (e.g., puncture, aspiration, culture) for repeated therapy failure

Consider consulting with an **allergist** for allergic rhinitis that does not respond to antihistamines and nasal steroids.

Substance Abuse and Dependency

Jerry A. Friemoth • James Short •
Susan Louisa Montauk

OBJECTIVES

■ Differentiate between the characteristics of the use and abuse of tobacco, alcohol, and illicit drugs based on the stages of change model

■ Illustrate models for the work-up of substance dependency and abuse in a family practice

■ Describe pharmacologic and psychosocial interventions that may be useful when managing substance abuse in a family practice

 INTRODUCTION

This chapter explores the chemical dependency issues you will likely encounter during your family medicine rotation. Substance abuse encompasses a broad range of psychoactive materials. Although the substances may differ, increasing and important evidence is showing that most addictions have neurobiologic pathways in common. Therefore, the work-up, psychologic issues, and modes of treatment underlying dependency are often the same.

TERMINOLOGY

Many terms used in this chapter have variable meanings throughout the medical literature. Several of the following definitions were chosen for their ability to clarify concepts and interrelationships discussed later, not for their unique truth.

Abuse, substance: using a chemical in such a way that it causes social, physical, or mental problems

Addiction: a pattern of compulsive substance (i.e., drug or chemical) use associated with psychologic and physical dependence, evidenced by repeated failures to refrain from use of the substance

Alcoholic blackout: a time period (e.g., minutes, hours, days) during which an intoxicated individual cannot form or store new memories, even though he or she appears to be awake and alert and can perform activities of daily living; most common in individuals with a long history of alcoholism

Dependence, physical: a state that repeatedly requires a substance, which may or may not be healthful, to remain in or return to relative physical homeostasis

Dependence, psychologic: a continued, psychologically perceived need for a substance that may or may not be healthful

Dependence, substance: a physiologic need or craving for a substance; often, but not always, associated with tolerance that is evidenced by a need to increase the dose of the substance to achieve the effect once brought about by a lower dose

Discontinuation syndrome: symptoms and signs that arise because of the lag time between stopping a medication and the full physiologic readjustment of the body to functioning without the medication; not a direct result of addiction or tolerance, although either may be present; often avoided by tapering rather than abruptly discontinuing the dose

Fetal alcohol syndrome: a diagnosis describing a specific set of birth defects caused by a woman's excessive consumption of alcohol during pregnancy; such defects include slow weight and height progression, microcephaly, brain damage, epicanthal folds (presents as small eyes or short eye openings), a flat midface, an indistinct (i.e., flattened) philtrum above a thin upper lip, and micrognathia (i.e., a small jaw)

Holiday heart: a term used to describe a major, acute heart problem (e.g., myocardial infarction, atrial fibrillation) that resulted from short-term, excessive use of alcohol

Poor control of use: intake of a substance in larger amounts or over a longer period than was intended

Relapse: the return of symptoms and signs of a disease after convalescence has begun

Tolerance: the phenomenon of experiencing 1) a decrease in the desired response when repeated doses of a substance are held constant and/or 2) the need to increase doses to maintain constancy of the desired response

Wernicke's encephalopathy: an encephalopathy associated with thiamin deficiency, chronic alcohol abuse, loss of memory, and confabulation

Withdrawal symptoms: symptoms and signs that can be associated with stopping a chemical, which one has become physically or psychologically dependent (Table 25–1)

⚙ BACKGROUND

In the United States, mortality rates from chemical dependency are staggering. Each year, 400,000 deaths result from tobacco use, 100,000 deaths result from alcohol use, and 20,000 deaths result from the use of illicit

TABLE 25–1. **Withdrawal Symptoms Associated with Various Substances**

Substance	Symptoms
Sedative-hypnotics (e.g., alcohol)	Tremulousness with elevated heart rate, respiratory rate, blood pressure, and temperature; grand mal seizures; hallucinations (usually auditory or visual); delirium tremens characterized by marked tremulousness, disorientation, unstable cardiovascular status, and severe diaphoresis
Stimulants (e.g., cocaine, nicotine)	Depression, anhedonia, hyperphagia, initial extreme cravings
Opiates	Intense drug craving, muscle cramps, anxiety, arthralgias, vomiting, malaise

Having one or more of the above responses after stopping a chemical does not always imply addiction.

drugs. If you consider persons injured because of their own abuse and the effects on friends, family, and significant others, the true enormity of the problem starts to emerge.

Prevalence is approximately 5% for illegal drug use, 15% for alcohol use, and 30% for tobacco use. The medical literature suggests that approximately 15% to 20% of the patients seen in your preceptor's office have alcohol or illicit drug problems and approximately 25% to 30% are current tobacco users.

> **NOTE**
>
> In the United States, the lifetime incidence of having at least one substance use disorder is 50% or higher.

 PREVENTION

Primary and secondary prevention of chemical dependencies can be addressed in clinical encounters using the "8 A's" (Table 25–2).

 DIAGNOSIS

When attempting to diagnose chemical dependency, all the following are evidence of a problem:

- One or more positive responses to the CAGE questions (Table 25–3) in the last year
- Compulsion or preoccupation with use

TABLE 25–2. The "8 A's" of Substance Abuse Prevention

ANTICIPATE that all can be vulnerable to chemical abuse. Giving anticipatory guidance to all patients, especially younger patients, is the most important primary prevention strategy.	ANTICIPATE
ASK about the use of tobacco, alcohol, and illicit drugs. Revisit the question periodically when their use is denied. Revisit the question at most visits when their use is admitted or highly suspected.	ASK
ASSESS patients who are chemically dependent for amount of use and related medical and psychosocial problems.	ASSESS
ACCEPT patient information in a nonjudgmental manner. This does not mean that you do not give your opinion about right and wrong actions (e.g., "It is wrong to hit your child, and alcohol puts you in that position"). Rather, accept that your patient's disease is the problem, not your patient.	ACCEPT
ADVISE all users to stop. Make use of general and patient-specific reasons, personal and family histories of substance-related diseases, physical examination findings, and social roles (e.g., scout troop leader, deacon, parent).	ADVISE
ASSIST patients in stopping use according to their current stage of change. When the abused substance can have dire consequences if used just once (e.g., street heroin that could contain unknown ingredients), encourage immediate cessation and offer immediate detoxification assistance. For substances that only have severe effects from chronic use, assist patients in identifying their own quit date.	ASSIST
ARRANGE follow-up visits to continue your support, encouragement, and assessment for about 1 to 2 weeks after 1) an agreed upon quit date, 2) a patient has agreed to immediate abstinence, or 3) a patient has attended a detoxification program. If the patient has relapsed, review what happened (e.g., what was the patient doing at the time, where did the first cigarette or drink come from). Revisit ASSIST when necessary.	ARRANGE
APPLAUD all patients attempting recovery or continuing in recovery at every visit for the first 2 years, then at frequent intervals.	APPLAUD

- Inability to stop use when started
- Use to avoid withdrawal symptoms
- Increased tolerance
- Related medical or behavioral problems (e.g., blackouts, depression, hypertension, trauma, chronic abdominal pain, liver dysfunction, sexual dysfunction, sleep disorders, problems with family, work, or school)

Presentation

Tobacco

Patients commonly complain of a cough, shortness of breath, mouth sores, stomach pain, frequent bronchitis, leg pain, and chest pain.

TABLE 25–3. **The CAGE Questions**

- Have you ever felt that you should **cut** down on your drinking or using?
- Have people **annoyed** you by criticizing your use?
- Have you ever felt bad or **guilty** about your use?
- Have you ever had a drink or used a drug first thing in the morning to steady your nerves or get rid of a hangover (i.e., as an **eye opener**)?

Alcohol and illicit drugs

Patients who abuse alcohol or illicit drugs often present with one or more concerns.

Psychosocial complaints include:

- Anxiety
- Depression
- Irritability
- Insomnia
- Family distress or violence
- Job problems or frequent requests for work excuses
- Legal problems

NOTE

Assess parents and children for substance abuse if parents complain of significant behavioral problems in one or more of their children.

Physical complaints include:

- Trauma
- Gastrointestinal problems (e.g., nausea, abdominal pain)
- Weight changes
- Palpitations or chest pain
- Sexual dysfunction
- Depression
- Insomnia
- Anxiety
- Family dysfunction

History

History of present illness

Tobacco

- Do you smoke or chew tobacco? If so, how much and for how long?

- Have you ever tried to quit? If so, how long did it work, and why did it stop working?
- Are you interested in quitting now?

Alcohol and illicit drugs

In addition to the assessment questions suggested below, Table 25–4 includes questions that may be helpful when assessing for alcohol abuse in women. Although the following questions focus on alcohol, they can be used for suspected abuse of any substance.

- How long have you been drinking?
- How do you define "a drink?"
- How many days per week do you drink?
- How many beers and shots do you have most days? How many do you have on the weekends?
- What time of day do you drink?
- What is the earliest time you might drink on a day off?
- What is the most you have drunk in 1 day during the last 6 months?
- What is the most you have drunk on one occasion in the last year?
- When you drink alcohol, how does it make you feel?
- How much can you drink before you feel "drunk?"
- How do others perceive you when you are drunk? What have they said?
- How much can you drink and still drive safely?
  - □ Do not mistake an answer to this as an accurate assessment! Any answer other than "none" deserves further investigation.
- What is the longest time you have gone without any alcohol in the last year?
- What amount of drinking do you feel is the maximum you should do during 1 day or 1 week?

TABLE 25–4. The TWEAK Questions for Female Alcohol Drinkers

	Question	Points*
Tolerance	How many drinks does it take before you begin to feel the first effects of alcohol?†	2
Worried	Have close friends or relatives worried or complained about your drinking in the last year?	2
Eye opener	Do you sometimes take a drink in the morning when you first get up?	1
Amnesia	Has a friend or family member ever told you about things you said or did while you were drinking that you could not remember?	1
Kut down	Do you sometimes feel the need to cut down on your drinking?	1

Reprinted with permission from Bradley KA, Boyd-Wickizer J, et al: Alcohol screening questionnaires in women: a critical review. *JAMA* 280:166–171, 1998.
*A positive screen is a score of 2 or more.
†Three or more drinks indicates tolerance.

- Are you experiencing any current problems with:
  - □ Family (e.g., neglecting the children, frequently arguing or fighting with spouse)
  - □ School (e.g., absences, suspensions, expulsions)
  - □ Work (e.g., absences, poor performance)
  - □ The legal system (e.g., disorderly conduct, driving an automobile or operating machines when under the influence of a substance)

Past medical history

Ask about problems associated with substance abuse (Table 25–5).

Family history

Ask about family history of substance abuse. Also ask about conditions for which substance abuse can be a risk factor (see Table 25–5).

> **NOTE**
>
> A family history of bipolar disorder is a significant risk factor for abuse of alcohol and other substances.

Social history

- Can you smoke at work?
- What are the current stressors in your life?
- Do you drink alcohol (often a smoking trigger)?

TABLE 25–5. Problems Associated With Substance Abuse

System	Associated Problems
Constitutional	Accidents, falls
Dermatologic	Postsurgical or other wound complications
Cardiovascular	Coronary artery disease, stroke, high blood pressure, peripheral vascular disease
Respiratory	COPD, frequent asthma exacerbations
Gastrointestinal	Liver problems, hepatitis, pancreatitis
Musculoskeletal	Muscle cramps, multiple fractures
Neurologic	Dementia, peripheral neuropathy, seizures
Psychologic	Depression, anxiety, alcohol withdrawal syndrome, partner violence, family dysfunction
Hematologic	Anemia, dyslipidemias
Endocrine	Diabetes

COPD = chronic obstructive pulmonary disease.

- Do you smoke cigarettes (often an alcohol trigger)?
- What coping mechanisms do you use?

Review of Systems (Table 25–6)

Physical Examination (Table 25–7)

Laboratory Tests

In general, laboratory tests are not helpful for the diagnosis of substance abuse.

Tobacco

An arterial blood gas may help to identify pulmonary problems associated with excessive use of tobacco.

Alcohol

In cases of alcohol abuse, complete blood count findings often include anemia. Microcytic anemia suggests gastrointestinal bleeding. Macrocytic anemia suggests vitamin B_{12} or folate deficiency.

Hepatic profile findings include:

- Elevated alanine aminotransferase (ALT) and aspartate aminotransferase (AST) with an AST:ALP ratio greater than 1.5
- Elevated prothrombin time and partial thromboplastin time
- Decreased albumin (liver failure)
- Elevated γ-glutamyltransferase (GGT), which is often seen but is not very specific for abuse

Alcohol abuse may also result in elevated levels of amylase and lipase (pancreatitis), triglycerides, and uric acid.

TABLE 25–6. Review of Systems in the Diagnosis of Substance Abuse

System	Common Patient Complaints
Constitutional	Significant weight change, insomnia, lethargy
Cardiovascular	Chest pain, high blood pressure, leg pain with activity
Pulmonary	Shortness of breath, chronic cough, sinus problems, chest cold
Gastrointestinal	Abdominal pain, diarrhea, constipation
Musculoskeletal	Muscle cramps, multiple fractures, gout
Neurologic	Attention deficits, poor memory, peripheral neuropathy
Psychologic	Depression, anxiety, mood swings, rage reactions, insomnia, blackouts
Genitourinary	Nocturia

TABLE 25–7. **Physical Examination Findings in Substance Abuse**

System	Findings
Vital signs	High blood pressure (anxiety, withdrawal, arteriosclerosis), weight loss, obesity or patient weight concerns (address before smoking cessation)
Dermatologic	Palmar erythema, spider angiomas (liver disease), rosacea, other facial redness (alcohol), tobacco stains on fingers, significantly wrinkled skin
HEENT	Sinus pain with palpation and upper respiratory infection symptoms (sinusitis), oral lesions (leukoplakia, cancer), facial edema (alcohol), parotid swelling (vomiting), conjunctival injection, pale palpebral conjunctiva (anemia), dilated pupils, dry mucous membranes, pharyngeal erythema (marijuana), nasal irritation, septum perforation (cocaine)
Cardiovascular	Poor peripheral pulse and pretibial venous stasis (peripheral vascular disease), arrhythmias (especially supraventricular "holiday heart"), signs of cardiomyopathy or ischemia (alcohol, cocaine), tachycardia (marijuana, alcohol withdrawal)
Respiratory	Cough, tachypnea (lung disease), black sputum (smoked substances)
Urogenital	Testicular atrophy (testosterone dysfunction from alcohol)
Gastrointestinal	Tenderness (gastritis, hepatitis, peptic ulcer disease, pancreatitis), enlarged liver or spleen (hepatitis)
Musculoskeletal	Muscle tenderness or weakness
Neurologic	Poor memory, peripheral neuropathy, aphasia (alcohol), constellations of mental status changes*, numbness and weakness of extremities (alcohol polyneuropathy), symptoms of seizures or cerebrovascular accidents (cocaine, alcohol)

*Mental status changes can include Wernicke-Korsakoff syndrome (alcohol); elevated mood, depression, agitation, confusion, or paranoid ideation (marijuana); and euphoria, depression, irritability, anxiety, or acute psychotic symptoms (cocaine).

Illicit drugs

A toxicology screen performed on urine, serum, or both can demonstrate recently used drugs.

Imaging Studies

A chest radiograph may reveal an increase in the anteroposterior diameter, a flat diaphragm, or bleb (tobacco).

Additional Studies

Peak expiratory flow can help quantify certain pulmonary problems. Spirometry may show an elevated forced expiratory volume in 1 second/forced vital capacity ratio or an elevated peak expiratory flow (i.e., 25% to 75%) [marijuana and tobacco]. An electrocardiogram may show signs of ischemia, arrhythmia, or myocardial infarction (cocaine).

Spirometry follow up

If spirometry testing was done and was normal, stress the importance of stopping use now before damage is done. If the results were abnormal, stress the importance of stopping now to limit further damage.

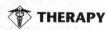 THERAPY

Nonpharmacologic Therapy

Support

Nicotine

Smoking cessation programs are available at low cost through the American Cancer Society, American Heart Association, American Lung Association, and Nicotine Anonymous. Behavioral programs are critical to most persons trying to quit.

Alcohol and illicit drugs

Recovery from alcohol and other drugs is often punctuated by relapse and a substance-related problem before stable recovery is achieved. With alcoholism, there is a 70% success rate (defined as abstinence and improvement in functioning 1 year after treatment) if treatment is obtained in an early stage (i.e., while the patient is employed and has family support).

Alcoholic's Anonymous (AA) is the most widely used program in the world for nonpharmacologic treatment of alcoholism and is based on a core of 12 steps. Although almost all AA groups emphasize the inclusion of "God" in the 12 steps, the way they emphasize this component varies. A few AA groups consciously try to appeal to those who have difficulty working within a framework that accepts the existence of a supreme being. Nevertheless, for most AA followers, the belief in a supreme being is key. Therefore, consider the patient's cultural and spiritual beliefs before suggesting AA.

Various other 12-step programs exist for other drugs, including Cocaine Anonymous and Narcotics Anonymous.

> **NOTE**
>
> Recommending a 12-step program for relatives and friends of people with substance abuse problems [e.g., Al-Anon (alcohol), Nar-Anon (drugs)] often is important.

Pharmacotherapy

For many persons with substance abuse problems, medication must be used in conjunction with a behavioral program to be successful.

Nicotine and tobacco

Nicotine replacement during the period of acute nicotine withdrawal allows the smoker to concentrate on other aspects of cessation. Smokers who are highly dependent on nicotine benefit the most. Three forms of nicotine replacement are available: patches, inhalers, and gum. All are ideally used for about 8 weeks. The main adverse effect of the patch is skin irritation. The gum may aggravate jaw or dental problems, may cause nausea if excessive chewing causes nicotine to be swallowed, and must be chewed in a specific manner. The inhaler may cause minor irritation.

Bupropion, initially marketed as an antidepressant, has shown benefit in enhancing tobacco cessation rates. It is usually contraindicated in patients with eating disorders (e.g., anorexia, bulimia) because it is associated with weight loss in a significant number of patients. It is also contraindicated in patients with seizure disorders because the seizure threshold can be decreased if used in doses greater than 200 mg or if doses are less than 8 hours apart. The more common side effects include restlessness, insomnia, and nausea. A target quit date for smoking cessation is usually set, but not until 1 week after beginning bupropion treatment.

NOTE

Patients who combine nicotine replacement or bupropion with cessation counseling or a behavior modification program have the most success.

Alcohol

Disulfiram inhibits alcohol dehydrogenase and is most useful in patients who repeatedly relapse. It can be used daily or when one anticipates a particularly tempting situation (e.g., a party). Inhibition of alcohol dehydrogenase results in high levels of acetaldehyde, which can produce reactions such as cutaneous flushing, headache, nausea, and vomiting. Although uncommon, reactions may also include myocardial infarction, seizures, arrhythmias, and congestive heart failure. Thus, disulfiram is contraindicated in patients who are pregnant or those with severe coronary artery disease, cognitive dysfunction, liver failure, or hypothyroidism.

Naloxone is an opioid antagonist found to be useful in reducing relapse in patients with alcoholism. It is contraindicated in patients who are opioid dependent, receiving opioid analgesics, or in acute opioid withdrawal as well as in patients with acute hepatitis or liver failure.

URGENCIES AND EMERGENCIES

Withdrawal

The most common emergency of chemical dependency is withdrawal (see Table 25–1).

Other Common Emergencies

Other common emergencies in alcohol and drug-abusing patients include **severe intoxication, seizures, coma or obtundation,** and **severe agitation.** In such cases, one would generally call for emergency transport. Whenever possible, while waiting for transport obtain:

- A physical examination to rule out (or in) the need for emergent treatment before transport
- Intravenous (IV) access
  - If feasible, get screening blood tests, including toxicology, when access is begun.
- As much history as possible, including history from ancillary sources

Emergency Measures in the Outpatient Office

Severe intoxication with seizures

- Lorazepam: 2 to 4 mg IV push or
- Diazepam: 5 to 10 mg IV push

Coma or obtundation with suspected chemical abuse

- Naloxone: 0.4 mg IV every 3 to 5 minutes; give 3 doses, if needed
- Glucose: 50 mg IV if hypoglycemia cannot be ruled out

Severe agitation

- Diazepam: 5 to 10 mg IV or
- Haloperidol: 2 to 5 mg IV

 SPECIAL POPULATIONS

Children

Among adolescents, alcohol and tobacco are currently the most popular drugs, with marijuana, stimulants, inhalants, and lysergic acid diethylamide also very prevalent. Assuring confidentiality for adolescents is critical. Focus on any changes in functioning at home, at school, and with friends. Ask about use of tobacco, alcohol, and other drugs among peers and family.

In addition, ask adolescents if they agree with any of the following statements:

- Drinking helps me forget.
- Drinking helps me be friendly.
- Drinking helps me feel good about myself.
- Drinking helps me relax.
- Drinking helps me be friends with others who drink.

A positive response to three or more items indicates a need for further evaluation.

Seniors

About two-thirds of older adult alcoholics are early-onset alcoholics, having been alcoholic from early adulthood. The remaining one-third of older adult alcoholics are late-onset alcoholics, with increased drinking secondary to loneliness and losses. Older patients may also use alcohol to self-medicate for insomnia, pain, or depression. Many older patients with alcoholism are "hidden," with the patient or family covering up presentations and the physician reluctant to identify the problem. The CAGE questions (see Table 25–3) are a useful screening tool, and AA is an excellent treatment resource for those whose spiritual beliefs suit it.

Pregnancy

Use of alcohol, tobacco, and illicit drugs in pregnancy is strictly contraindicated. Use of alcohol during pregnancy is associated with negative effects on the fetus (e.g., fetal alcohol syndrome). Use of cocaine during pregnancy increases the risk of spontaneous abortion, abruptio placentae, premature delivery, stillbirth, and sudden infant death syndrome. In addition, there is convincing evidence of long-term developmental delays, distractability, and behavioral problems in these children.

◀▶ CONSULTS

Depending on your preceptor's interest, experience, and training, she may use several options for managing patients with chemical dependency. Brief assessment and intervention without active counseling for chemical dependency, which generally requires additional training, and the use of medications can be extremely effective if the appropriate referrals are made and followed up. In such cases, knowledge of local treatment resources is essential. Resources include outpatient and inpatient chemical dependency programs and individual therapists (e.g., psychiatrist, psychologist, social worker, psychiatric nurse) knowledgeable about chemical dependency.

Vaginal Discharge

Maria M. Sandvig

OBJECTIVES

- Distinguish between normal presentations and common pathologic diagnoses that present with a vaginal discharge
- Describe the physical signs and symptoms of vaginal discharge that should be observed and charted
- Recognize when immediate therapy is necessary to prevent major complications
- Be familiar with the general categories of therapy for vaginal discharge

 INTRODUCTION

The characteristics of healthy, normal vaginal discharge vary with age and hormonal balance. Prepubertal girls generally have no vaginal discharge when they are young, but often develop a white discharge several years before puberty, when their estrogen levels begin to increase. Post-menopausal women not taking hormone replacements often have little to no vaginal discharge.

Most women (i.e., women between puberty and menopause) have a discharge that varies across each menstrual cycle. Just before and just after menses, the discharge may appear light brown. During ovulation the consistency may be sticky and viscous. When placed between the thumb and forefinger, the discharge often stretches in an intact "string" formation for 1 to 2 inches before breaking. This characteristic, known as spindlekieten, has been used for family planning in various cultures to determine when to seek or avoid vaginal-penile intercourse.

Factors that provide a balance in the vaginal ecosystem include host metabolic products, bacterial flora and their metabolic products, estrogen, and pH level. Many things can alter this equilibrium, including:

- Sexually transmitted diseases (STDs)
- Medications such as antibiotics, oral contraceptives, and hormones
- Irritants such as chemicals and foreign bodies
- Activities such as douching and sexual intercourse

TERMINOLOGY

Bacterial vaginosis: an overgrowth of *Haemophilus vaginalis* (previously called *Gardnerella vaginalis*) and anaerobic bacteria that leads to a malodorous discharge with clue cells

Cervical ectropion: an erythematous, ectocervical surface composed of glandular epithelium that has not yet encountered the normal process of metaplasia

Cervical erosion: an erythematous, ectocervical surface composed of denuded squamous epithelium

Cervicitis: inflammation of the cervical mucosa that is commonly associated with one or more of the following:

- A mucopurulent cervical discharge with more than 10 white blood cells (WBCs) per high-power field
- A cervix that is friable when manipulated (e.g., may bleed easily if touched with a speculum, cotton swab, cytobrush, or spatula)
- A positive test for *Chlamydia trachomatis* or *Neisseria gonorrhoeae*
- An erythematous, edematous cervix (sometimes difficult to differentiate from erosion or ectropion)

Chemical irritation: an inflammatory reaction to a foreign substance (e.g., soap, perfume, douche solution, minipads, latex condoms, spermicide)

Clue cell: an epithelial cell covered by the small Gram-negative bacilli called *Haemophilus vaginalis* and associated with bacterial vaginosis

Discharge, vaginal: mucus from the vagina that can originate from the vaginal walls or the cervical os and is often described in terms of:

- Color (translucent, white, greenish, yellowish, brownish, blood-tinged)
- Amount (copious, moderate, scant)
- Consistency (frothy, watery, homogenous, curd-like, thin, leukorrhea)
- Smell (fishy, malodorous, normal)

Lesion, gynecologic: excoriations, ulcers, blisters, or papillary structures seen on the vulva, vaginal wall, or cervix

Leukorrhea: an abnormal vaginal discharge made up of viscous fluid containing mucus and pus

Metaplasia: in relation to cervical cytology, the cellular process that replaces the glandular cells with squamous cells and results in the "movement" of the transition zone into the endocervix

Strawberry cervix: a term used to describe a cervix with classical punctate hemorrhagic lesions related to *Trichomonas vaginalis*

Urethritis: inflammation of the urethra that, when present in women, is most often associated with a Gram-negative bacterial cystitis; can also be associated with *Chlamydia, Trichomonas* vaginitis, or atrophic changes

Vaginitis: inflammation of the vaginal mucosa

Vaginitis, atrophic: irritation associated with a low-estrogen state that is marked by thinning and drying of the mucous membranes and is most often noted in perimenopausal and postmenopausal women

Vaginitis, *Candida*: a vaginal yeast infection that often leads to a thick, curd-like white discharge with intense pruritus

Vaginitis, *Monilia:* see *vaginitis, Candida*
Vaginitis, *Trichomonas:* a urogenital, protozoal infection that can lead to a vaginal discharge
Vaginitis, yeast: see *vaginitis, Candida*
Vaginosis: infection of the vaginal mucosa
Vulvovaginitis: inflammation of the vulva and vagina

 ## BACKGROUND

In the United States, an abnormal vaginal discharge is the most common gynecologic complaint physicians encounter, leading to approximately 10 million office visits per year.

 ## PREVENTION

Teaching patients about symptom recognition, risk factors, and primary prevention techniques (e.g., condoms, diaphragms, spermicides, abstinence) can help avoid vaginitis and cervicitis.

Screening

Some authorities advocate screening populations at high risk for gonorrheal and chlamydial infections every 6 months, while other authorities advocate screening every year. Regardless, screening for STDs and other abnormal discharges should be considered for all of the following:

- Pregnant women
- Nonmonogamous sexually active individuals
- Women with a history of a previous STD (screen during routine pelvic examination)

Primary Prevention

Information on pathology-specific primary prevention for various causes of an abnormal vaginal discharge can be found in Table 26–1.

Secondary Prevention

When gonorrhea is diagnosed, patients should be treated empirically for *Chlamydia* and vice versa, because they are often found together.

If the patient's sexual partner is diagnosed with *Chlamydia,* gonorrhea, or *Trichomonas* vaginalis, the patient should be treated empirically for the diagnosed disease because the likelihood that it has been transmitted is high.

TABLE 26–1. **Primary Prevention for Various Causes of Abnormal Vaginal Discharge**

Cause of Discharge	Primary Prevention Techniques
Atrophic vaginitis	Consider hormone replacement a few years before or during menopause
Bacterial vaginosis	Suggest avoiding frequent douching (e.g., no more than once a month), using an acidic solution if douching, using condoms during intercourse*, wearing cotton underwear
Chemically induced vaginitis	Assess bubble baths, vulvar and vaginal deodorants, lubricants, spermicides, and other hygiene products as possible causes of inflammation (individual specific)
Gonorrhea, *Chlamydia* cervicitis, *Trichomonas* vaginitis	Suggest knowing sexual partners well, treat all who are infected and their sexual partners, suggest using condoms 100% of the time when not in an ongoing monogamous relationship
Herpes simplex cervicitis	Suggest knowing sexual partners well, using condoms 100% of the time when not in an ongoing monogamous relationship, not having intercourse with a partner with an active genital lesion, not receiving oral-genital stimulation from a partner with any active oral lesion
Yeast vaginitis	Suggest control of glucose in diabetics, changing underclothes after working out to the point of perspiring, wearing cotton underwear, minimizing steroid use, and, for women on oral contraceptives, using the lowest estrogen dose possible

*Using condoms during intercourse can be helpful when the alkalotic pH induced by ejaculate is part of the problem.

DIAGNOSIS

Table 26–2 covers key information that may save you time and effort when diagnosing an abnormal vaginal discharge.

Presentation

Common presenting complaints include:
- "I have a discharge."
- "My boyfriend has a discharge."
- "It hurts to pee."
- "I itch down there."
- "My stomach hurts a lot."
- "I have this terrible smell when I have sex."
- "I want a Pap smear" (some patients mistakenly think "Pap smear" means gynecologic examination to rule out infection).

TABLE 26–2. Associated Characteristics and Therapy of Abnormal Vaginal Discharges

	Yeast Vaginitis	Gonnorhea and Chlamydia Cervicitis	Trichomoniasis	HSV Cervicitis	Bacterial Vaginosis	Chemically Induced Vaginitis	Atrophic Vaginitis	Normal Reproductive Age Discharge
Discharge color	White	Yellow or green-yellow	Yellow or gray	Translucent	Yellow or off-white	Off-white to yellow	Whitish, may be blood tinged	Translucent to white
Discharge consistency	Thick, curd-like	Leukorrhea	Frothy	Watery	Homogenous	Leukorrhea	Thin	Stringy
Discharge amount	Variable but often copious	Moderate	Variable but often copious if advanced	Scant to copious	Scant to moderate	Scant to copious	Scant	Scant to copious
Discharge microscopic findings	Yeast particles (budding yeast, pseudohyphae, hyphae); few or no WBCs	WBCs TNTC	>10 WBCs/HPF; mobile protozoa are larger than a WBC, much larger than sperm, but smaller than epithelial cells	WBCs TNTC	>20% of epithelial cells are clue cells, no lactobacilli, many small cocci	>10 WBC/HPF to TNTC, no lactobacilli	Epithelial cells, few to many WBCs, diverse flora	Lactobacilli and epithelial cells

(continued)

TABLE 26–2. Associated Characteristics and Therapy of Abnormal Vaginal Discharges (*Continued*)

	Yeast Vaginitis	Gonorrhea and Chlamydia Cervicitis	Trichomoniasis	HSV Cervicitis	Bacterial Vaginosis	Chemically Induced Vaginitis	Atrophic Vaginitis	Normal Reproductive Age Discharge
Discharge pH	3.8–4.2	<4.5	6–7	Not diagnostic	>4.5	Not diagnostic	5.5–7	3.8–4.2
Commonly associated signs	Mild to severe erythema, dry vaginal walls	Cervicitis, endometritis	Cervical micro-hemorrhages	Very common with primary HSV (80%); less common with secondary HSV (20%)	Vaginal inflammation is minimal	Vulvovaginal inflammation	Thin, pale to erythematous vaginal mucosa that may have petechiae	Pink vaginal walls and introitus, changes with stage of menstrual cycle
Commonly associated symptoms	Vulvovaginal itching and irritation	Pelvic pain, dysuria, irregular bleeding, dysmenorrhea	Vulvar itching, dyspareunia, dysuria, pelvic/low abdominal pain, malodorous*	Vulvar itching or burning in a discrete area that recurs along a dermatome	Amine "fishy" odor is common, 50% are asymptomatic	May or may not be malodorous, vulvovaginal burning	Dysuria, urine frequency, urgency or urge incontinence, vulvar itching or burning, dyspareunia, spotting, may or may	Absence of foul odor

Other							
KOH prep for microscopy can help with visualization of yeast particles	STD	STD, fomites (warm moist towels, counters) may harbor live organisms for many hours	STD, symptoms more common if perimenstrual	KOH added to a microscopic specimen will enhance the fishy smell	Associated with spermicides, douching, bath water products, laundry detergent, vaginal contraceptives, perfumed or dyed toilet paper, hot tub or swimming pool chemicals, synthetic clothing	Associated with low-estrogen states and, therefore, with pelvic laxity and stress incontinence	OCs thicken and whiten discharge, ectropions increase a translucent discharge, cervical erosion can cause leukorrhea

not be malodorous

HPF = high-power field; HSV = herpes simplex virus; KOH = postassium hydroxide; OC = oral contraceptive; STD = sexually transmitted disease; TNTC = too numerous to count; WBC = white blood cell.

*Trichomoniasis may be asymptomatic, but almost 50% become symptomatic in 6 months.

History

Patients are often concerned about being labeled with an STD. Thus, learning to obtain the history in a respectful, nonjudgmental manner can be key to building a relationship that will allow for the most accurate diagnosis, the most cost-effective and expedient therapy, and the best likelihood for future prevention. Work toward taking the history with the same attitude and facial expression that you would have if asking questions about a sinus infection.

History of present illness

- How much discharge have you noticed? Does the discharge soak through your underpants?
- What color is the discharge? On toilet paper or underpants?
  - □ Protein even from a normal discharge can yellow in oxygen (i.e., on underwear).
- How many days have you noticed the discharge?
- What is the texture of the discharge? Is it thick or thin?
- Do you have burning with urination, fever, or abdominal pain?
- Could you be pregnant? When did your last menstrual period begin?
- Do you douche? If so, how often and with what agent?
- Is the discomfort at the opening of the vagina or inside?

Past medical history

- Have you recently been using antibiotics?
- Have you been diagnosed with an immune deficiency disorder [e.g., human immunodeficiency virus infection]?
- Do you have uncontrolled diabetes?
- Do you have a history of STDs or other vaginal discharge complaints or diagnoses?

Social history

- Are you sexually active?
- What is the approximate date of your last sexual intercourse?
- Do you have intercourse or other sexual relations with men, women, or both?
- How often do you use condoms (never, sometimes, 99%, 100%)?
  - □ Many patients will easily admit to not using condoms 1% of the time, yet even 1% is an important reason for additional education.
- How many partners have you had intercourse with in the past 6 months? How long have you been with your present partner(s)?
- Do you know if your partner has had sexual contact with others since the two of you have been sexually active?
- Have you been involved with oral or rectal sex in the last few months?

Review of Systems (Table 26–3)
Physical Examination (Table 26–4)

Although the standard of care still includes the use of a speculum, and likely will for some time, several early studies have suggested that a speculum may be unnecessary. Researchers who inserted a cotton swab blindly into the vaginal pool to collect vaginal secretions for phenaphthazine pH paper and for microscopy have found diagnostic sensitivities comparable to those of speculum collection for *Trichomonas* vaginitis, bacterial vaginosis, and *Candida* vulvovaginitis. In addition, urine-based nucleic acid amplification tests have been found to be very sensitive for both gonorrhea and *Chlamydia*.

Using a speculum has important advantages, such as that visualization may allow for a more accurate presumptive diagnosis. In many cases, however, particularly in younger women, use of a speculum may negate their willingness to agree to testing.

Laboratory Tests

The **wet prep** is often a key component in the diagnosis of an abnormal vaginal discharge. The procedure consists of five steps.

- **Step 1:** Using a cotton-tipped applicator, retrieve a specimen of discharge from the vaginal wall, posterior fornix, or cervix. Place the specimen into a test tube that contains a few drops of saline, then stir it a few times.
- **Step 2:** When near the microscope, place a drop of the test tube contents onto a slide. Place a coverslip over the slide, and place it on the microscope under the lens. Immediately proceed to the next step.

NOTE

Trichomonads cannot "swim" on a dry slide. If the initial test tube specimen or the slide specimen becomes dry, all trichomonads are likely to be mistaken for white blood cells (WBCs).

TABLE 26–3. **Review of Systems for Abnormal Vaginal Discharge**

System	Common Patient Complaints
Constitutional	Fever
Gastrointestinal	Stomach pain, cramping
Urogenital	Pelvic area or lower abdominal cramping, itching, burning, irritation, pain with intercourse or urination, urgency to urinate, increased frequency of urination, inability to urinate when feel the urge, mucus vaginal discharge
Musculoskeletal	Low back pain

TABLE 26–4. **Physical Examination Findings with Abnormal Vaginal Discharge**

System	Findings
Vital signs	Fever
Gastrointestinal	Suprapubic or lower gradient tenderness
Urogenital	
External examination	Excoriations, papules, pustules, vesicles, ulcerations, and erythema on the labia majora and minora; pubic lice; tender inguinal lymph nodes
Internal inspection	Abnormal color, consistency, or amount of mucus in the vagina; mucus coming from the cervical os (cervicitis); dry, moist, erythematous, or pink vaginal walls
Bimanual examination	Cervical motion tenderness (pelvic inflammation, endometriosis), adnexal mass (tubo-ovarian abscess, ectopic pregnancy)
Musculoskeletal	Nonradicular low back pain or ache

- **Step 3:** Scan under low power for WBCs, red blood cells (RBCs), hyphae, and epithelial cells.
- **Step 4:** Scan under high power for lactobacilli, clue cells, intracellular cocci, and trichomonads. If yeast is suspected but yeast particles are not visualized, proceed to step 5.
- **Step 5:** Place another drop of the test tube contents onto a new slide. Add a drop of potassium hydroxide to the slide specimen to lyse the epithelial cells. Place a coverslip over the slide, and place it under the high-power lens. With the epithelial cell walls out of the picture, hyphae are usually much more visible. In clinical practice, many physicians use only one slide for steps 2 through 5. Many preceptors prefer that you prepare a second slide for potassium hydroxide, however, so that the first can be saved for visualization of the epithelial cells.

A **DNA probe or cultures** for gonorrhea and *Chlamydia* should be performed in most cases of abnormal vaginal discharge.

Urine-based nucleic acid amplification tests can diagnose chlamydial and gonorrheal infections with urine alone. Unfortunately, they are not yet easily available.

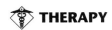 **THERAPY**

Nonpharmacologic Therapy

To prevent yeast vaginitis:

- Wear cotton underwear to encourage absorption of perspiration
- Avoid daily use of minipads

To prevent bacterial vaginosis:

- Avoid douching more than once a month and douche with a mild vinegar solution (i.e., 10% vinegar in 90% water)

In cases of chemical irritation:

- Use a mild soap
- Use a sodium bicarbonate sitz bath and topical vegetable oils for comfort

Pharmacotherapy (Table 26–5)

Atrophic vaginitis

Estrogen replacement is generally the therapy of choice for atrophic vaginitis. It is available in oral, transdermal, and intravaginal preparations (Table 26–6). Metabolism and excretion of all preparations occurs through similar pathways. Depending on the vaginal dose applied, systemic and local

TABLE 26–5. Pharmacotherapy for Various Diagnoses of Abnormal Vaginal Discharge

Diagnosis	Suggested Dose	Alternates
Bacterial vaginosis	Metronidazole 500 mg orally twice daily or 750 mg once daily for 7 days; administer 1 hour before or 2 hours after meals	Metronidazole 0.75% gel applied twice daily into the vagina for 5–7 days OR Clindamycin 2% topical cream* applied once daily for 7 days
Gonorrhea[†]	Ceftriaxone 125 mg IM in a single dose	Ciprofloxacin 500 mg orally in a single dose
Chlamydia[†]	Azithromycin 1 g orally once	Doxycycline 100 mg orally twice daily for 7 days
Trichomonas vaginitis[†]	Metronidazole 2 g orally (tablets come in 500 mg) in a single dose	Metronidazole 500 mg orally twice a day for 7 days
Yeast vaginitis	Clotrimazole 1% cream, one applicator full vaginally at bedtime for 7 days	Terconazole 0.8% cream, one applicator full vaginally at bedtime for 3 days[‡] OR Fluconazole 150 mg orally in a single dose OR OTC medications (clotrimazole 1% or miconazole 2%)

IM = intramuscular; OTC = over the counter.
*Topical creams do not work well for urinary infections.
[†]Treat the patient's partner as well.
[‡]Terconazole is often reserved for resistant cases.

TABLE 26–6. **Estrogen Replacement Preparations for the Treatment of Atrophic Vaginitis**

Preparation	Suggested Dose	Special Instructions
Intravaginal estrogen cream	4 g daily for 2 weeks, then titrate as needed; as an alternate, consider 2–4 g daily, 3 weeks on and 1 week off for 3–6 months	Advise patient to lie down for 30 minutes after applying intravaginal estrogen
Intravaginal estrogen ring	One ring lasts 90 days	Rings can be removed for cleaning, then replaced, throughout their use
Transdermal estrogen	0.05–0.1 mg patches changed twice weekly	Transdermal estradiol does not go through first-pass metabolism and is delivered continuously, avoiding the fluctuations that are sometimes clinically significant when using other formulations; if changing from oral to the skin patch, wait 1 week after stopping the oral form before beginning the new delivery system
Oral estrogen*	0.625–2.5 mg once daily	If patient complains of nausea, administer with food or on a full stomach

*Systemic estrogen therapy works well at alleviating the urogenital signs and symptoms of atrophic vaginitis.

tissue effects may occur, although they are normally of short duration (i.e., 5 to 6 hours). Even vaginal creams and suppositories are absorbed well enough through the vaginal mucosa that chronic daily administration in any patient with a uterus necessitates progesterone replacement to avoid endometrial hyperplasia.

Chemically induced vaginitis

Avoid the irritant and consider mild, short-term, topical steroids (e.g., hydrocortisone 1%).

 ## URGENCIES AND EMERGENCIES

There are serious potential sequelae of cervicitis, including pelvic inflammatory disease (PID), pelvic organ scarring, infertility, and increased risk of ectopic pregnancy. A woman with PID usually has copious vaginal discharge, a fever higher than 101°F, abdominal pain, and tenderness (i.e., cervical motion and adnexal tenderness) on bimanual examination. If left untreated, complications such as tubo-ovarian abscesses and fallopian tube adhesions can develop, leading to infertility and increased risk of ectopic pregnancy. Uncomplicated PID can be treated with intramuscular ceftriaxone, azithromycin, and close follow up. Women with PID who are pregnant, immunocompromised, or unable to tolerate oral fluids should be considered for inpatient treatment.

SPECIAL POPULATIONS

Children

A white vaginal discharge can be seen in newborns within the first few days of birth as a result of *in utero* exposure to high maternal hormone levels.

One-fourth of sexually active adolescents are infected each year with an STD. A careful history and examination to exclude sexual abuse is imperative for any child who presents with a vaginal discharge or an STD.

A vaginal discharge unrelated to sexual abuse is common in young girls, however, usually from soap or poor hygiene. For example, soap use can cause irritation that disappears within a few days of using a milder product. Poor hygiene (e.g., wiping back to front after urination) can result in itching and dysuria combined with a yellow or green vaginal discharge. After verifying that there is no foreign matter in the introitus, prescribe 15-minute tub soaks a few times a day for a few days. Instruct the patient to use warm bath water without any chemicals (e.g., soap, bubble bath), except for a quarter of a cup of household vinegar.

Seniors

Yeast vaginitis is rare in any low-estrogen state. Menopause induces an alkalotic environment in the vagina, however, decreasing some of the normal protection of the premenopause hormone cycle, leading to increased risk of other vaginal infections.

Pregnancy

During pregnancy, increased hormone levels affect the glycogen content and normal flora of the vagina, thus making the environment more conducive to yeast growth, especially during the third trimester. Treatment with nystatin vaginal tablets is one of the safest treatments because it has little systemic absorption.

Metronidazole is contraindicated in the first trimester; therefore, treatment of *Trichomonas* vaginitis is problematic. Referral to a gynecologist or obstetrician should be considered.

✺ COMPLEMENTARY/ALTERNATIVE MEDICINE

Culture-positive yogurt in the vagina is thought by some to decrease the vaginal pH by introducing lactobacilli. Most yogurts available in grocery stores contain live cultures, but patients should be advised to read the packaging to verify.

Many herbal preparations are used in the vagina for various complaints. Such products include tree oil, pulsatilla, kreosotum, borax, hydrastis, sepia, and calcarea carb.

◆◗ CONSULTS

A patient with a recalcitrant vaginal discharge that does not respond to conventional treatment should be referred to a gynecologist. This can be an unusual presentation for a genital tract carcinoma.

Any pediatric patient with a suspected STD or sexual abuse requires complete evaluation by a professional trained in sexual abuse identification and treatment.

Complementary/ Alternative Medicine

Bruce Gebhardt • Therese Zink

DEFINITION

OBJECTIVES

■ Describe the basic trends in the population of patients making use of complementary/alternative medicine

■ Define and describe the distinguishing characteristics of several major therapies currently used in complementary/alternative medicine

In 1993, a landmark article on alternative medicine was published in the New England Journal of Medicine. In the article, alternative medicine was defined as any therapy that is not routinely taught in allopathic or osteopathic medical schools or is not practiced in hospitals. Yet, to many, the term "alternative" implies a modality not only separate from but antagonistic to conventional Western medicine. Thus, terms such as "complementary" and "integrative" have also been used. For this book, we have chosen the terminology used by the Society of Teachers of Family Medicine—complementary/alternative medicine (CAM).

HISTORY

Many CAM therapies, such as traditional Chinese medicine and Ayurvedic medicine, have existed for thousands of years. Hippocrates, the traditional father of Western medicine, used herbs and skeletal manipulation.

In the 19th century, medicine was often dangerous; blood letting and heavy metals were common treatments. Doctors searching for less harmful treatments began to use other forms of therapy, such as homeopathy, chiropractic medicine, naturopathy, and osteopathy. Although these approaches differed greatly, they all had a common theme—the body contains a "vital force" that must be addressed in healing. The goal was to assist the body's innate ability to heal itself by correcting the flow of the "vital force."

In the late 1800s and the early 1900s, the scientific approach to medicine met with many successes. Meticulously defined gross anatomy and microscopic anatomy and the science of microbiology came to the forefront. Scientists identified the role of cleanliness in health and began to identify the organisms that caused disease.

In the 1920s, the Flexner report, a product of the United States Senate and the American Association of Medical Colleges, was released. It attempted to assure standardization of medical education by outlining curricular needs using a biomedical model. Medical schools were accredited using this model, and "nonscientific" modalities fell out of favor. The Flexner report remains the backbone of medical school curricula today.

By the 1960s, the purely biomedical model was scrutinized more closely. It was extremely successful when a specific cause of a disease process could be elucidated. However, it was less successful for chronic diseases with no cure, illnesses with multiple causes, and symptoms that could not be defined as a known disease process. Some patients felt dehumanized (i.e., felt they were being treated as a collection of organs and cells) and looked for ways to take control of their own health. Other patients with medical problems for which no cause could be found were told they had no disease, in spite of how they felt. Soon, often without physician consultation, patients began to try CAM therapies. Recognizing that paternalism did not work well with patients who wanted control over their bodies and that psychologic and social concerns play a large role in patients' interpretations of health, some physicians began to change their approach.

Interest and research in CAM has mushroomed. Currently, at least one in three Americans use some form of CAM therapy. More dollars are spent directly on these modalities than on primary care services. Most people pay cash for CAM therapies without receiving insurance reimbursement. Books about CAM have become bestsellers, the national media has put many spotlights on the topic, and many medical schools have begun to address CAM. In response to the growing use of CAM therapies, the National Center for Complementary and Alternative Medicine (NCCAM) was created within the National Institutes of Health (NIH) to sponsor research and grants and to act as a public information clearinghouse.

SEMANTICS

Language often differs between CAM providers and allopathic practitioners. Allopathic terms stem from a historic tradition with a heavy military influence, which is why militaristic terms (e.g., painkillers, antibiotics, orders, treatment armamentarium) are common. CAM historically has attempted a broad convergence of multiple forces; thus, a different language is used (e.g., balance, gentle, natural). Most CAM providers speak of total body harmony, both biologic and spiritual.

WORKING WITH PATIENTS WHO USE CAM

Several studies have examined which patients use CAM and why. Although patients from all walks of life use CAM, it is most common among white, educated, high-income women. Not surprisingly, CAM is generally not used for diseases that conventional medicine treats effectively (e.g., bacterial meningitis). However, patients with chronic conditions (e.g., arthritis, headache, back pain) that have no "cure" often turn to CAM. Patients afflicted with terminal illnesses (e.g., cancer, AIDS) also experiment with CAM to augment conventional treatments or as a "last ditch" effort.

Many of us fear that patients will use CAM in place of conventional treatments. We shudder to think of cancer patients turning to CAM without proper diagnosis and treatment with conventional methods. Although this fear is real, studies demonstrate that few patients use CAM without also seeking a physician's services. Unfortunately, 70% of patients do not tell their physicians about using CAM therapies because they feel they will be reproached. In addition, many physicians neglect to ask about CAM and feel uncomfortable discussing it because they know little about the various techniques.

The key is to realize that your patients may be using CAM. If a patient is using CAM, find out what therapies and thoroughly research the available data (the NIH is a good source). Discuss CAM therapies in an open and nonjudgmental way with your patients. Educate your patients about therapy that is in their best interest, and be sure they understand what conventional medicine has to offer. Strongly consider contacting CAM practitioners who are working with your patients. Be involved!

POPULAR THERAPIES USED IN COMPLEMENTARY/ALTERNATIVE MEDICINE

NOTE

Many current CAM treatment modalities have not been proved beneficial by well-designed (i.e., evidence-based) studies, just as the effectiveness of some conventional practices has not been rigorously documented.

Acupuncture

In this ancient healing art, the body is described as being composed of conduits or pathways of Qi. Qi, defined as "life force," is said to be balanced by acupuncture. Acupuncture has been practiced for thousands of years in Asia, where it is used in combination with herbs, nutrition, and martial arts to keep people well.

Unlike in Asia, acupuncture in the United States is predominately used for tertiary care, not prevention. In 1971, it debuted for use in mainstream medicine anesthesia. Its therapeutic role in pain control has been well researched, and acupuncture is now being studied as a treatment for substance abuse and other illnesses.

Chiropractic Medicine

Chiropractic philosophy includes the principle that disease is related to the blockage of energy flow. Therefore, this therapeutic approach involves aligning the spine to remove blockages. Chiropractors are best known for treatment of back pain, but many treat other medical conditions with spinal manipulation, including asthma, otitis media, and menorrhagia.

Chiropractors have been practicing for 100 years in the United States. They receive postgraduate training and are eligible for license in all 50 states. Chiropractic care with a focus on the neuromuscular and skeletal systems is the CAM therapy that has been the most accepted and researched by allopathic medicine. Use of chiropractic medicine for the treatment of low back pain has been extensively studied and is included in the Agency for Health Care Research and Quality guidelines. Other well-researched chiropractic treatments include those for cervical spine pain and headaches. Uses outside of these have not been well researched or proved beneficial.

Homeopathy

Homeopathy originated in Germany in the 1700s and is currently used extensively in Europe. This clinical approach views illness as an imbalance between several internal and external forces acting on the body. Treatment is said to work by rebalancing forces, reinforcing the body's defenses, and allowing the body to heal itself. Treatments are based on the concept of "like with like," or the "law of similars." For example, a very dilute solution of bee venom is used to treat inflammatory conditions characterized by burning and stinging pain.

Homeopathic medications are licensed by the FDA for over-the-counter distribution. These solutions are diluted more than 10^6 times. Although a few well-conceived studies suggest some benefit and no adverse effects in the treatment of arthritis, allergic rhinitis, and cyclic breast pain, quality research is limited.

Biofeedback

Biofeedback is used to train patients in relaxation by monitoring respiration, heart rate, and skin temperature. Research has documented success in the use of biofeedback in the treatment of headaches, fecal incontinence, and pain.

Herbal Medicine

Herbal medicine uses plant parts in an attempt to treat and prevent disease. According to the World Health Organization, over 80% of the world's population incorporate herbal medicine into routine health care. In Europe and China, herbs (i.e., "phyto-medicines") have been studied in clinical settings. In the United States, herbs are marketed as food products and are available over the counter with only limited government regulation. Although the herbal market in the United States is several billion dollars a year, only a small amount of good research exists that documents safety and efficacy. Of the many studies conducted, most lack standardization of the concentration or dosage of the active ingredients.

> **NOTE**
>
> Many patients, even well-educated patients, falsely assume that herbs are safe because they are available over the counter and are labeled "natural."

It is important to ask patients about what herbs they are taking. Some may interfere with prescription and over-the-counter medications. Several good sources of information on herbal remedies are included in Appendix III.

Naturopathy

Naturopathy dates back to the 4th century BC during the time of Hippocrates. Naturopaths attempt to enhance the body's inherent ability to heal with diet, lifestyle adjustments, bodywork, hydrotherapy, acupuncture, and herbs.

The use of naturopathy declined rapidly from the 1940s to the 1950s with the advancement of pharmaceuticals and medical technology. Since 1986, the year the American Association of Naturopathic Physicians incorporated in Oregon, naturopaths trained at postgraduate programs may take national and state licensing exams in some areas of the country. In nine states, they are even considered primary care providers. The state of Washington mandates that health insurance must pay for the services of a naturopath.

Research suggests that naturopathic treatments may be less costly than treatments prescribed by physicians. Unfortunately, there is currently no well-done research that shows naturopathy to be effective.

Complementary/Alternative Medicine Therapies Recognized by the National Institutes of Health

Reflecting the growing use of CAM therapies, the NIH has published a list of CAM techniques eligible for research funding (Table 1).

THE FUTURE OF COMPLEMENTARY/ALTERNATIVE MEDICINE

Physicians are now taking an interest in CAM for various reasons. Treating chronic illnesses is often frustrating, and some CAM therapies hold

TABLE 1. **Categories for CAM Identified by the NIH**

Category	Included Modalities
Diet, nutrition, and lifestyle changes	Macrobiotics diet, megavitamins, changes in lifestyle (e.g., Dr. Dean Ornish's program for lowering cardiac risk factors)
Mind–body interventions	Relaxation exercises, prayer, guided imagery, art therapy, counseling
Traditional ethno-medicine	Acupuncture, Asian medicine, Ayurvedic medicine (India), Native American medicine, Hispanic medicine, African-American medicine
Manual healing	Acupressure, chiropractic medicine, massage, reflexology, therapeutic touch, rolfing
Pharmacologic and biologic treatments	Herbs, antioxidizing agents, chelation, metabolic therapy
Bioelectromagnetic therapy	TENS units (for pain relief), capacitor or electrode stimulation of bone, soft tissue, or wounds (to enhance cytogenesis)

CAM = complementary/alternative medicine; NIH = National Institutes of Health; TENS = transcutaneous electrical nerve stimulation.

promise. For example, some research indicates that chiropractic therapy for the treatment of back pain and acupuncture for the treatment of chemotherapy-induced nausea may work. In addition, patients are using CAM, and physicians need to be educated about CAM to best serve their patients. Finally, hospital systems and HMOs are investing in CAM as a way to increase revenue and decrease cost. Physician involvement is needed to ensure quality of care through appropriate studies.

Scientific Validation

We need to approach CAM as we would approach any other medical treatment—looking toward research and documentation of effectiveness and safety. What really works and how? What are the long-term outcomes of CAM? What role does the placebo effect play? (Many studies show that the placebo effect can give positive outcomes in over 30% of problems.) Does it matter if a therapy works as a placebo if it helps when conventional therapy does not?

Possible Paradigm Shift

Currently, scientific proof concerning the efficacy of CAM is scarce, and many question if current research methods can appropriately be used for such an assessment. In Western medicine, the current model used as the gold standard of research is the double-blind, placebo-controlled trial. We like to identify the one chemical in an herb that exerts a favorable effect.

We generally want one treatment, preferably in pill form, for a given diagnosis.

CAM practitioners approach problems using a different model. They often want to use the whole herb for its effect, not a distilled fraction. They use multiple herbs or other therapies (e.g., massage, dietary changes) to enhance health. They are not interested in testing each therapy to find a single effective factor; it is the combination that works. For that matter, for a given disease, the therapies chosen may be different for each patient.

These differences in paradigms make research about CAM difficult. How does one do placebo massage? If a patient has multiple therapies at once, which one is effective, or is it the combination that is responsible for the positive effect? How do we measure energy work or auras? We need to identify the individual needs of our patients, not treat them only as the "average" patient, and use therapies that valid research supports. A combination of traditional Western medicine and CAM may prove to be our best approach.

COMPLEMENTARY/ALTERNATIVE MEDICINE IN THIS MANUAL

This appendix is only meant to provide a brief overview of CAM. CAM is a vast field that is difficult to grapple with, even in a full text. Many chapters in this book contain a section at the end describing CAM therapies that may be considered for the particular focus of that chapter. Evidence is detailed if it exists.

Pharmaceuticals

TABLE 1. Generic to Trade Name Cross References with Availability Status*

Common Generic Name	Trade Name and Availability Status	Description
Acarbose	Rx: Precose	α-Glucosidase inhibitor, hypoglycemic
Acetaminophen	OTC: Numerous preparations	Antipyretic, analgesic
Acetaminophen + caffeine	OTC: Excedrin Aspirin Free	Analgesic, antimigraine
Acetaminophen + caffeine + aspirin	OTC: Excedrin Extra Strength, Excedrin Migraine	Analgesic, antipyretic, antimigraine
Acetic acid + aluminum acetate	OTC: Domeboro, Pedi-Boro	Otic antibiotic and antifungal solution
Acetic acid + propylene glycol	Rx: Vosol, Acetasol, Burow's Otic	Otic antibiotic and antifungal solution
Acetylcysteine	Rx: Mucomyst	Mucolytic
Albuterol + ipratropium inhaler	Rx: Combivent	Combination β_2-agonist and anticholinergic
Amitriptyline	Rx: Elavil, Endep[†]	Tricyclic antidepressant
Amoxicillin	Rx: Amoxil, Polymox[†]	Third-generation penicillin
Amoxicillin + clavulanate	Rx: Augmentin	Third-generation penicillin + β-lactamase inhibitor
Ardeparin	Rx: Normiflo	Anticoagulant
Aspirin	OTC: Numerous preparations	Antiplatelet, analgesic, anti-inflammatory
Aspirin + caffeine + butalbital ± codeine	Rx: Fiorinal, Fiorinal + Codeine	Narcotic analgesic
Atorvastatin	Rx: Lipitor	HMG-CoA reductase inhibitor, dyslipidemic
Azelastine	Rx: Astelin	Nasal antihistamine
Azithromycin	Rx: Zithromax	Macrolide
Beclomethasone	Rx: Beconase, Vancenase[†]	Steroid

(continued)

This appendix was compiled by James O'Dea, Christine O'Dea, and Susan Louisa Montauk.

TABLE 1. Generic to Trade Name Cross References with Availability Status* (*Continued*)

Common Generic Name	Trade Name and Availability Status	Description
Benzocaine + antipyrine	Rx: Auralgan	Topical otic anesthetic
Benzonatate	Rx: Tessalon Perles	Non-sedating antitussive
Benzoyl peroxide	OTC: Numerous preparations Rx: Numerous preparations†	Antibacterial, keratolytic (acne)
Bupropion	Rx: Wellbutrin	Antidepressant, nicotine receptor agonist
Cefpodoxime	Rx: Vantin	Third-generation cephalosporin
Ceftibuten	Rx: Cedax	Third-generation cephalosporin
Ceftriaxone	Rx: Rocephin	Injectable third-generation cephalosporin
Cefuroxime	Rx: Ceftin, Kefurox, Zinacef	Second-generation cephalosporin
Celecoxib	Rx: Celebrex	Cox-2 inhibiting NSAID, analgesic, antipyretic
Cerivastatin	Rx: Baycol	HMG-CoA reductase inhibitor, dyslipidemic
Cetirizine	Rx: Zyrtec	Nonsedating antihistamine
Chlorpheniramine	OTC: Numerous preparations	Sedating antihistamine
Chlorpropamide	Rx: Diabinese	First-generation sulfonylurea, hypoglycemic
Cholestyramine	Rx: Questran, Questran Light, Prevalite	Bile acid sequestrant, dyslipidemic
Ciprofloxacin	Rx: Cipro	Fluoroquinolone
Ciprofloxacin ± hydrocortisone	Rx: Cipro HC Otic	Antibacterial + anti-inflammatory otic suspension
Clarithromycin	Rx: Biaxin	Macrolide
Clindamycin	Rx: Cleocin†	Antianaerobe antibiotic
Clonidine	Rx: Catapres†	Central-acting α-adrenergic blocker
Clotrimazole	OTC: Numerous vaginal preparations Rx: Lotrisone cream and lotion, Mycelex Troches, and vaginal tablets	Imidazole antifungal
Codeine	OTC: Available in some states in a cough syrup Rx: Numerous preparations	Narcotic antitussive

(*continued*)

TABLE 1. **Generic to Trade Name Cross References with Availability Status*** (*Continued*)

Common Generic Name	Trade Name and Availability Status	Description
Codeine + acetaminophen	Rx: Tylenol + codeine[†]	Narcotic analgesic, antitussive
Colestipol	Rx: Colestid	Bile acid sequestrant, dyslipidemic
Cromolyn	OTC: Intal Rx: Intal	Mast cell stabilizer
Crotamiton	Rx: Eurax	Scabicide
Dalteparin	Rx: Fragmin	Anticoagulant
Dapsone	Rx: Dapsone[†]	Antibiotic
Dextromethorphan	OTC: Numerous preparations Rx: Numerous preparations	Antitussive
Diazepam	Rx: Valium[†]	Anxiolytic, muscle relaxant
Dihydroergotamine	Rx: D.H.E. 45	Vasoconstrictor for migraine
Diltiazem	Rx: Cardizem CD, Dilacor XR[†]	Calcium channel blocker
Diphenhydramine	OTC: Benadryl[†]	Sedating antihistamine
Disulfiram	Rx: Antabuse	Alcohol dehydrogenase inhibitor
Doxycycline	Rx: Doryx, Vibramycin	Tetracycline antibiotic
Econazole	Rx: Spectazole	Topical imidazole antifungal
Enoxaparin	Rx: Lovenox	Injectable anticoagulant
Ephedrine	OTC: Numerous diet and asthma preparations Rx: Broncholate, Marax, Rynatuss	Anorectic, vasoconstrictor, bronchodilator
Epinephrine	Adrenaline[†]	Adrenergic bronchodilator
Ergotamine + caffeine	Rx: Cafergot, Ercaf, Wigraine, Ergomar	Vasoconstrictor for migraines
Erythromycin	Rx: E.E.S., E-Mycin, Eryc, Ilosone[†]	Macrolide antibiotic
Erythromycin	Rx: A/T/S, Erycette, Eryderm, Erygel	Topical macrolide antibiotic
Estrogen	Rx: Estrace, Ogen, Ortho Dienestrol, Premarin[†]	Hormone
Fenofibrate	Rx: TriCor	Fibric acid dyslipidemic
Fexofenadine	Rx: Allegra	Nonsedating antihistamine
Fluconazole	Rx: Diflucan	Oral antifungal
Fluoxetine	Rx: Prozac[†]	SSRI antidepressant
Fluvastatin	Rx: Lescol	HMG-CoA reductase inhibitor, dyslipidemic

(continued)

TABLE 1. Generic to Trade Name Cross References with Availability Status* (*Continued*)

Common Generic Name	Trade Name and Availability Status	Description
Folic acid	OTC: Numerous preparations Rx: Folvite	Vitamin
Furosemide	Rx: Lasix	Loop diuretic
Gemfibrozil	Rx: Lopid	Fibric acid dyslipidemic
Glimepiride	Rx: Amaryl	Second-generation sulfonylurea
Glipizide	Rx: Glucotrol	Second-generation sulfonylurea
Glyburide	Rx: Diabeta, Glynase, Micronase	Second-generation sulfonylurea
Grepafloxacin	Rx: Raxar	Fluoroquinolone antibiotic
Griseofulvin	Rx: Fulvicin-U/F, Grifulvin V	Oral antifungal
Guaifenesin	OTC: Breonesin, Guaituss, Robitussin† Rx: Humibid	Antitussive, mucolytic
Halperidol	Rx: Haldol	Dopamine-2 agonist antipsychotic
Heparin	Rx: Heparin	Injectable anticoagulant
Hydralazine	Rx: Apresoline	Vasodilator, antihypertensive
Hydrochlorothiazide (HCTZ)	Rx: Esidrix, HydroDIURIL, Microzide, Oretic†	Thiazide diuretic, antihypertensive
Hydrocodone	Rx: Hycodan	Narcotic antitussive, analgesic
Hydrocodone + acetaminophen	Rx: Vicodin	Narcotic antitussive, analgesic
Hydrocortisone	OTC: Numerous preparations Rx: Numerous preparations	Antipruritic, anti-inflammatory
Hydroxyzine	Rx: Atarax, Vistaril†	Sedating antihistamine
Ibuprofen	OTC: Advil, Motrin, Nuprin Rx: Motrin	NSAID, analgesic, antipyretic
Insulin	OTC: Humulin, Novolin Rx: Humalog	Hypoglycemic
Ipecac syrup	OTC: Ipecac	Emetic
Ipratropium	Rx: Atrovent	Anticholinergic bronchodilator
Isoniazid	Rx: Rifamate, Rifater†	Antimycobacterial
Isotretinoin	Rx: Accutane	Oral retinoid for acne
Itraconazole	Rx: Sporanox	Imidazole antifungal
Ketoconazole	Rx: Nizoral	Imidazole antifungal

(*continued*)

TABLE 1. Generic to Trade Name Cross References with Availability Status* (*Continued*)

Common Generic Name	Trade Name and Availability Status	Description
Labetalol	Rx: Normodyne, Trandate	Nonselective adrenergic blocker, antihypertensive
Leucovorin	Rx: Leukovorin	Folate agonist
Levofloxacin	Rx: Levaquin	Fluoroquinolone antibiotic
Lidocaine	Rx: Xylocaine	Injectable local anesthetic
Lindane	Rx: Kildane, Kwell, Scabene	Scabicidic lotion, shampoo
Lithium	Rx: Eskalith, Lithane, Lithobid, Lithonate	Antimanic agent, mood stabilizer
Loracarbef	Rx: Lorabid	Second-generation cephalosporin
Loratadine	Rx: Claritin	Nonsedating antihistamine
Lorazepam	Rx: Ativan	Anxiolytic
Lovastatin	Rx: Mevacor	HMG-CoA reductase inhibitor, dyslipidemic
Meperidine	Rx: Demerol[†]	Narcotic analgesic
Metformin	Rx: Glucophage	Biguanide, hypoglycemic
Methylcellulose	OTC: Citrucel	Bulk-forming fiber (GI)
Methyldopa	Rx: Aldomet[†]	Central α-adrenergic blocker
Methylprednisolone	Rx: Depo-Medrol, Medrol, Medrol dosepak, Solu-Medrol	Corticosteroid
Metoclopramide	Rx: Reglan	Antiemetic, promotes bowel motility
Metronidazole	Rx: Flagyl, MetroCream, MetroGel, MetroGel-Vaginal, Noritate	Antiprotozoal and antibacterial
Miconazole	OTC: Desenex, Lotrimin Monistat 7 Rx: Monistat 3	Imidazole antifungal
Miconazole	OTC: Monistat-Derm cream Rx: Monistat-Derm lotion	Imidazole antifungal
Miglitol	Rx: Glyset	α-Glucosidase inhibitor hypoglycemic
Misoprostol	Rx: Cytotec	Mucosal-protective prostaglandin
Montelukast	Rx: Singulair	Leukotriene inhibitor, bronchodilator
Morphine	Rx: Kadian, MSIR, Oramorph, Roxanol[†]	Narcotic analgesic
Nadolol	Rx: Corgard	Selective β-adrenergic blocker

(*continued*)

TABLE 1. Generic to Trade Name Cross References with Availability Status* (*Continued*)

Common Generic Name	Trade Name and Availability Status	Description
Naloxone	Rx: Narcan	Narcotic antagonist
Naltrexone	Rx: ReVia	Narcotic antagonist
Naproxen	OTC: Aleve Rx: Anaprox, Naprosyn	NSAID, analgesic, antipyretic
Nasal saline	OTC: Ocean Mist	Isotonic nasal solution
Nedocromil	Rx: Tilade	Mast cell stabilizer
Niacin	OTC: Numerous preparations Rx: Niaspan†	Vitamin, dyslipidemic
Nicotine	OTC: Numerous preparations	Nicotine withdrawal aid
Nitroglycerin	Rx: Numerous preparations	Vasodilator and venodilator
Nystatin	Rx: Mycostatin, Mytrex	Antifungal cream, ointment, pastilles, oral, powder
Ofloxacin	Rx: Floxin Otic	Otic fluoroquinolone antibiotic
Orlistat	Rx: Xenical	Lipase inhibitor
Oxiconazole	Rx: Oxistat	Topical imidazole antifungal
Oxycodone	Rx: OxyContin, Roxicodone	Narcotic analgesic
Oxycodone + aspirin	Rx: Percodan	Narcotic analgesic
Oxymetazoline	OTC: Afrin, Neo-Synephrine	Decongestant nasal spray
Pentamidine	Rx: Nebupent, Pentam	Antibiotic for *Pneumocystis carinii* pneumonia
Permethrin	OTC: Nix, Acticin Rx: Elimite	Scabicide cream, rinse, and lotion
Phentermine	Rx: Adipex-P, Fastin, Ionamin	Sympathomimetic amine anorectic
Phenytoin	Rx: Dilantin†	Anticonvulsant
Pioglitazone	Rx: Actos	Thiazolidinedione hypoglycemic
Polymixin B sulfate + neomycin + hydrocortisone	Rx: Cortisporin Otic	Antimicrobial, anti-inflammatory
Pravastatin	Rx: Pravachol	HMG-CoA reductase inhibitor dyslipidemic
Prazosin	Rx: Minipress	Peripheral α-adrenergic blocker antihypertensive
Prednisone	Rx: Deltasone, Sterapred†	Oral corticosteroid
Prochlorperazine	Rx: Compazine	Antiemetic
Promethazine	Rx: Phenergan	Antiemetic

(*continued*)

TABLE 1. **Generic to Trade Name Cross References with Availability Status* (Continued)**

Common Generic Name	Trade Name and Availability Status	Description
Propoxyphene + acetaminophen	Rx: Darvocet	Narcotic analgesic
Propranolol	Rx: Inderal[†]	Selective β-adrenergic blocker
Pseudoephedrine	OTC: Numerous preparations, including Sudafed Rx: Numerous preparations	Sympathomimetic decongestant
Psyllium	OTC: Numerous preparations, including Metamucil	Bulk-forming fiber (GI)
Pyrimethamine	Rx: Daraprim	Antiparasitic
Repaglinide	Rx: Prandin	Oral meglitinide hypoglycemic
Rifabutin	Rx: Mycobutin	Antimycobacterial
Rofecoxib	Rx: Vioxx	Cox-2 inhibiting NSAID, analgesic, antipyretic
Rosiglitazone	Rx: Avandia	Oral thiazolidinedione, hypoglycemic
Salmeterol	Rx: Serevent	Long-acting β_2-agonist, bronchodilator
Sibutramine	Rx: Meridia	Serotonin, norepinephrine, and dopamine reuptake inhibitor; anorectic
Simvastatin	Rx: Zocor	HMG-CoA reductase inhibitor, dyslipidemic
Sumatriptan	Rx: Imitrex	Vasoconstrictor for migraine
Terbinafine	Rx: Lamisil	Allylamine antifungal
Terbutaline	Rx: Brethaire, Brethine, Bricanyl	Subcutaneously administered β-adrenergic agonist, bronchodilator
Terconazole	Rx: Terazol	Topical antifungal
Tetracycline	Rx: Sumycin	Tetracycline antibiotic
Theophylline	Rx: Elixophyllin, Slo-Phyllin, Uni-Dur	Oral bronchodilator
Tobramycin + dexamethasone	Rx: TobraDex	Ophthalmic antibiotic + anti-inflammatory
Tolazamide	Rx: Tolinase	First-generation sulfonylurea hypoglycemic
Tolbutamide	Rx: Orinase	First-generation sulfonylurea hypoglycemic

(continued)

TABLE 1. Generic to Trade Name Cross References with Availability Status* (*Continued*)

Common Generic Name	Trade Name and Availability Status	Description
Tretinoin	Rx: Renova, Retin-A	Retinoid for acne
Triamcinolone	Rx: Aristocort, Kenalog	Topical steroid
Trimethoprim + sulfamethoxazole	Rx: Bactrim, Cotrim, Septra, Sulfatrim	Combination sulfonamide + folate antagonist
Tripelennamine	Not applicable	Sedating antihistamine
Troglitazone	Rx: Rezulin	Thiazolidinedione, hypoglycemic
Trovafloxacin	Rx: Trovan	Fluoroquinolone
Verapamil	Rx: Calan, Isoptin, Verelan†	Calcium channel blocker antihypertensive
Warfarin	Rx: Coumadin	Oral anticoagulant
Zafirlukast	Rx: Accolate	Leukotriene inhibitor
Zileuton	Rx: Zyflo	Leukotriene inhibitor

Cox-2 = cyclooxygenase-2; GI = gastrointestinal; HMG-CoA = 3-hydroxy-3-methylglutaryl coenzyme A; NSAID = nonsteroidal anti-inflammatory drug; OTC = over the counter; Rx = prescription; SSRI = selective serotonin reuptake inhibitor; + = with; ± = with or without.

*We attempted to designate all available formulations. Absence of a brand name does not imply it is a less desirable product.

†The generic version is available.

References for Further Study

CHAPTER 1: WHAT IS FAMILY MEDICINE?

Golden RL: William Osler at 150: an overview of a life. *JAMA* 282(23):2252–2258, 1999.

Stanard JR: *Caring for America: The Story of Family Practice.* Virginia Beach, The Donning Company/Publishers, 1997.

Stephens GG: Family medicine as counterculture. 1979. *Fam Med* 30(9):629–636, 1998.

Stephens GG: *The Intellectual Basis of Family Practice.* Tucson, Winter Publishing Company, Inc., 1982, p 237.

CHAPTER 2: CHANGING HEALTH BEHAVIORS IN A FAMILY PRACTICE

Cockerham WC: *Medical Sociology,* 5th ed. Englewood Cliffs, New Jersey, Prentice Hall, 1992.

Glanz K, Lewis FM, Rimer BK (eds): *Health Behavior and Health Education: Theory, Research and Practice.* San Francisco, Jossey-Bass Inc., 1997.

Gropper RC: *Culture and the Clinical Encounter.* Yarmouth, Maine, Intercultural Press, 1996.

Prochaska JO, Goldstein MG: Process of smoking cessation: implications for clinicians. *Clin Chest Med* 12:727–734, 1991.

Zimmerman GL, Olsen CG, Bosworth MF: A "stages of change" approach to helping patients change behavior. *Am Fam Physician* 61:1409–1422, 2000.

CHAPTER 3: PREVENTION AND SCREENING GUIDELINES FOR ADULTS

Age Charts for Periodic Health Examination. Leawood, Kansas, American Academy of Family Physicians, 1994 (reprint #510).

American Cancer Society report on the cancer related checkup. *CA Cancer J Clin* 30:194–232, 1980.

Guide to Clinical Preventive Services: Report of the United States Preventive Services Task Force, 2nd ed. Baltimore, Williams & Wilkins, 1996.

Healthy People, The Surgeon General's Report on Health Promotion and Disease

Prevention. Washington, DC: Government Printing Office; 1979. US Dept of Health, Education, and Welfare publication PHS 79-55071A.

Rudy DR, Zdon MJ: Update on colorectal cancer. *Am Fam Physician* 61:1759–1770, 2000.

Mahoney M: Screening for colorectal cancer. *Am Fam Physician* 61:3477–3482, 2000.

CHAPTER 4: PREVENTION AND SCREENING GUIDELINES FOR SENIORS

Goldberg TH, Chavin SI: Preventive medicine and screening in older adults. *J Am Geriatr Soc* 45:344–354, 1997.

Kennie DC, Warshaw GA: *Clinical Aspects of Aging*, 3rd ed. Baltimore, Williams & Wilkins, 1990.

Miller KE, Zylstra RG, Standridge JB: The geriatric patient: a systematic approach to maintaining health. *Am Fam Physician* 61:1089–1092, 2000.

Sox HC: Preventive health services in adults. *N Engl J Med* 330:1589–1595, 1994.

CHAPTER 5: PREVENTION AND SCREENING GUIDELINES FOR CHILDREN AND ADOLESCENTS

Broderick P: Pediatric vision screening for the family physician. *Am Fam Physician* 58:691–702, 1998.

Care of Infants and Children: Recommended Curriculum Guidelines for Family Practice Residents. Leawood, Kansas, American Academy of Family Physicians, 1998 (reprint #260).

Ellis MR, Kane KY: Lightening the lead load in children. *Am Fam Physician* 62:545–54 and 559–560, 2000.

Hofmann AD, Greydanus DE (eds): *Adolescent Medicine*, 3rd ed. New York, McGraw-Hill, 1997.

Mahoney MC: Screening for iron deficiency anemia among children and adolescents. *Am Fam Physician* 62:671–673, 2000.

Spegelblatt LS: Alternative medicine: should it be used by children? *Curr Probl Pediatr* July:180–188, 1995.

Strasburger VC, Brown RT: *Adolescent Medicine: A Practical Guide*, 2nd ed. Philadelphia, Lippincott Williams & Wilkins, 1998.

Washington RL: Interventions to reduce cardiovascular risk factors in children and adolescents. *Am Fam Physician* 59:2211–2220, 1999.

CHAPTER 6: ACNE VULGARIS

Leyden JJ: Therapy for acne vulgaris. *N Engl J Med* 336(16):1156–1162, 1997.

Russell JJ: Topical therapy for acne. *Am Fam Physician* 61:357–365, 2000.

CHAPTER 7: ALLERGIC RHINITIS

Balon J: A comparison of active and simulated chiropractic manipulation as adjunctive treatment for childhood asthma. *N Engl J Med* 339(15):1013–1020, 1998.

Lewith GT: Unconventional therapies in asthma: an overview. *Allergy* 51(11):761–769, 1996.

Noble SL, Forbes RC, Woodbridge HB: Allergic rhinitis. *Am Fam Physician* 51(4):837–846, 1995.

CHAPTER 8: ASTHMA

Gross KM, Ponte CD: New strategies in the medical management of asthma. *Am Fam Physician* 58(1):89–100 and 109–112, 1998.

Guidelines for the Diagnosis and Management of Asthma: Clinical Practice Guidelines. Bethesda, Maryland: US Department of Health and Human Services, National Institutes of Health; 1997. NIH publication 97–4051.

Mellins RB, Evans D, Clark N, et al: Developing and communicating a long-term treatment plan for asthma. *Am Fam Physician* 61:2419–2425, 2000.

CHAPTER 9: BRONCHITIS

Hafner JP, Ferro TJ: Acute bronchitis in adults: a modern approach to management. *Hosp Med* 34(8):41–44 and 47–50, 1998.

Hueston WJ, Mainous AG: Acute bronchitis. *Am Fam Physician* 57:1270–1280, 1998.

CHAPTER 10: CHRONIC OBSTRUCTIVE PULMONARY DISEASE—CHRONIC BRONCHITIS AND EMPHYSEMA

Celli BR, Snider GL, Heffner J, et al: Standards for the diagnosis and care of patients with chronic obstructive pulmonary disease. *Am J Respir Crit Care Med* 152(suppl 5, pt 2):S77–S121, 1995.

Ferguson GT: Management of COPD. *Postgrad Med* 103(4):129–142, 1998.

Heath JM, Mongia R: Chronic bronchitis: primary care management. *Am Fam Physician* 57(10):2365–2372, 1998.

Martinez FJ: Diagnosing chronic obstructive pulmonary disease: the importance of differentiating asthma, emphysema, and chronic bronchitis. *Postgrad Med* 103(4):112–128, 1998.

CHAPTER 11: CORONARY ARTERY DISEASE

Morey SS: AHA and ACC outline approaches to coronary disease risk assessment. *Am Fam Physician* 61:2534–2537, 2000.

Myers J, Voodi L, Umann T, et al: A survey of exercise testing: methods, utilization, interpretation, and safety in the VAHCS. *J Cardiopulm Rehabil* 20(4):251–258, 2000.

Pearce KA, Boosalis MG, Yeager B: Update on vitamin supplements for the prevention of coronary disease and stroke. *Am Fam Physician* 62(6):1359–1366, 2000.

Zanger DR, Solomon AJ, Gersh BJ: Contemporary management of angina, part II: medical management of chronic stable angina. *Am Fam Physician* 61:129–140, 2000.

CHAPTER 12: DIABETES MELLITUS

American Diabetes Association: clinical practice recommendations 2000. *Diabetes Care* 23(suppl 1):S1–S116, 2000.

Gray H, O'Rahilly S: Toward improved glycemic control in diabetes. *Arch Intern Med* 155:1137–1142, 1995.

Reaven GM: Pathophysiology of insulin resistance in human disease. *Physiol Rev* 75:473–485, 1995.

Reaven GM: Role of insulin resistance in human disease (syndrome X): an expanded definition. *Annu Rev Med* 44:121–131, 1993.

Williams G: Management of non-insulin dependent diabetes mellitus. *Diabetes Care* 21(suppl 1):S37, 1998.

Woolf SH, Davidson MB, Greenfield S, et al: Controlling blood glucose levels in patients with type 2 diabetes mellitus. An evidence-based policy statement by the American Academy of Family Physicians and American Diabetes Association. *J Fam Pract* 49(5):453–460, 2000.

CHAPTER 13: DYSLIPIDEMIAS

Downs JR, Clearfield M, Weis S, et al: Primary prevention of acute coronary events with lovastatin in men and women with average cholesterol levels: results of AFCAPS/TexCAPS. Air Force/Texas Coronary Atherosclerosis Prevention Study. *JAMA* 279(20):1615–1622, 1998.

Morelli V, Zoorob RJ: Alternative therapies, part II: congestive heart failure and hypercholesterolemia. *Am Fam Physician* 62(6):1325–1332, 2000.

National Institutes of Health: Second report of the National Cholesterol Education Program expert panel on detection, evaluation, and treatment of high blood cholesterol in adults. *JAMA* 269:3015–3023, 1993.

Safeer RS, Lacivita LC: Choosing drug therapy for patients with hyperlipidemia. *Am Fam Physician* 61:3371–3384, 2000.

Shamir R, Fisher EA: Dietary therapy for children with hypercholesterolemia. *Am Fam Physician* 61:675–684, 2000.

CHAPTER 14: HEADACHE

Coutin IB, Glass SF: Recognizing uncommon headache syndromes. *Am Fam Physician* 54(7):2247–2255, 1996.

Giammarco R, Edmeads J, Dodick D: *Critical Decisions in Headache Management.* Hamilton, Ontario, B.C. Decker Inc., 1998.

Logemann C, Rankin LM: Newer intranasal migraine medications. *Am Fam Physician* 61:180–188, 2000.

Moore KL, Noble SL: Drug treatment of migraine: Part I. Acute therapy and drug-rebound headache. *Am Fam Physician* 56(8):2039–2051, 1997.

Moore KL, Noble SL: Drug treatment of migraine: Part II. Preventive therapy. *Am Fam Physician* 56(9):2279–2288, 1997.

Morey SS: Guidelines on migraine: Part I. Headache. *Am Fam Physician* 62(7):1699–1701, 2000.

Morey SS: Guidelines on migraine: Part II. General principles of drug therapy. *Am Fam Physician* 62(8):1915–1917, 2000.

Morey SS: Guidelines on migraine: Part III. Recommendations for individual drugs. *Am Fam Physician* 62(9):2145–2149, 2000.

Morey SS: Guidelines on migraine: Part IV. General principles of preventive therapy. *Am Fam Physician* 62:2359–2363, 2000.

Silberstein S, Lipton RB, Goadsby PJ: *Headache in Primary Care.* Oxford, Isis Medical Media, 1999.

CHAPTER 15: HUMAN IMMUNODEFICIENCY VIRUS INFECTION

McPherson-Baker S, Malow RM, Penedo F, et al: Enhancing adherence to combination antiretroviral therapy in nonadherent HIV-positive men. *AIDS Care* 12(4):399–404, 2000.

Montauk SM, Gebhardt B: Opportunistic infections and psychosocial stress in HIV. *Am Fam Physician* 56:87–97, 1997.

Sullivan LM, Stein MD, Savetsky JB, et al: The doctor-patient relationship and HIV-infected patients' satisfaction with primary care physicians. *J Gen Intern Med* 15(7):462–469, 2000.

United States Public Health Service/Infectious Disease Society of America. USPHS/IDSA 1999 guidelines for the prevention of opportunistic infections in persons infected with HIV, part I: prevention of exposure. *Am Fam Physician* 61:163–179, 2000.

United States Public Health Service/Infectious Disease Society of America. USPHS/IDSA 1999 guidelines for the prevention of opportunistic infections in persons infected with HIV, part II: prevention of the first episode of disease. *Am Fam Physician* 61:441–477, 2000.

United States Public Health Service/Infectious Disease Society of America. USPHS/IDSA 1999 guidelines for the prevention of opportunistic infections in persons infected with HIV, part III: prevention of disease recurrence. *Am Fam Physician* 61:771–788, 2000.

CHAPTER 16: HYPERTENSION

Joint National Committee on Prevention, Detection, Evaluation and Treatment of High Blood Pressure. Sixth report of the Joint National Committee on Prevention, Detection, Evaluation and Treatment of High Blood Pressure. *Arch Intern Med* 157:2413–2446, 1997.

Kannel WB, Wolf PA, Verter J, et al: Role of blood pressure in stroke: the Framingham study. *JAMA* 214:301–310, 1970.

Skolnik NS, Beck JD, Clark M: Combination antihypertensive drugs: recommendations for use. *Am Fam Physician* 61:3049–3056, 2000.

CHAPTER 17: KNEE INJURIES

Clemente CD: *Anatomy: A Regional Atlas of the Human Body*, 3rd ed. Baltimore, Urban and Schwarzenberg, 1987.

Johnson MW: Acute knee effusions: a systematic approach to diagnosis. *Am Fam Physician* 61:2391–2400, 2000.

Moore KL: *Clinically Oriented Anatomy*, 2nd ed. Baltimore, Williams & Wilkins, 1985.

Paluska SA, McKeag DB: Knee braces: current evidence and clinical recommendations for their use. *Am Fam Physician* 61:411–421, 2000.

Snider RK (ed): *Essentials of Musculoskeletal Care*. Rosemont, Illinois, American Academy of Orthopaedic Surgeons, 1997.

CHAPTER 18: LOW BACK PAIN

Acute Low Back Problems in Adults: Clinical Practice Guideline Number 14. Rockville, Maryland: Agency for Health Care Policy and Research; 1994. US Dept of Health and Human Services publication 95-0643.

Cherkin DC, Deyo RA, Battie M, et al: A comparison of physical therapy, chiropractic manipulation, and provision of an educational booklet for the treatment of patients with low back pain. *N Engl J Med* 339(15):1021–1029, 1998.

Patel AT, Ogle AA: Diagnosis and management of acute low back pain. *Am Fam Physician* 61:1779–1788, 2000.

Rosomoff HL, Rosomoff RS: Low back pain: evaluation and management in the primary care setting. *Med Clin North Am* 83(3):643–662, 1999.

Travell JG, Simons DG: *Myofascial Pain and Dysfunction: The Trigger Point Manual*, vol 2. Baltimore, Williams & Wilkins, 1992.

CHAPTER 19: MENTAL HEALTH AND ILLNESS— ANXIETY AND DEPRESSION

American Psychiatric Association: *Diagnostic and Statistical Manual of Mental Disorders, 4th ed.* Washington, DC, American Psychiatric Press, Inc., 2000.

Depression in Primary Care: Clinical Practice Guideline Number 5, vol 1. Rockville, Maryland: Agency for Healthcare Policy and Research; 1993. US Dept of Health and Human Services publication 93-0550.

Depression in Primary Care: Clinical Practice Guideline Number 5, vol 2. Rockville, Maryland: Agency for Healthcare Policy and Research; 1993. US Dept of Health and Human Services publication 93-0551.

Epperly TD, Moore KE: Health issues in men, part II: common psychosocial disorders. *Am Fam Physician* 62:117–126, 2000.

Goldberg RJ: The P-450 system. Definition and relevance to the use of antidepressants in medical practice. *Arch Fam Med* 5(7):406–412, 1996.

Griswold KS, Pessar LF: Management of bipolar disorder. *Am Fam Physician* 62:1343–1356, 2000.

Lange JT, Lange CL, Cabaltica RBG: Primary care treatment of post-traumatic stress disorder. *Am Fam Physician* 61:1035–1045, 2000.

Preboth M: Clinical review of recent findings on the awareness, diagnosis and treatment of depression. *Am Fam Physician* 61:3158–3169, 2000.

Servan-Schreibern D, Kolb R, Tabas G: Somatizing patients, part I: practical diagnosis. *Am Fam Physician* 61:1073–1079, 2000.

Servan-Schreibern D, Kolb R, Tabas G: Somatizing patients, part II: practical management. *Am Fam Physician* 61:1423–1430, 2000.

CHAPTER 20: OBESITY

Berke EM, Morden NE: Medical management of obesity. *Am Fam Physician* 62(2):419–426, 2000.

Dickerson LM, Carek PJ: Drug therapy for obesity. *Am Fam Physician* 61:2131–2142, 2000.

Expert Panel on the Identification, Evaluation, and Treatment of Overweight in Adults. Clinical guidelines on the identification, evaluation, and treatment of overweight and obesity in adults: executive summary. *Am J Clin Nutr* 68(4):899–917, 1998.

Morelli V, Zoobor RJ: Alternative therapies, part I: depression, diabetes, obesity. *Am Fam Physician* 61:1051–1061, 2000.

Poston WSC, Foreyt JP: Successful management of the obese patient. *Am Fam Physician* 61:3615, 2000.

Rosenbaum M, Liebel RL, Hirsch J: Obesity. *N Engl J Med* 337(6):396–407, 1997.

Weinsier RL, Hunter GR, Heini AF, et al: The etiology of obesity: relative contribution of metabolic factors, diet, and physical activity. *Am J Med* 105:145–150, 1998.

CHAPTER 21: OTITIS MEDIA AND OTITIS EXTERNA

Pichichero ME: Acute otitis media, part I: improving diagnostic accuracy. *Am Fam Physician* 61:2051–2060, 2000.

Pichichero ME: Acute otitis media, part II: treatment in an era of increasing antibiotic resistance. *Am Fam Physician* 61:2410–2418, 2000.

CHAPTER 22: PARTNER VIOLENCE

American Medical Association. American Medical Association diagnostic and treatment guidelines on domestic violence. *Arch Fam Med* 2:39–47, 1992.

Eyler AE, Cohen M: Case studies in partner violence. *Am Fam Physician* 60(9):2569–2577, 1999.

Ferris LE, Norton PG, Dunn EV, et al: Guidelines for managing domestic abuse when male and female partner are patients of the same physician. *JAMA* 278:851–857, 1997.

Zink TM: Domestic violence: reality for some of your toughest patients. *Minn Med* 80:26–32, 1997.

CHAPTER 23: PRURITIC SKIN—COMMON DERMATOSES

Committee on Infectious Diseases. *Red Book: Report of the Committee on Infectious Diseases*, 25th ed. Elk Grove Village, Illinois, American Academy of Pediatrics, 2000.

Correale CE, Walker C, Murphy L, et al: Atopic dermatitis: a review of diagnosis and treatment. *Am Fam Physician* 60(4):1191–1197, 1999.

Diehl KB: Topical antifungal agents: an update. *Am Fam Physician* 54(5):1687–1692, 1996.

Johnson BA, Nunley JR: Treatment of seborrheic dermatitis. *Am Fam Physician*, 61(9):2703–2712, 2000.

Noble SL, Frobes RC: Diagnosis and management of common tinea infections. *Am Fam Physician* 58:163–174, 1998.

Peterson CM, Eichenfield LF: Scabies. *Pediatr Ann* 2:97–100, 1996.

CHAPTER 24: SINUSITIS

Fagnan LJ: Acute sinusitis: a cost-effective approach to diagnosis and treatment. *Am Fam Physician* 58(8):1795–1802, 1998.

Spector SL, Bernstein IL, Li JT, et al: Parameters for the diagnosis and management of sinusitis. *J Allergy Clin Immunol* 102(suppl 6, pt 2):S107–S144, 1998.

CHAPTER 25: SUBSTANCE ABUSE AND DEPENDENCE

Bradley KA, Boyd-Wickizer J, Powell SH, et al: Alcohol screening questionnaires in women: a critical review. *JAMA* 280:166–171, 1998.

Christophersen AS: Amphetamine designer drugs: an overview and epidemiology. *Toxicol Lett* 112,113:127–131, 2000.

DuRant RH, Smith JA: Adolescent tobacco use and cessation. *Prim Care* 26(3):553–575, 1999.

Giannini AJ: An approach to drug abuse, intoxication and withdrawal. *Am Fam Physician* 61:2763–2782, 2000.

Glynn TJ, Manley MW. *How to Help Your Patients Stop Smoking: A National Cancer Institute Manual for Physicians.* Baltimore, MD: National Cancer Institute; 1990. NIH publication 90-3064.

Lewis DC: The role of the generalist in the care of the substance-abusing patient. *Med Clin North Am* 81(4):831–843, l997.

Longo LP, Johnson B: Addiction, part I: benzodiazepines—side effects, abuse risk and alternatives. *Am Fam Physician* 61:2121, 2000.

Longo LP, Parran T, Johnson B, et al: Addiction, part II: identification and management of the drug-seeking patient. *Am Fam Physician* 61:2401–2409, 2000.

McIlvain HE, Bobo JK: Tobacco cessation with patients recovering from alcohol and other substance abuse. *Prim Care* 26(3):671–689, 1999.

Rigler SK: Alcoholism in the elderly. *Am Fam Physician* 61: 1710–1724, 2000.

Rustin TA: Assessing nicotine dependence. *Am Fam Physician* 62:579–590, 2000.

The Physicians' Guide to Helping Patients With Alcohol Problems. Washington, DC: National Institute of Alcohol Abuse and Alcoholism; 1995. US Dept of Health and Human Services publication NIH 95-3769.

CHAPTER 26: VAGINAL DISCHARGE

Bachmann GA, Nevadunsky NS: Diagnosis and treatment of atrophic vaginitis. *Am Fam Physician* 61:3090–3096, 2000.

Egan ME, Lipsky MS: Diagnosis of vaginitis. *Am Fam Physician* 61:1095–1108, 2000.

Haefner H: Current evaluation and management of vulvovaginitis. *Clin Obstet Gynecol* 42(2):184–195, 1999.

Majeroni B: Bacterial vaginosis: an update. *Am Fam Physician* 57(6):1285–1289, 1998.

Ringdahl EN: Treatment of recurrent vulvovaginal candidiasis. *Am Fam Physician* 61:3306–3315, 2000.

Sobel JD: Vulvovaginitis in healthy women. *Compr Ther* 25(6,7):335–346, 1999.

Woodward C: Drug treatment of common STDs, part I: herpes, syphilis, urethritis, chlamydia and gonorrhea. *Am Fam Physician* 60(5):1387–1394, 1999.

Appendix I: COMPLEMENTARY/ALTERNATIVE MEDICINE

Astin JA: Why patients use alternative medicine. *JAMA* 279(19): 1548–1553, 1998.

Calixto JB: Efficacy, safety, quality control, marketing and regulatory guidelines for herbal medicines (phytotherapeutic agents). *Braz J Med Biol Res* 33(2):179–189, 2000.

Drivdahll CE, Miser WF: The use of alternative care by a family practice population. *Journal of the American Board of Family Practice* 11:193–199, 1998.

Eisenberg D: Advising patients who seek alternative medical therapies. *Ann Intern Med* 127:61–69, 1997.

Fugh-Berman A: *Alternative Medicine: What Works.* Baltimore, Williams & Wilkins, 1997.

Rosa LB, Rosa E, Sarner L, et al: A close look at therapeutic touch. *JAMA* 279(13):1005–1010, 1998.

Zink T, Chaffin J: Herbal 'health' products: what family physicians need to know. *Am Fam Physician* 58(5):1133–1140, 1998.

GENERAL INFORMATION

Practice Guidelines (Books)

Committee on Infectious Diseases. *Red Book: Report of the Committee on Infectious Diseases*, 25th ed. Elk Grove Village, Illinois, American Academy of Pediatrics, 2000.

United States Preventive Services Task Force. *Guide to Clinical Preventive Services: An Assessment of the Effectiveness of 169 Interventions.* Baltimore, Williams & Wilkins, 1995.

Evidence-Based Medicine (Books)

Greenhalgh T: *How to Read a Paper: The Basics of Evidence-Based Medicine.* London, BMJ Publishing Group, 1997.

McKibbon A, Eady A, Marks S: *PDQ Evidence-Based Principles and Practice.* Hamilton, Ontario, B.C. Decker Inc., 1999.

Silagy C, Haines A: *Evidence-Based Practice in Primary Care.* London, BMJ Publishing Group, 1998.

Evidence-Based Medicine (Journal Series)

How to Read a Paper. *British Medical Journal* Series. (Each article in this 1997 series by Greenhalgh describes a different aspect of how to read a paper.)

Users' Guides to the Medical Literature. *JAMA* Series. (Since 1993, JAMA has published several articles every year in this series.)

Evidence-Based Medicine (Journal Articles)

Shaughnessy AF, Slawson DC, Becker L: Clinical jazz: harmonizing clinical experience and evidence-based medicine. *J Fam Pract* 47:425–428, 1998.

Shaughnessy AF, Slawson DC, Bennet JH: Becoming an information master: a guidebook to the medical information jungle. *J Fam Pract* 39:489–499, 1994.

Slawson DC, Shaughnessy AF, Bennett JH: Becoming a medical information master: feeling good about not knowing everything. *J Fam Pract* 38:505–513, 1994.

INFORMATION TECHNOLOGY RESOURCES

Resource	Web address
Agency for Healthcare Research and Quality	www.ahcpr.gov
Agency for Healthcare Research and Quality: Clinical Practice Guidelines Online	www.ahcpr.gov/clinic/cpgonline.htm
American Academy of Family Physicians	www.aafp.org
American Academy of Family Physicians: Index to algorithms published in *AFP*	www.aafp.org/afp/algorithms/
American Academy of Family Physicians: Recommended Curriculum Guidelines for Family Practice Residents	www.aafp.org/edu/guide
American Family Physician	www.aafp.org/afp/
American Psychiatric Association	www.psych.org
American Psychological Association	www.apa.org
CDC: National Immunization Program	www.cdc.gov/nip
Food Guide Pyramid	www.nal.usda.gov:8001/py/pmap.htm
Health Oasis Mayo Clinic	www.mayohealth.org
MEDLINE*plus* Health Information	www.nlm.nih.gov/medlineplus
National Center for Biotechnology Information	www.ncbi.nlm.nih.gov
National Clearinghouse for Alcohol and Drug Information	www.health.org/catalog/index.htm
National Guideline Clearinghouse	www.guidelines.gov
National Institute of Diabetes & Digestive & Kidney Diseases	www.niddk.nih.gov
National Institute on Drug Abuse	www.nida.nih.gov
National Institutes of Health	www.nih.gov
National Library of Medicine	www.nlm.nih.gov
Nutrition and Your Health: Dietary Guidelines for Americans	www.nal.usda.gov/fnic/dga/dguide95.html
Society of Teachers of Family Medicine	www.stfm.org
University of Cincinnati College of Medicine	www.med.uc.edu
Weight-control Information Network	www.niddk.nih.gov/health/nutrit/win.htm

AFP = *American Family Physician;* CDC = Centers for Disease Control.

Index

Page numbers in *italics* denote figures and "t" denote tables